MANAGING PAIN

MANAGING PAIN

Essentials of Diagnosis and Treatment

Edited by

Chad M. Brummett, MD
ASSISTANT PROFESSOR OF ANESTHESIOLOGY
DIRECTOR, PAIN RESEARCH
DEPARTMENT OF ANESTHESIOLOGY
UNIVERSITY OF MICHIGAN
ANN ARBOR, MICHIGAN

AND

Steven P. Cohen, MD
PROFESSOR OF ANESTHESIOLOGY
JOHNS HOPKINS SCHOOL OF MEDICINE, BALTIMORE, MD &
UNIFORMED SERVICES UNIVERSITY OF THE HEALTH
SCIENCES, BETHESDA, MD
DIRECTOR OF PAIN RESEARCH, WALTER REED NATIONAL
MILITARY MEDICAL CENTER, BETHESDA, MD
CHIEF, ANESTHESIA & OPERATIVE SERVICES, 48TH COMBAT
SUPPORT HOSPITAL, FORT MEADE, MD
COLONEL, US ARMY RESERVE

OXFORD
UNIVERSITY PRESS

OXFORD
UNIVERSITY PRESS

Oxford University Press is a department of the University of Oxford.
It furthers the University's objective of excellence in research, scholarship,
and education by publishing worldwide.

Oxford New York
Auckland Cape Town Dar es Salaam Hong Kong Karachi
Kuala Lumpur Madrid Melbourne Mexico City Nairobi
New Delhi Shanghai Taipei Toronto

With offices in
Argentina Austria Brazil Chile Czech Republic France Greece
Guatemala Hungary Italy Japan Poland Portugal Singapore
South Korea Switzerland Thailand Turkey Ukraine Vietnam

Oxford is a registered trademark of Oxford University Press
in the UK and certain other countries.

Published in the United States of America by
Oxford University Press
198 Madison Avenue, New York, NY 10016

Library of Congress Cataloging-in-Publication Data
Managing pain : essentials of diagnosis and treatment/[edited by] Chad M. Brummett, Steven P. Cohen.
p. ; cm.
Includes bibliographical references and index.
ISBN 978-0-19-985943-6 (alk. paper)—ISBN 978-0-19-993149-1 (alk. paper)—
ISBN 978-0-19-997829-8 (alk. paper)
I. Brummett, Chad M. II. Cohen, Steven P. (Steven Paul), 1963-
[DNLM: 1. Pain Management. 2. Pain—diagnosis. 3. Pain—drug therapy. WL 704.6]
LC Classification not assigned
616'.0472—dc23
2012030925

ISBN 978-0-19-985943-6

9 8 7 6 5 4 3 2 1
Printed in the United States of America
on acid-free paper

From Chad

To my wife Kate and my children Christopher and Annabelle for their love, patience and understanding.

To my mother Anita for her unwavering love and support, and to my father Jack for teaching me integrity, hard work and dedication.

To my many mentors, collaborators, clinical colleagues, trainees, and students who continue to push me to ask clinically important questions and make it possible to seek the answers. Special thanks to my chairman Kevin Tremper for taking a chance on me.

From Steve

To my wife Karen, and my children Berklee, Zared and Seffrah, for their patience and understanding during the many hours I spent writing and editing this book.

To my mother Harriet, and in memory of my father Allen, who guided me onto a path of inquiry and knowledge.

To my mentors, and physician and nurse colleagues at Johns Hopkins, the 48th Combat Support Hospital, and Walter Reed, including my research nurse Connie, whose collective feedback and assistance have made me a better doctor.

To all of the trainees I've collaborated with over the years at Johns Hopkins and Walter Reed, whose questions have kept me attuned to the need for better research and books such as this.

To all my patients, especially the wounded service members, who have entrusted their care to me.

ACKNOWLEDGMENTS

"The authors gratefully acknowledge Andrea Seils and Rebecca Suzan from Oxford University Press for their support, guidance and assistance throughout the production process.

We would also like to extend our most genuine thanks to the authors for delivering high-quality, clinically oriented chapters in a timely fashion.

Finally, we are indebted to our departments for their patience and and assistance in helping us bring this project to fruition."

CONTENTS

PART THREE
ADDITIONAL CONSIDERATIONS IN THE PAIN PATIENT

PART FOUR
CASE-BASED PAIN CHAPTERS

PREFACE

Pain is a fascinating subject that affects nearly everyone at some time. To find proof of this, one need only open up a newspaper, read a magazine, or turn on the TV set. Our knowledge about the mechanisms and treatment of pain is growing so rapidly that much of the material published only a few years ago is now obsolete. It is such an important topic that people whose lives it consumes will sometimes go to incredible lengths to learn about it and try to eradicate it. Yet there is still so much misinformation and conflicting data out there that it is sometimes difficult to know the right course of action. The reason we know this is that we see it every day.

In the most recent Institute of Medicine report on pain, it was estimated that more than 100 million Americans live with chronic pain. Pain is the leading cause of disability in the world, and the second most common reason people visit healthcare providers. It should therefore come as no surprise that there are countless books available to doctors and patients alike focused on pain medicine, with more and more being published every month. These books are almost all written by "pain management doctors," physicians who have trained in "pain medicine," and they are virtually all targeted to a "pain management" audience. However, the burden of pain extends to all doctors, not just those who treat it every day.

We both have been asked to edit books many times, and for the most part we have declined nearly all offers. Raising children, running a clinical practice, and overseeing clinical trials can be very time consuming. Why, then, did we accept this assignment? Because we both felt there was—and still is—a strong need for a book designed to assist frontline healthcare providers with one of the most challenging problems in medicine: how to effectively treat chronic pain.

This book is one of the few that caters to non-pain practitioners, designed to include not just primary care doctors but non-pain specialty physicians and ancillary healthcare providers. The chapters were carefully chosen to reflect those conditions and scenarios most frequently encountered by primary care providers, and they were designed to maximize "clinical relevance." It is written in simple, readily understandable language, with germane case-based presentations that might be encountered in everyday non-specialty care practice. In fact, the authors who wrote the chapters compiled the cases from the cases of real-life individuals. Importantly, though the book is edited by experts in pain medicine, many of the chapters are written by non-pain physicians who are experts in their respective specialties—doctors who have trained in neurology, surgery, physical medicine and rehabilitation, internal medicine, anesthesiology, and other areas. This serves to enhance its usefulness to the non-pain-trained healthcare provider, who must battle the chronic pain epidemic every day of every week. Sometimes the battle is won (e.g., a patient with shingles is treated and fully recovers), but more often it is lost, or perhaps fought to a stalemate, as there are many dilemmas (e.g., when to prescribe opioids, when to send a patient to a spine surgeon), pitfalls (e.g., adverse effects and non-compliance), and obstacles (e.g., addiction) that need to be overcome. It is our hope that with this book, the scales will tilt a little more toward the side of "battles won."

Finally, we would like to thank our families for their support and patience, and the authors and publisher for providing us with the opportunity to help fill this critical gap in pain education. It is our hope that this book will be part of a larger overall effort in the medical community that aims to enhance clinicians' understanding of chronic pain and their ability to treat it.

Steven Cohen & Chad Brummett

CONTRIBUTORS

Kalyna Apkarian
Undergraduate Student
John Hopkins University
Baltimore, Maryland

Sawsan As-Sanie, MD, MPH
Department of Obstetrics and Gynecology
University of Michigan
Ann Arbor, Michigan

Charles E. Argoff, MD
Professor of Neurology
Albany Medical College
Albany, New York

Helen A. Baghdoyan, PhD
Professor of Anesthesiology
University of Michigan
Ann Arbor, Michigan

Thomas H. Brannagan III, MD
Director of Peripheral Neuropathy Center, Neurological Institute
and
Professor of Clinical Neurology
Columbia University Medical Center
New York, New York

Chad M. Brummett, MD
Director of Pain Research
Department of Anesthesiology
University of Michigan Health System
Ann Arbor, Michigan

Lucy Chen, MD
Assistant Professor
Massachusetts General Hospital
Harvard Medical School
Boston, Massachusetts

Srinivas Chiravuri, MD
Director of Neuromodulation and Implantable Device Program
and
Director of Pain Medicine Fellowship
University of Michigan Health System
Ann Arbor, Michigan

Sigrun Chrubasik, PhD, MD
Professor
Research Coordinator of the Herbal Drug Unit
Institute of Forensic Medicine
University of Freiburg
Freiburg, Germany

Daniel J. Clauw, MD
Director
Chronic Pain and Fatigue Research Center
and
Professor
Departments of Anesthesiology, Internal Medicine (Rheumatology), and Psychiatry
and
Vice Chair for Research Department of Anesthesiology
University of Michigan
Ann Arbor, Michigan

Steven P. Cohen, MD
Professor
Walter Reed National Military Medical Center
Bethesda, Maryland
and
Associate Professor of Anesthesiology and Critical Care Medicine
Johns Hopkins School of Medicine
Baltimore, Maryland

Wade Cooper, DO
Clinical Assistant Professor of Neurology
University of Michigan Health System
Ann Arbor, Michigan

Roy Dekel, MD
Department of Gastroenterology
Tel-Aviv Medical Center
Tel-Aviv, Israel

Guy D. Eslick, DrPH, PhD, FACE, FFPH
Associate Professor of Surgery and Cancer Epidemiology
The Whiteley-Martin Research Centre
and
Discipline of Surgery
The University of Sydney
Nepean Hospital
Penrith, Australia

Artemus Flagg, MD
Department of Anesthesiology
Johns Hopkins School of Medicine
Baltimore, Maryland

Richard E. Harris, PhD
Assistant Professor of Anesthesiology
and
Research Assistant Professor of Internal Medicine
University of Michigan
Ann Arbor, Michigan

Afton L. Hassett, PsyD
Associate Research Scientist
Department of Anesthesiology
University of Michigan Medical School
Chronic Pain & Fatigue Research Center
Ann Arbor, Michigan

Salim M. Hayek, MD, PhD
Professor, Department of Anesthesiology and Perioperative Medicine
Case Western Reserve School of Medicine
and
Chief, Division of Pain Medicine
University Hospitals Case Medical Center
Cleveland, Ohio

Mark Hoffman, MD
Department of Obstetrics and Gynecology
University of Michigan
Ann Arbor, Michigan

Sharon X. H. Hu, MB, BS, BSc
The Whiteley-Martin Research Centre
Discipline of Surgery
The University of Sydney, Nepean Hospital,
Penrith, New South Wales
Australia

Julie H. Y. Huang, MD, MBA
Department of Anesthesiology and Critical Care Medicine
Johns Hopkins School of Medicine
Baltimore, Maryland

Robert W. Hurley, MD, PhD
Chief of Pain Medicine
and
Associate Professor of Anesthesiology, Neurology, Orthopaedics and Rehabilitation
University of Florida
Gainesville, Florida

Tomas Kucera, MD, MS
Department of Anesthesiology
University of Florida
Gainesville, Florida

Caleb Kroll, MD
Fellow in Pain Medicine
Johns Hopkins School of Medicine
Baltimore, Maryland

Ralph Lydic, PhD
Bert La Du Professor of Anesthesiology
University of Michigan
Ann Arbor, Michigan

Jianren Mao, MD, PhD
Richard J. Kitz Professor of Anesthesia Research
Harvard Medical School
Boston, Massachusetts

Kristine Phillips, MD, PhD
Division of Rheumatology
University of Michigan
Ann Arbor, Michigan

Srinivasa N. Raja, MD
Professor of Anesthesiology and Critical Care Medicine
and
Director of Pain Research and the Division of Pain Medicine
Johns Hopkins School of Medicine
Baltimore, Maryland

Andrei D. Sdrulla, MD, PhD
Department of Anesthesiology and Critical Care Medicine
Johns Hopkins School of Medicine
Baltimore, Maryland

Devon Shuchman, MD
Department of Anesthesiology
University of Michigan
Ann Arbor, Michigan

Howard S. Smith, MD
Professor and Academic Director of Pain Management
Albany Medical College
Albany, New York

Ami D. Sperber, MD, MSPH
Department of Gastroenterology
Tel-Aviv Medical Center
Tel-Aviv, Israel
and
Faculty of Health Sciences
Ben-Gurion University of the Negev
Beer-Sheva, Israel

Michael Sternberg, BS
University of Michigan
Ann Arbor, Michigan

Glenn Treisman, MD, PhD
Professor of Psychiatry and Behavioral Sciences
Johns Hopkins School of Medicine
Baltimore, Maryland

Christina M. Ulane, MD, PhD
Assistant Professor of Neurology
Columbia University Medical Center
New York, New York

Julia Vlachojannis, MSc, MD
Institute of Forensic Medicine
University of Freiburg
Freiburg, Germany

Henry E. Vucetic, MD
Department of Anesthesiology and Perioperative Medicine
Division of Pain Management
University Hospitals Case Medical Center
Case Western Reserve School of Medicine
Cleveland, Ohio

Mark Wallace, MD
Division of Pain Medicine
Department of Anesthesiology
University of California at San Diego
San Diego, California

Brian G. Wilhelmi, MD
Johns Hopkins School of Medicine
Baltimore, Maryland

David A. Williams, PhD
Professor of Anesthesiology
University of Michigan Medical School
Chronic Pain & Fatigue Research Center
Ann Arbor, Michigan

Suzanna M. Zick, ND, MPH
Research Assistant Professor of Family Medicine
University of Michigan
Ann Arbor, Michigan

PART I

PHARMACOLOGIC PAIN THERAPIES

1

Opioids

LUCY CHEN, STEVEN P. COHEN, AND JIANREN MAO

Opioids have been successfully used over many decades to treat acute, chronic, and cancer-related pain. Despite extensive efforts in search of new pharmacological drugs for pain treatment, opioids remain the most efficacious among clinically available pain medications. Opioid analgesics are generally divided into three groups: (1) naturally occurring alkaloids derived from poppy seeds (e.g., heroin, morphine, and codeine) and their semi-synthetic derivatives (e.g., oxycodone, oxycontin, hydromorphone, and oxymorphone), (2) synthetic phenlypiperidines (e.g., meperidine and fentanyl), and (3) synthetic pseudopiperidines (e.g., methadone, propoxyphene). Based on their mechanisms of action, opioids also can be categorized as pure agonists (e.g., morphine, hydromorphone, meperidine, fentanyl, methadone, levorphanol, oxycodone) or agonist-antagonists (e.g., pentazocine, dezocine, butorphanol, nalbuphine, buprenorphine). The doses and formulations of commonly used opioids are summarized in Table 1.1.[1]

Opioids act on three major classes of endogenous receptors to achieve their analgesic effects: μ, κ, and δ (mu, kappa, and delta receptors). These receptors are widely distributed throughout the body, including in the central and peripheral nervous systems, as well as throughout internal organs and structures such as the gastrointestinal tract. Activation of opioid receptors produces analgesia, euphoria, respiratory depression, decreased gastrointestinal (GI)

Table 1.1 FORMULATIONS, DOSAGES, AND PHARMACOLOGICAL INFORMATION FOR COMMONLY PRESCRIBED OPIOIDS

OPIOID AGONIST				
Drug	*Equianalgesic Dosage*	*Administration Route*	*Duration of Action*	*Comments*
Morphine	30 mg	IV, IM, PO, PR; SR formulation	3 to 6 h for short-acting, 8 to 12 h for SR	Reference standard for all opioids; renally excreted active metabolite
Oxycodone (percocet)	20 mg	PO, PR; SR formulation	3 to 6 h for short-acting, 8 to 12 h for SR	Widely available in combination form with non-opioid analgesics; SR form popular among recreational users
Hydromorphone (dilaudid)	3 to 6 mg	PO, PR, IV, IM	3 to 6 h	Higher PO:IV conversion ratio than other opioids
Hydrocodone (vicodin)	30 to 60 mg	PO	3 to 6 h	Wide variation in morphine equivalent dose. Most commonly prescribed opioid in United States. Typically used in combination form with non-opioid analgesic. Formulations containing <15 mg hydrocodone are schedule III in United States

Oxymorphone (opana)	10 mg	IV, IM, PO, PR, SR formulation	4-8 hours, 12 h for SR	10% oral bioavailability results in high PO: IV conversion ratio. Longer elimination half-life than morphine or oxycodone. Absorption of oral formulation varies greatly in the presence of alcohol.
Methadone (dolophine)	2 to 20 mg	PO, PR, IV	6 to 12 h for pain	Morphine: methadone conversion varies according to dose and length of opioid use, ranging from 2:1 to >20:1 in patients on very high doses. Any physician with a schedule II Drug Enforcement Agency license may prescribe for pain. May take 5 to 7 days to reach steady state because of the extended half-life (i.e., accumulation). Electrocardiogram monitoring recommended with higher doses. Other properties such as NMDA receptor antagonism and reuptake inhibition of serotonin and norepinephrine might slow the development of tolerance and increase efficacy for neuropathic pain.
Fentanyl (Duragesic)	12.5 mcg/h (TD) 800 to 1000 mcg (TM) 200 to 400 mcg (B)	TD, TM, B	72 hours for TD; 10 min to 2 h for TM and B	TD, TM, and B formulations may be useful in patients with poor bowel function. TD: Wide variation in conversion ratios. Delivery system might be associated with fewer gastrointestinal side effects. TM and B: delivery systems associated with more rapid (10 min) onset than immediate release oral opioids. Approved by the U.S. Food and Drug Administration for breakthrough cancer pain in opioid-tolerant patients.

(continued)

Table 1.1 *(CONTINUED)*

OPIOID AGONIST				
Drug	*Equianalgesic Dosage*	*Administration Route*	*Duration of Action*	*Comments*
Codeine	200 mg	PO, PR	3 to 6 h	Often used in combination with non-opioid analgesics. Efficacy and side effects might be affected by rate of metabolism to morphine. Popular as a cough suppressant.
Propoxyphene (Darvon)	200 mg	PO, PR	3 to 6 h	Wide variation in morphine equivalent dose. Often used in combination form with non-opioid analgesic. Toxic metabolite might accumulate with excessive use, especially in elderly patients. Weak antagonist at NMDA receptor.
Meperidine (Demerol)	300 mg	PO, PR, IV	2 to 4 h	Toxic metabolite might accumulate with excessive use, especially in patients with renal insufficiency. Associated with tachycardia and hypertension. Might cause more "euphoria" than other opioids. Concurrent use with monoamine oxidase inhibitors might result in fatal reactions.

Drug Name	*Dosage*	*Administration Route*	*Duration of Action*	*Comments*
Buprenorphine (Butrans patch) **Suboxone (4:1 ratio of buprenorphine to naloxone)**	0.3 to 24 mg (SL) 5 to 70 mcg/h (TD) 2 to 24 mg/d	SL, PR, IV, TD	6 to 8 h (7 days for patch)	Partial μ agonist and κ antagonist that might precipitate withdrawal in opioid-dependent patients on high doses. Lower abuse potential and fewer psychomimetic effects than pure agonists. Not readily reversed by naloxone. Schedule III drug in United States. Primary use of SL preparation is to treat addiction. Used in combination with naloxone (Suboxone, Subutex) for opioid dependence. Might prolong QT interval.
Butorphanol (Stadol)	1 mg/spray, repeat after 60 to 90 min (NS) 1 to 2 mg (IV/IM)	NS, IM, IV, PO	3 to 4 h	Partial agonist and antagonist at μ receptor and antagonist at κ receptor. Commonly used as nasal spray to treat migraine headache, and less commonly for labor pain. Significant abuse potential.
Nalbuphine (Nubain)	10 to 20 mg	SC, IM, IV	3 to 6 h	Mixed agonist-antagonist, often used for labor and delivery. Sometimes used to treat refractory opioid-induced pruritis.

(continued)

Table 1.1 (CONTINUED)

Drug Name	Dosage	Administration Route	Duration of Action	Comments
AGONIST-ANTAGONISTS, PARTIAL AGONISTS				
Pentazocine **Pentazocine/ Naloxone (Talwin)**	30 to 60 mg parenteral 50 to 100 PO	PO, SC, IM, IV	3 to 4 h parenteral, 8 h PO	Mixed agonist-antagonist. Naloxone added in 1970s to prevent abuse. Also prescribed in preparation with acetaminophen.
ANTAGONISTS				
Drug Name	*Dosage*	*Administration Route*	*Duration of Action*	*Comments*
Naloxone (Narcan)		**(Narcan)**		
	0.01 to 2 mg	IV	30 to 60 min	0.01 to 0.04 mg IV for pruritus; 0.4 to 2 mg q2 minutes up to 10 mg total for respiratory depression emergency.

PO, oral; PR, rectal; IM, intramuscular; IV, intravenous; TD, transdermal; TM, transmucosal; B, buccal; SL, sublingual; NMDA, *N*-methyl-D-aspartate; SR, sustained release; NS, nasal spray; SC, subcutaneous.

Adapted from Howard F. Chronic Pelvic Pain. *Obstetrics & Gynecology.* 2003;101(3):594–611.

motility, and cardiovascular effects. In addition, the development of tolerance and dependence with opioid analgesics presents practical challenges in the clinical setting. Concerns over side effects, tolerance, dependence, addiction, and, more recently, opioid-induced hyperalgesia (OIH) have limited the use of opioids for the management of pain.[2,3]

CENTRAL NERVOUS SYSTEM

Analgesia

Opioids are considered to be the most powerful class of analgesics according to the World Health Organization guidelines for pain management. Opioids induce profound analgesia, mainly through their actions at spinal and supraspinal regions. (1) Opioids act on the central terminal of primary nociceptive afferents, thereby reducing the release of neurotransmitters (e.g., substance P, excitatory amino acids such as glutamate) involved in the transmission of nociceptive pain signals from the periphery. This effect is related to the ability of opioids to reduce calcium influx into presynaptic afferent terminals. (2) In addition to presynaptic actions, opioids directly inhibit postsynaptic neuronal activity by hyperpolarizing cell membranes through potassium channel opening, making it more difficult for postsynaptic neurons to become excited. Reduced excitability of second-order neurons within the spinal cord dorsal horn helps block the transmission of spinal nociceptive signals to supraspinal regions in the brain. (3) Opioids may also activate supraspinal descending inhibitory systems and/or induce the release of endogenous opioid peptides, leading to further inhibition of nociceptive transmission within the central nervous system.[4,5]

Several important features of opioid-induced analgesia provide the rationales for using opioid therapy in pain management.

(1) Interactions between spinal and supraspinal opioid actions can lead to additive or synergistic analgesic effects, thereby reducing the total dose of opioids required in order to achieve effective analgesia. (2) Interactions between different opioid receptor subtypes, such as μ and δ receptors, may produce synergistic analgesic effects and/or prevent the development of opioid tolerance and dependence. Accordingly, it is possible that a combination of two opioids acting at different receptors might be more effective than either opioid alone.[6] (3) Although tolerance to individual opioid analgesics can develop clinically, incomplete tolerance to each opioid is often present despite the fact that different opioid receptor agonists may act at the same opioid receptor subtype. This provides a practical reason for switching opioids (i.e., opioid rotation) in those patients who have developed tolerance. (4) Besides their central analgesic effects, opioids also produce analgesia when applied at peripheral sites under certain circumstances (e.g., during inflammation secondary to trauma or surgery). This could significantly reduce the side effects associated with systemic opioid administration, and it provides an impetus to search for more specific peripherally acting opioid receptor agonists.[7]

Euphoria, Dysphoria, and Sedation

Opioids, particularly μ-opioid receptor agonists, produce profound euphoria, as well as sedation, at high doses. Mechanistically, the ventral tegmental dopaminergic system is thought to be a site of interest, as it might be responsible for positive reinforcement following the repeated use of opioids. Although κ-opioid receptor agonists have been postulated to produce dysphoria via the inhibition of the dopaminergic system, their role in clinical opioid therapy remains unclear.

Effects on the Neuroendocrine System

It is well recognized that opioids may regulate the secretion and/or release of several hypothalamic hormones by their direct actions in this region. For example, morphine can inhibit the release of gonodotropin-releasing hormone and corticotropin-releasing hormone from the hypothalamus, leading to the decreased release of adrenocorticotropic hormone from the pituitary. A low level of adrenocorticotropic hormone can cause a decline in the plasma cortisol concentration, which might manifest as fatigue, weakness, loss of appetite, and weight loss with long-term opioid administration. Long-term opioid use might also result in a decrease in luteinizing hormone and follicle-stimulating hormone in women and testosterone in men. As a result, female patients might experience a disrupted menstrual cycle, reduced fertility and sex drive, and accelerated osteoporosis when on opioids.[8]

Effects on Sleep

An opioid's effect on sleep patterns varies according to the opioid use stage (acute use, chronic use, or opioid withdrawal). During the acute phase of opioid use, there might be diminished rapid eye movement (REM) sleep, decreased deep sleep, and increased arousal and wakefulness. As a result, the patient's overall sleep efficiency and total sleep time might be decreased. During chronic opioid use, there are reductions in REM and deep sleep as well. However, the arousal index might also decrease, and this might be accompanied by an increase in total sleep time and sleep efficiency. Studies have shown that acute heroin abstinence induces an increase in wakefulness and decreased and disrupted REM sleep. Total sleep time is also decreased and has been observed to remain below the normal range for up to a week after abstinence. Chronic opioid withdrawal, however, presents with significant insomnia, frequent arousals, and decreased REM sleep that can persist for prolonged time periods. Between 13 and 22 weeks following chronic methadone withdrawal, total sleep time is increased with a rebound in REM sleep.[9]

Opioids and Cognitive Function

Opioids produce adverse effects in the central nervous system, including changes in cognitive function. Opioids affect consciousness, which manifests clinically as sedation, drowsiness, and sleep disturbance. Opioids can also affect thinking processes and the ability to react to stimuli, which might present clinically as cognitive impairment, psychomotor impairment, delirium, hallucinations, dreams, and nightmares. Studies have shown that patients receiving immediate-release morphine for palliative care displayed significant anterograde and retrograde memory impairment, delayed recall of verbal information, and reduced performance on a complex tracking task. However, the long-term effects of opioids on neuropsychological performance in patients with chronic noncancer pain remain a subject of controversy. For example, a 12-month course of treatment with oral sustained-release morphine in patients with noncancer pain does not seem to significantly disrupt cognitive function. In contrast, opioids appear to cause a moderate improvement in some aspects of cognitive function in select patients, possibly due to pain relief and a concomitant improvement in feelings of well-being and mood. Other studies have shown that patients who are on long-term oral opioid therapy performed statistically significantly poorer than controls in tests measuring vigilance/attention, psychomotor speed, and working memory. Cognitive deficits are more prominent in methadone maintenance patients being treated for drug addiction. Their performances are significantly poorer than those of controls on all neuropsychological domains measured: information processing, attention, short-term visual memory, delayed visual memory, short-term verbal memory, long-term verbal memory, and problem solving. Possible factors that might influence opioid-related effects on cognitive functions include advanced age, advanced disease, dosage, and overall physical condition. Therefore, optimal opioid therapy requires careful clinical assessment, identification of risk factors, objective monitoring of cognition function, and maintenance of adequate hydration. When there is significant cognitive impairment, either dose reduction or a switch to a different opioid is needed.[10–13]

Convulsions

High doses of opioids have been shown to cause convulsions in animals. This side effect appears to be rare in humans unless excessively high doses are used, often in combination with drugs that lower the seizure threshold (e.g., tricyclic antidepressants). In low doses, opioids may actually raise the seizure threshold. Possible mechanisms of opioid-induced convulsions might include excitation of the hippocampus and spinal cord ventral horn, either directly or indirectly through disinhibition. An important characteristic of opioid-induced convulsions is that opioid receptor antagonists such as naloxone might be more effective than conventional anticonvulsants such as benzodiazepines in their treatment.

Respiratory Depression

Opioids affect all regulatory mechanisms of respiration, including rate, rhythm, and minute volume, through their interactions with brainstem respiratory centers. The most significant effect of opioids on respiration is the attenuated responsiveness of the central respiratory centers to carbon dioxide. Although the degree of respiratory depression is related to the dose, timing, and specific pharmacological characteristics of an opioid, respiratory depression can occur within the analgesic dose range, and as early as in the first few minutes after administration of a single dose of systemic opioids. In comparison, agonist-antagonist opioids appear to be less likely to cause respiratory depression, whereas fentanyl (a potent opioid) and its derivatives (e.g., sufentanil) can cause serious chest rigidity after a single dose, further compromising the respiratory effort. Although opioid-induced respiratory depression does not generally result in significant clinical consequences in most contexts, life-threatening respiratory depression can occur in those patients who are elderly, concomitantly use other respiratory suppression drugs (e.g., sedatives, muscle relaxants, alcohol), and have underlying respiratory diseases. Opioids can also cause or exacerbate obstructive sleep apnea, especially during initiation or dose titration, and should be used with caution in this population. Naloxone can reverse opioid-induced respiratory depression, but its short half-life often requires re-dosing.

Temperature Regulation

The hypothalamic temperature regulatory point can be reset by opioids, leading to a decrease in body temperature. However, opioids such as meperidine in combination with monoamine oxidase inhibitors can paradoxically result in life-threatening hyperthermia and coma.

Antitussive Effects

Opioids such as codeine have long been used as effective antitussive agents. Opioids' antitussive effect is mainly due to their action on the medullary cough center. In general, the antitussive effects of opioids occur at much lower doses than the respiratory depressant effects. Some opioid derivatives such as dextromethorphan possess antitussive properties with negligible analgesic and respiratory depression effects, and are extensively used in over-the-counter cough medicines.

Nausea and Vomiting

Distinct from their inhibitory effects on peristalsis, which might also cause nausea and vomiting, opioids can cause nausea and emesis via their direct action on the central chemoreceptor trigger zone located in the area postrema of the medulla. Although all opioids have the potential to cause nausea and vomiting, the capacity of each opioid to elicit these side effects differs (i.e., oral morphine may be associated with a higher incidence than other opioids). Because sustained-release transdermal formulations such as the fentanyl patch do not cause as much slowing of the GI tract and are generally associated with lower peak blood levels than shorter-acting oral or transmucosal formulatons, the incidence of nausea and vomiting caused by such formulations might also be lower. Similar to other opioid-related side effects, patients usually develop tolerance to these adverse effects. Employing opioid rotation can effectively reduce the occurrence of nausea and vomiting.

Pruritus

Opioid-related pruritus might be centrally mediated, although its exact mechanisms remain to be elucidated. Pruritus may occur with any route of opioid administration; however, it does appear to be more likely following intrathecal or epidural administration. Some opioids such as morphine are more likely to cause this problem, possibly as a result of histamine release. Thus, changing to a different opioid or switching to an opioid agonist-antagonist might alleviate this side effect. In severe cases, a small dose of naloxone can reduce opioid-related pruritus without substantially reversing the analgesic effects.

Miosis

Severe constriction of the pupils is a hallmark sign of opioid overdose, particularly in association with μ- and κ-opioid toxicity. Although tolerance to the miotic effect of opioids can develop, miosis persists even in opioid addicts. This effect is largely due to the excitatory effects of opioids on the parasympathetic system innervating the pupil.

GI SYSTEM

Opioids exert many GI effects via their action on GI motility, tone, and secretions, causing either therapeutic effects or significant side effects.

GI Motility

In patients on regular opioid therapy, the incidence of opioid-related bowel dysfunction ranges from 40 percent to 50 percent, increasing in the elderly and individuals on high doses. Most opioids reduce motility at multiple GI sites, including the stomach and the small and large intestines. Gastric emptying times might be delayed by as much as 12 hours. These actions increase the risk of gastric reflux and aspiration, particularly in those patients who already have a compromised gag reflex. In the small and large intestines, the propulsive peristaltic waves are diminished or abolished, and resting tone and spasm are increased by opioids. The delayed passage of bowel contents leads to considerable desiccation of the feces, which is a major cause of opioid-related constipation. This side effect can be particularly detrimental in elderly patients treated with opioids. Although opioid-induced constipation is generally an unwanted side effect, opioids have been used to treat hypersecretion and hypermotility associated with diarrhea.[14]

GI Tone

Opioids cause increased tone at the antral portion of the stomach and other parts of the GI tract with periodic spastic activities. In particular, morphine-induced spastic constriction of the sphincter of Oddi is well documented in patients with biliary tract disease, which can result in pain and occasionally nausea, vomiting, fevers, and diarrhea. Some opioids such as meperidine, fentanyl, and butorphanol might produce less biliary spasm than morphine. Besides their effects on the GI tract, opioids also act on other smooth muscle groups such as those in the urinary tract and uterus. The voiding reflex is reduced, and external sphincter tone is increased, causing urinary retention. This adverse effect is more common in the elderly, males with prostatic hypertrophy, and those on analgesic drugs with anticholinergic effects, such as antidepressants and antipsychotics. In severe cases, treatment might require bladder catheterization.

GI Secretion

μ-opioid receptor agonists reduce the secretion of hydrochloric acid in the stomach and decrease biliary, pancreatic, and intestinal secretions. Although the direct effect of opioid receptor activation in parietal cells of the stomach is increased secretions, the indirect effects of opioids, through increased release of somatostatin and decreased release of acetylcholine, are often dominant, thereby counteracting opioid's direct effects on gastric secretions.

CARDIOVASCULAR SYSTEM

Myocardium

Cardiovascular functions are affected by opioids as well. Although severe opioid-related myocardial depression is rare in healthy individuals, in patients with coronary artery disease, opioids can reduce cardiac oxygen consumption and left ventricular end-diastolic pressure. This, in combination with their sedative and analgesic effects, is why opioids such as morphine can be beneficial in patients with acute myocardial infarction. However, the potential consequences of vasodilatation via an opioid's effects on the vascular system should always be taken into consideration in the clinical setting.

Vascular System

Opioids can cause significant peripheral vasodilatation. This can produce profound hypotension, particularly in patients with decreased blood volume, which occurs in patients with hypertension and other cardiovascular problems and in the elderly. Histamine release promoted by opioids is largely responsible for opioids' vasodilatory effects. Some opioids cause less histamine release (e.g., fentanyl, sufentanil) than others (e.g., morphine) and might be useful in such cases. H_1-receptor antagonists do not completely reverse or prevent morphine-induced hypotension. Instead, naloxone appears to be more effective.

TOLERANCE, DEPENDENCE, ADDICTION, AND OIH

The development of tolerance and dependence is an intrinsic pharmacological property of all opioid receptor agonists. Opioid use can also lead to OIH. Opioid addiction is a psychiatric substance abuse disorder.

Tolerance

Opioid tolerance is a pharmacological phenomenon in which repeated exposure to an opioid results in a decreased therapeutic effect or the need for a higher dose in order to maintain the same effect. Mechanisms responsible for tolerance can include desensitization due to decreased interaction with the G-protein second messenger system, and internalization of opioid receptors.

Dependence

Physical dependence manifests as a constellation of clinical symptoms and signs upon inappropriate withdrawal (abstinence) from opioids following their use. Withdrawal symptoms and signs might include the following:

fatigue	coryza	lacrimation
yawning	pupillary dilation	piloerection
diaphoresis	increased anxiety	tachycardia
nausea	diarrhea	abdominal cramping
vomiting	insomnia	increased sensitivity to pain

Addiction

Opioid addiction is a substance abuse disorder characterized by persistent use despite significant adverse consequences. In the context of pain treatment, patients with opioid addiction might demonstrate any of the following: (1) impaired ability to control opioid use, (2) using opioids for a purpose other than pain relief, (3) requesting opioids or opioid dose escalation despite adequate analgesia, and/or (4) drug-seeking behaviors (e.g., multiple opioid prescription providers, unexplainable loss of opioid prescriptions, multiple episodes of early refills). Whereas doctor shopping tends to occur more commonly in women, diversion appears to be more common in men. Opioid addiction must be differentiated from pseudoaddiction, which can present with similar behaviors.

Recently, several abuse-resistant (abuser is less able to abuse) or abuse-deterrent (abuser would not want to abuse) formulations of long-acting opioids have been introduced in clinical practice. Whereas abuse-resistant formulations incorporate physical barriers designed to reduce the ability of someone to physically (e.g., crushing or chewing) or chemically (e.g., extracting) alter the compound, abuse-deterrent formulations such as Embeda contain an opioid antagonist (e.g., naloxone) that is release when the drug is physically manipulated, thereby blocking the rapid euphoric (and analgesic) effect. Although these drugs can theoretically prevent or reduce the incidence of recreational drug abuse, they cannot prevent patients from overdosing from taking more drug than prescribed.

Pseudoaddiction

Pseudoaddiction refers to "abnormal behaviors" that occur as a direct consequence of inadequate pain control. Many of these behaviors are similar to those seen with addiction. Some physicians consider this phenomenon as an iatrogenic cause of inadequate pain management with opioid analgesics. The development of pseudoaddiction might be related to (1) the inadequate prescription of analgesics to treat pain, (2) demands for opioid prescription by the patient to overcome inadequate pain relief, and/or (3) mistrust between the patient and the healthcare team. In contrast to addiction, the aberrant behaviors associated with pseudoaddiction disappear when a trial of opioid dose escalation adequately alleviates pain.

OIH

Opioid administration can induce a paradoxical increase in pain sensitivity, including hyperalgesia (enhanced painful response to noxious stimuli) and/or allodynia (painful response elicited by innocuous stimuli). This might be seen with acute or chronic administration of opioids, particularly in high doses. It is difficult to distinguish pharmacological tolerance from hyperalgesia when analgesic effects are assessed via subjective pain scores, but several features of OIH observed in animal and human studies can be helpful in making this distinction. (1) Because OIH conceivably exacerbates a preexisting pain condition, pain intensity should be increased above the level of preexisting pain following opioid treatment in the absence of apparent disease progression. (2) OIH is less well-defined in terms of quality and often extends beyond the distribution of a preexisting pain state because the underlying mechanisms of OIH involve neural circuits and extensive cellular and molecular changes. (3) Quantitative sensory testing might reveal changes in pain threshold, tolerability, and distribution patterns in subjects with OIH. (4) Whereas the undertreatment of a preexisting pain condition or the development of pharmacological tolerance can be overcome by a trial of opioid dose escalation, OIH is typically worsened following opioid dose escalation.[15–17]

PRACTICAL ISSUES REGARDING OPIOID THERAPY

Opioid administration and dosing are clearly outlined in many pharmacological handbooks and textbooks. Several practical issues are outlined as follows.

Dose Titration

Start with a small dose of opioid, and then slowly titrate up to achieve pain control. The principle behind this practice is to administer the lowest possible dose that produces adequate analgesia in order to minimize side effects.

Choice of Opioid

Many short-acting opioids such as codeine, hydrocodone, and oxycodone are found in combination with non-opioid compounds (usually acetaminophen or, less commonly, a non-steroidal anti-inflammatory drug), including Tylenol #3, Vicodin, and Percocet. Many physicians are familiar with the use of these compounds in the short-term for mild to moderate pain. However, toxicity from acetaminophen overdose in these compounds might be a limiting factor for patients who need to use high doses of opioids for their pain control, especially in patients who already have impaired liver function. Similarly, morphine might not be a good choice in patients with renal dysfunction because of the risk of accumulation of morphine's active metabolite products, such as morphine-6-glucuronide, which has a longer half-life and is more potent than morphine, and morphine-3-glucuronide, which is inactive but possesses neuroexcitatory effects (i.e., opioid hyperalgesia, myoclonus, or even seizures with high doses). In patients with renal failure, the buildup of active or toxic metabolites and the dialyzability of the parent drug and its metabolites have to be considered. Current recommendations are that methadone and fentanyl are relatively safe, morphine and codeine are best avoided if possible, and oxycodone and hydromorphone should be used with caution in patients with renal failure.[18] The potential for abuse of different opioids is another factor that might influence drug selection, with sustained release transdermal fentanyl and long-acting methadone being associated with less euphoria and possibly abuse potential than other opioids.

Short-acting versus Long-acting Opioids

In the acute pain setting, a short-acting opioid alone will be appropriate for pain management. Patient-controlled analgesia is frequently used in post-surgical or other trauma patients to provide quick and easy access for pain control, with studies showing superior pain relief and fewer side effects than observed with intermittent opioid administration. After intravenous medications are discontinued, short-acting oral opioids can be continued and slowly tapered for pain control. In individuals with constant, chronic pain, sustained-release opioids might provide superior pain relief with fewer side effects than comparable doses of short-acting preparations. Because most chronic pain patients experience some breakthrough pain, short-acting opioids can be used as supplementation.

Opioid Contract/Agreement

Opioid agreements have become a tool for providing better communication between physicians and patients regarding the side effects and risks of long-term opioid treatment. They can reduce the likelihood that patients will receive prescriptions from multiple prescribers (doctor shopping), request early refills, and call physicians after hours. Opioid agreements can provide grounds for a physician to terminate opioid treatment, but they will not necessarily serve as a reliable tool for identifying patients who are abusing opioids. Some experts advocate three-way opioid agreements involving the patient, the prescribing physician, and the primary care provider. Although opioid agreements might increase the physician's comfort level with opioid therapy, it is debatable whether or not they provide any legal protection.[19]

MANAGING SIDE EFFECTS

Respiratory Side Effects

(1) Carefully selecting the right opioid agent based on a patient's age, concomitant use of other respiratory depressant drugs, and underlying respiratory diseases is the first measure used to prevent a complication. (2) Slow opioid dose titration and close monitoring of the patient are needed, especially in elderly patients. (3) The opioid receptor antagonist naloxone can be used in incremental doses to effectively reverse opioid-induced respiratory depression should it occur. Histamine release from opioid therapy also causes bronchial constriction and can further compromise respiratory status in patients with obstructive pulmonary disease. Under such circumstances, agents such as fentanyl or oxycodone might be less troublesome than morphine (Table 1.2).

Table 1.2 THE TREATMENT OF COMMON OPIOID-RELATED SIDE EFFECTS

Side Effect	*Tolerance*	*Treatment*
Euphoria, sedation	Yes	Stimulants such as methylphenidate and modafinil
Neuroendocrine effects	No	Testosterone supplementation in men; less research has been done in woman, but oral contraceptives or dehydroepiandrosterone might be beneficial
Sleep disturbances	No	Appropriate sleep hygiene

(continued)

Table 1.2 (*CONTINUED*)

Side Effect	*Tolerance*	*Treatment*
Cognitive effects	Yes	Refrain from complex tasks requiring cognitive and psychomotor function such as driving during acute dose increases. Stimulants might be beneficial in some people.
Respiratory depression	Yes	μ receptor antagonists such as naloxone
Constipation	No	Avoid dehydration and encourage activity and a diet rich in fiber. Transdermal formulations (e.g., fentanyl) might have a lower incidence. If ineffective, consider peristalsis-stimulating opioids and stool softeners. Consider magnesium preparations and peripherally acting opioids (e.g., methylnaltrexone) for refractory cases.
Nausea and vomiting	Yes	Consider use of a co-analgesic (e.g., non-steroidal anti-inflammatory medication or adjuvant) or opioid rotation. If ineffective, dopamine antagonists (e.g., metoclopramide or prochlorperazine), 5-hydroxytryptamine-3 (5-HT-3) antagonists, or anticholinergics (scopolamine) can be helpful.

(continued)

Table 1.2 *(CONTINUED)*

Side Effect	*Tolerance*	*Treatment*
Pruritis	Yes	The strongest evidence supports μ antagonists, but the parenteral formulations limit their utility. Antihistamines such as diphenhydramine are first-line oral treatments. Dopamine and 5-HT-3 antagonists may be considered as alternatives.
Urinary retention	No	Consider use of co-analgesics without urinary retention properties (e.g., gabapentin, acetaminophen) and discontinuing concomitant drugs with anticholinergic effects (antidepressants). μ receptor antagonists might provide some benefit but are limited by their lack of a readily available oral formulation. Straight catheterization might be required in refractory cases.
Opioid-induced hyperalgesia	No	Important to distinguish from tolerance; this can be accomplished with a trial of dose escalation or dose reduction. If suspected, consider a drug holiday, reducing the opioid dose until hyperalgesia improves, or switching to a different opioid. The addition of adjuvants might help dose tapering. The use of NMDA receptor antagonists (e.g., dextromethorphan) might be helpful in some cases.

Constipation and Other GI Side Effects

An aggressive bowel regimen should be initiated at the same time as opioid therapy in order to prevent constipation. Fluid hydration, maintaining a high activity level, and consuming a diet high in fiber are simple measures that can decrease opioid-related bowel dysfunction in patients who take opioids. Oral laxatives can be divided into two major categories: softening agents and peristalsis-inducing drugs. Stool softeners such as docusate sodium can be used prophylactically and are associated with few side effects. These serve to increase secretions in the GI tract, as well as the absorption of these secretions by hard stool. Stool softeners by themselves are largely ineffective when administered in individuals who are dehydrated.

Bulk-forming laxatives such as fiber and psyllium are often considered as first-line therapy for constipation. When these are ineffective, osmotic laxatives such as lactulose (15 to 30 ml BID) might be effective. These agents produce an influx of fluid into the small bowel, thereby increasing peristalsis and softening stool. Peristalsis-inducing agents such as senna and bisacodyl act via direct stimulation of the mesenteric plexus. As with other drugs that enhance peristalsis, abdominal pain, diarrhea, and flatulence are potential side effects. Suppositories and enemas might be unpalatable to some patients and are generally reserved for refractory cases.

Stimulant laxative suppositories work predominantly via a local effect and therefore might be ineffective when feces are impacted high in the GI tract. Severe opioid-related constipation that is unresponsive to conservative management can be reversed by oral naloxone. However, high doses of μ-antagonists can counteract the analgesic effects when absorbed systemically. Methylnaltrexone is a recently approved peripherally acting opioid receptor antagonist that does not cross the blood–brain barrier, and it has been shown to be effective in around 50 percent of patients with opioid-induced constipation. Because of its peripheral mechanism of action, in addition to maintaining analgesia, methylnaltrexone will also not reverse centrally mediated opioid adverse effects (including the central contribution to bowel dysfunction). For morphine-induced biliary spasm, naloxone remains the gold standard, though atropine or nitroglycerine (0.6 to 1.2 mg) can also be effective.[20]

Nausea and Vomiting

Opioid dose reduction and opioid rotation can reduce the incidence of opioid-induced nausea and vomiting. This side effect also can be treated with dopaminergic antagonists (droperidol, metoclopramide, prochlorperazine), anticholinergics (scopolamine), and/or serotonin antagonists (ondansetron). The successful treatment of constipation can also be helpful in reducing nausea and vomiting.

Pruritus

Antihistamine drugs such as diphenhydramine can be used to treat pruritus caused by opioid therapy. When this is unsuccessful, μ-antagonists (e.g., naloxone) can provide relief in refractory cases. Opioid rotation also might be helpful.

Opioid Tolerance

When opioid tolerance is suspected in a clinical setting, the following measures offer a reasonable treatment algorithm. (1) Increase the opioid dose by 15 percent to 20 percent at each dose adjustment until a good analgesic effect is achieved. The interval of such dose adjustments might depend on the half-life of the opioid used, as well as on the disease state. (2) Opioid rotation may be considered. Empirically, the equianalgesic dose for a new opioid might be decreased by 30 percent to 50 percent because of incomplete cross-tolerance (i.e., although people on long-standing morphine will be tolerant to all opioids, they are somewhat less tolerant to non-morphine opioids). (3) Because tolerance might be partially mediated through a mechanism involving *N*-methyl-D-aspartate (NMDA) receptors, a clinically available NMDA receptor antagonist (e.g., dextromethorphan, memantine, amantadine, or ketamine) may be employed in conjunction with an opioid. Dextromethorphan (30 to 60 mg every 6 to 8 hours, titrated to effect) can retard the progression of tolerance. Other drug classes that might potentially decrease tolerance include calcium channel blockers and cholecystokinin antagonists.

Methadone is a unique long-acting opioid that can inhibit the reuptake of norepinephrine and serotonin, as well as block NMDA receptors. Because serotonin and norepinephrine reuptake blockade and NMDA receptor antagonism can both alleviate neuropathic pain, methadone might be an ideal choice in individuals with a neuropathic component to their pain (which might require higher doses of opioids to treat) or those who have developed tolerance to other opioids. The potential for serious methadone-related side effects must be considered in the clinical setting. In patients on methadone, death might result from cardiotoxicity related to a prolonged QT interval or accidental overdose due to the slow accumulation resulting from methadone's long half-life (i.e., it might take up to a week in some patients for methadone to reach a steady-state blood level, which can lead noncompliant patients to increase the dose on their own). (4) The use of adjuvant medications to target different pain mechanisms is also recommended, including acetaminophen, non-steroidal anti-inflammatory drugs, antidepressants, anticonvulsants, topical agents, and neuropathic pain medications. For cancer-related pain, radiation therapy and/or chemotherapy are often effective adjunctive therapies.[21]

MANAGING OIH

Sometimes the only way to distinguish opioid hyperalgesia from tolerance is a trial of drug weaning. When OIH is suspected, several approaches may be considered. (1) Slowly decrease the opioid dose by 10 percent to 15 percent every 3 to 7 days until hyperalgesia is improved. (2) Consider opioid rotation; patients might get better pain relief with a different opioid analgesic, often at a lower equianalgesic dose. (3) Use adjuvant pain medications as stated above to minimize the amount of opioid, thereby reducing the risk of worsening hyperalgesia. (4) Use clinically available NMDA receptor antagonists such as dextromethorphan, memantine, and ketamine.

MANAGING PHYSICAL DEPENDENCE AND WITHDRAWAL SYMPTOMS

Depending on the dosage used and the duration of therapy, reductions in opioid doses of between 50 percent and 80 percent can be undertaken without precipitating withdrawal. When withdrawal symptoms and signs are observed, a number of approaches can be considered, including restarting the same opioid at the previous dose. If the goal is to discontinue opioid therapy, taper the dose at a rate of 15 percent to 20 percent every 3 to 7 days after initially reducing the starting dose by 33 percent to 50 percent. Clonidine is an α-2 agonist that is frequently used to prevent and treat withdrawal symptoms. It is typically dosed orally at 0.2 to 0.4 mg/day (or at a transdermal dose of 0.1 to 0.3 mg applied once per week). Treatment can be continued for 4 days for short-acting opioids, or for up to 14 days for long-acting opioids. Other medications that have been used to manage opioid withdrawal include methadone, lofexidine, and buprenorphine. A recent Cochrane review concluded that there was stronger evidence to support buprenorphine as an effective treatment for opioid withdrawal than clonidine or lofexidine,[22] but care must be taken to avoid withdrawal in patients on very high doses. Some experts have advocated the use of ultra-rapid opioid detoxification via naloxone challenges under general anesthesia as a means to rapidly discontinue opioid use in individuals who have failed high-dose opioid use secondary to tolerance, side effects, and OIH,[23] but this treatment has the potential for serious consequences.[24]

MANAGING PATIENTS WITH INADEQUATE PAIN RELIEF DESPITE OPIOID THERAPY

In evaluating a patient on opioids with inadequate pain relief, it is important to consider the possible reasons for the lack of response. The clinical assessment of opioid tolerance, physical dependence, or OIH should rely on (1) carefully evaluating the possibility of disease progression, (2) reviewing the details of the analgesic regimen and compliance with that regimen (i.e., failure to understand the directions, divergence), (3) documenting other medications that could potentially decrease the effectiveness of opioids (i.e., ranitidine, celecoxib, and isoniazid for codeine), and (4) exploring preexisting or newly developed psychosocial issues that can influence treatment (e.g., depression or posttraumatic stress disorder).

Although it might prove difficult to make a clear clinical distinction between true pharmacological tolerance and increased opioid demand secondary to other factors, every effort should be made to investigate the underlying causes. For example, increased pain due to disease progression can be curtailed by appropriate adjunctive therapies such as radiation therapy in cancer patients, rather than simply increasing the opioid dose. In general, opioid doses should not be escalated only to reduce subjective pain scores. In an effort to distinguish between pharmacological tolerance and OIH, a trial of dose escalation is not unreasonable. If the pain improves for more than a short time period, the cause of inadequate pain relief is likely to be opioid tolerance. However, if the pain worsens or does not consistently respond to dose escalation, OIH should be considered, and the opioid dose should be decreased or tapered off.

SUMMARY

Physician perspectives on opioid therapy for chronic pain run the gamut from extremely liberal (i.e., opioids for all chronic pain patients with no limit on dosage) to ultra-conservative (i.e., only for cancer pain after non-opioid treatments have failed). When considering opioid therapy, one must weigh the likelihood of treatment success against the potential adverse effects. Long-term success with opioid therapy is contingent on a multitude of factors, including genetics, psychological factors, clinical and disease-specific factors, and co-morbidities that can influence how well medications are tolerated. Young patients might be more likely to develop tolerance than older patients, and neuropathic pain (e.g., diabetic neuropathic, postherpetic neuralgia) might require higher doses than nociceptive pain (e.g., arthritis). Although virtually all guidelines advocate opioids as a reasonable treatment for malignant pain, it should be recognized that cancer patients are just as likely to experience side effects and exhibit aberrant behaviors as are other patients in the same demographic category. In contrast, there is little clinical evidence to support long-term opioid therapy in patients with long-standing functional pain syndromes (e.g., fibromyalgia, irritable bowel syndrome), although some well-selected patients with these disorders might benefit. In conclusion, successful opioid treatment depends on careful patient selection and opioid selection, slow dose titration to obtain adequate pain control using the lowest possible dose, and vigilance with regard to monitoring side effects.

REFERENCES

1. Howard F. Chronic pelvic pain. *Obstet Gynecol.* 2003;101(3):594–611.
2. Yaksh TL, Wallace MS. Opioids, analgesia, and pain management. In: Brunton LL, ed. *Goodman & Gilman's The Pharmacological Basis of Therapeutics.* 12th ed. New York, NY: McGraw-Hill; 2006; 481–526.
3. Dietis N, Rowbotham DJ, Lambert DG. Opioid receptor subtypes: fact or artifact? *Br J Anaesth.* 2011;107:8–18.
4. Heinricher MM, Morgan MM, Fields HL. Direct and indirect actions of morphine on medullary neurons that modulate nociception. *Neuroscience.* 1992;48:533–543.
5. Yaksh TL, Nouiehed R. Physiology and pharmacology of spinal opiates. *Ann Rev Pharmacol Toxicol.* 1985;25:433–462.
6. Rossi GC, Pasternak GW, Bodnar RJ. Mu and delta opioid synergy between the periaqueductal gray and the rostro-ventral medulla. *Brain Res.* 1994;665:85–93.
7. Stein C, Lang LJ. Peripheral mechanisms of opioid analgesia. *Curr Opin Pharmacol.* 2009;9:3–8.
8. Aloisi AM, Aurilio C, Bachiocco V, et al. Endocrine consequences of opioid therapy. *Psychoneuroendocrinology.* 2009;34 Suppl 1:S162–S168.
9. Paturi AK, Surani S, Ramar K. Sleep among opioid users. *Postgrad Med.* 2011;123:80–87.
10. Kamboj SK, Tookman A, Jones L, Curran HV. The effects of immediate-release morphine on cognitive functioning in patients receiving chronic opioid therapy in palliative care. *Pain.* 2005;117:388–395.
11. Tassain V, Attal N, Fletcher D, et al. Long term effects of oral sustained release morphine on neuropsychological performance in patients with chronic non-cancer pain. *Pain.* 2003;104:89–400.
12. Sjogren P, Thomsen AB, Olsen AK. Impaired neuropsychological performance in chronic nonmalignant pain patients receiving long-term oral opioid therapy. *J Pain Symptom Manage.* 2000;19:100–8.

13. Darke S, Sims J, McDonald S, Wickes W. Cognitive impairment among methadone maintenance patients. *Addiction.* 2000;95:687–695.
14. Thomas JR, Cooney GA, Slatkin NE. Palliative care and pain: new strategies for managing opioid bowel dysfunction. *J Palliat Med.* 2008;11 Suppl 1:S1–S19.
15. Trujillo KA, Akil H. Inhibition of morphine tolerance and dependence by the NMDA receptor antagonist, MK-801. *Science.* 1991;251:85–87.
16. Mao J. NMDA and opioid receptors: their interactions in antinociception, tolerance, and neuroplasticity. *Brain Res Rev.* 1999;30:289–304.
17. Mao J, Price DD, Mayer DJ. Mechanisms of hyperalgesia and morphine tolerance: a current view of their possible interactions. *Pain.* 1995;62:259–274.
18. Dean M. Opioids in renal failure and dialysis patients. *J Pain Symptom Manage.* 2004;28:497–504.
19. Arnold RM, Han PK, Seltzer D. Opioid contracts in chronic nonmalignant pain management: objectives and uncertainties. *Am J Med.* 2006;119:292–296.
20. Thomas J. Opioid-induced bowel dysfunction. *J Pain Symptom Manage.* 2008;35:103–113.
21. Uppington J. Opioids. In: Ballantyne J, ed. *The Massachusetts General Hospital Handbook of Pain Management.* 3rd ed. Lippincott, Williams & Wilkins; 2006; 104–126.
22. Gowing L, Ali R, White JM. Buprenorphine for the management of opioid withdrawal. *Cochrane Database Syst Rev.* 2009;3:CD002025.
23. O'Connor PG, Kosten TR. Rapid and ultrarapid opioid detoxification techniques. *JAMA.* 1998;279:229–234.
24. Gold CG, Cullen DJ, Gonzales S, Houtmeyers G, Dwyer MJ. Rapid opioid detoxification during general anesthesia: a review of 20 patients. *Anesthesiology.* 1999;91:1639–1647.

2

NSAIDs and Adjunctive Pain Medications

HOWARD S. SMITH, KALYNA APKARIAN, AND
CHARLES E. ARGOFF

Chronic pain is an extremely difficult and challenging clinical problem. Despite a relative lack of robust supporting evidence, it appears that a multimodal approach employing various combinations of pharmacologic, interventional, cognitive-behavioral, rehabilitative, neuromodulatory, complementary, and alternative therapies/techniques might currently represent the best treatment.[1]

NON-OPIOID PHARMACOLOGIC THERAPY

Non-opioid analgesics constitute an important group of agents for alleviating pain. Non-opioid analgesics may provide analgesia via a variety of different mechanisms. It is important to appreciate pharmacologic issues with respect to non-opioid analgesics concerning ceiling effects, adverse effects, synergistic effects, and drug–drug interactions, as well as the possible additive adverse effects of combination therapy.

Acetaminophen

Acetaminophen (known as paracetamol in Europe) is the most commonly administered over-the-counter analgesic, although its analgesic mechanisms remain uncertain.[2] Acetaminophen does not possess significant anti-inflammatory effects, but it continues to be a mainstay in guidelines for the treatment of osteoarthritis, especially in older adults who are more likely to experience adverse events with non-steroidal anti-inflammatory drugs (NSAIDs) and adjuvants.[3]

The maximum daily dose of acetaminophen has been 4 g/d; however, there is consideration of lowering that maximum to 3 or 3.2 g/d. In combination products containing acetaminophen and an opioid, the maximum dose of acetaminophen per pill will be limited to 325 mg. In many cases, there is little advantage in combining acetaminophen with traditional NSAIDs (tNSAIDs), and in some instances there might be increased adverse effects. However, in some people, the combination of acetaminophen and an NSAID might be better than either drug alone (as seen in human experimental data).[4] In head-to-head studies, NSAIDs are more effective analgesics than acetaminophen, so the main advantage of acetaminophen is a more favorable side effect profile, especially in the elderly. Intravenous acetaminophen (Ofirmev®) can be administered for acute pain or in the perioperative setting in doses of up to 1 g infusion.[5]

NSAIDs

NSAIDs contain anti-inflammatory, analgesic, and antipyretic properties. They are used widely to reduce pain, decrease morning stiffness, and improve function in patients with arthritis, in addition to their use as a treatment for as a host of other painful conditions, including headache, dysmenorrhea, and postoperative pain.[6] Although NSAIDs are one of the most commonly prescribed medications for neuropathic pain, there is little evidence in support of their use in this context. NSAIDs have been categorized into different classes based on their basic chemical structures (Table 2.1). Individual NSAIDs differ in potency with respect to their analgesic,

Table 2.1 CLASSIFICATION OF NONSTEROIDAL ANTI-INFLAMMATORY DRUGS BY CHEMICAL STRUCTURE CLASSES

Class	*Drug: Generic Name (Brand Name)*	*Indications and Supporting Evidence*
Propionic acids	Naproxen (Naprosyn, Anaprox, Aleve)	• Balanced inhibitory effects on both COX-1 and COX-2 • Might be among NSAIDs with the least increase in cardiovascular risk
	Flurbiprofen (Ansaid)	• An ophthalmic formulation exists • S-flurbiprofen appears to have both central and peripheral antinociceptive effects; R-flurbiprofen has only central effects
	Oxaprozin (Daypro)	• On initiation of therapy, can give three 600 mg tablets (1800 mg) for a loading dose • Once-daily dosing • No significant enterohepatic recirculation
	Ibuprofen (Motrin)	• Available as intravenous formulation, as well as in combination with hydrocodone or oxycodone

(continued)

Table 2.1 *(CONTINUED)*

Class	*Drug: Generic Name (Brand Name)*	*Indications and Supporting Evidence*
	Ketoprofen (Orudis, Oruvail)	• Might be effective in the prophylaxis of heterotopic calcification following hip or major pelvic intervention without affecting bone healing processes; available in topical formulation
	Ketorolac (Toradol)	• Oral and intravenous formulations available
Indoleacetic acids	Sulindac (Clinoril)	
	Indomethacin (Indocin)	• Drug of choice for chronic paroxysmal hemicrania headaches
	Etodolac (Lodine)	• Inhibits COX-2 preferentially more than COX-1
Phenylacetic acids	Diclofenac (Cataflam, Voltaren)	• Also available in topical formulations (e.g., gel, patch)
Salicylic acids (nonacetylated)	Salsalate (Disalcid)	
	Choline magnesium trisalicylate (CMT) (Trillsate)	• Might have fewer effects on platelet function and cause less GI mucosal insult than other compounds

(continued)

Table 2.1 (*CONTINUED*)

Class	*Drug: Generic Name (Brand Name)*	*Indications and Supporting Evidence*
Naphtylalkanone	Nabumetone (Relafen)	• The active component 6-methoxy-2-napthylactic acid inhibits COX-2 more preferentially than COX-1 • No enterohepatic recirculation
Oxicam	Piroxicam (Feldene)	• Once-daily dosing • Majority of effects appear to be peripheral
Anthranilic acid	Mefenamic acid (Ponstel)	
	Meclofenamate	• Potent inhibitor of 5-lipoxygenase and might be tolerated better by patients with aspirin-induced asthma; however, caution is advised in this context
Pyrroleacetic acid	Tolmetin (Tolectin)	• Half-life is biphasic-rapid (1 to 2 hours) and slow (~5 hours)
Pyrazolone	Phenylbutazone	

(*continued*)

Table 2.1 *(CONTINUED)*

Class	*Drug: Generic Name (Brand Name)*	*Indications and Supporting Evidence*
COX-2 Inhibitors	Celecoxib	• No effect on platelet function; can be utilized safely in perioperative period. Less GI toxicity than conventional NSAIDs. Might also have fewer adverse effects on bone formation (i.e., can be used after orthopedic surgery).

anti-inflammatory, and antipyretic properties, with the doses needed for anti-inflammatory activity being generally higher than those required in order to produce analgesia.[7] The anti-inflammatory effects of NSAIDs are thought to be due to the inhibition of cyclooxygenase (COX). There seems to be wide variation in the analgesic activity of various NSAIDs—even ones in the same class (or family; e.g., acetic acids)—such that large individual differences may exist. One NSAID might not work well for an individual patient, but another might work much better.[7]

tNSAIDs may be associated with multiple adverse effects; the three major ones are gastrointestinal mucosal insult, renal toxicity, and inhibition of platelet function. Risk factors for NSAID-induced gastroduodenal toxic effects include advanced age (>60 years); previous history of peptic ulcer, bleeding, or perforation of any type (or of past NSAID-induced gastrointestinal toxicity); multiple advanced co-morbid conditions; high-dose NSAIDs taken over prolonged periods; concomitant use of two or more NSAIDs; and concomitant use of gluocorticoids. Efforts to reduce the gastrointestinal toxicity of tNSAIDs include adding other separate agents such as proton pump inhibitors to NSAID therapy and using combination products (such as Arthotec® [a combination of diclofenac and misoprostol] or Prevacid® NapraPAC™ 500 [a combination of naproxen and lansoprazole]). Future efforts may include utilizing nitric oxide (NO)-releasing NSAIDs such as COX-inhibiting NO donators (CINODs).[8] Hybrid molecules generated by coupling an NO- or hydrogen sulfide–releasing moiety to aspirin or tNSAIDs are in development but are not yet ready for clinical use. Naproxcinod is a CINOD that has been investigated in clinical trials. Risk factors for NSAID-induced nephrotoxicity include hypovolemia, severe congestive heart failure, advanced hepatic cirrhosis, and preexisting chronic kidney disease.

Recently, the finding that conventional NSAIDs and COX-2 inhibitors might increase the risk of cardiovascular events in certain individuals has generated enormous attention. Prescribers of tNSAIDs and COX-2 inhibitors should use the lowest dose possible for control of symptoms for the shortest possible duration of time and conduct periodic surveillance for efficacy and adverse events. If NSAIDs are prescribed in patients with preexisting cardiovascular disease, one should consider adding aspirin (81 mg, enteric coated) in combination as a means to mitigate prothrombotic tendencies. Some NSAIDs (but not COX-2 inhibitors), when taken before aspirin, might thwart the potential cardioprotective effects of aspirin. In some patients with COX-1 gene variants, aspirin might not afford any cardiovascular protection.

Salicylates

Salicylates can be classified into two subgroups: acetylated and nonacetylated. Aspirin and benorylate are from the acetylated group, and drugs in the nonacetylated group include choline salicylate (Arthropan), choline magnesium trisalisylate (a combination of choline salicylate and magnesium salicylate; Trilisate), and salsalate or salicylsalicylic acid (hydrolyzed to two molecules of salicylate; Disalcid).

Nonacetylated salicylates are converted to salicylic acid and are much less potent inhibitors of COX than aspirin in vitro, which might explain why they seem to cause less gastrointestinal mucosal toxicity and have less of an inhibitory effect on platelets. Yet they exhibit comparable efficacy in invivo models of inflammation. Choline magnesium trisalicylate is available as 500 mg, 750 mg, and 1000 mg tablets and as a 500 mg/5 mL oral suspension. The usual adult dose is 500 to 750 mg orally three times per day (1500 to 2250 g/d).

Naproxen

Naproxen is marketed as the (S) isomer, which has 28 times the anti-inflammatory activity of the (R) isomer. Naproxen is available in both a salt form, naproxen sodium (Anaprox, Aleve), and a base form (Naprosyn). The main difference between the two is that the salt form is absorbed more rapidly (275 mg naproxen sodium is equivalent to 250 mg naproxen base). Prescription naproxen sodium is available as 275 mg and 550 mg (Anaprox DS) tablets. Naproxen base is available as 250 mg, 375 mg, and 500 mg tablets and as a 125 mg/15 mL oral suspension. Naproxen is also marketed as an enteric-coated formulation and in a long-acting formulation (Naprelan). Naprelan is available in 375 mg and 500 mg controlled-release tablets and uses proprietary Intestinal Protective Drug Absorption System technology. This technology entails a rapidly disintegrating tablet system combining an immediate-release component with a sustained-release component of microparticles that are widely dispersed. This facilitates the absorption of the NSAID throughout the gastrointestinal tract and results in relatively stable plasma levels for about 24 hours.

Diclofenac

Diclofenac is a phenylacetic acid. In addition to inhibiting COX, diclofenac diminishes the availability of arachidonic acid by stimulating its uptake and inhibiting its release. Diclofenac sodium is available in an enteric-coated formulation (Voltaren) and as a potassium salt (Cataflam). Voltaren is available in the United States as 25 mg, 50 mg, and 75 mg enteric-coated tables, with the adult dose ranging between 75 and 225 mg/d. A combination tablet containing diclofenac (50 mg [Arthrotec 50] or 75 mg [Arthrotec 75]) in an inner enteric-coated core with misoprostol (200 μg) in the outer mantle is available. Misoprostol, a prostaglandin E_1 analog, is added to minimize gastrointestinal mucosal injury. Although misoprostol in a dose of 800 μg/d might offer maximal gastrointestinal protection, it is not well tolerated by many patients. A dose of 400 μg/d seems to offer a reasonable balance between tolerability and gastrointestinal mucosal protection. Misoprostol should be avoided by women who are considering pregnancy. The major side effects are gastrointestinal, especially diarrhea, which might be explosive in nature.

Indomethacin

Indomethacin is an indole acetic acid that seems to inhibit membrane-bound phospholipase A-2 and C in polymorphonuclear cells, in addition to inhibiting COX. Along with its analgesic effects, it has been used to delay premature labor, reduce amniotic fluid volume in polyhydramnios, and close patent ductus arteriosus. Indomethacin is available as 25 mg and 50 mg capsules, 75 mg sustained-release capsules (25 mg uncoated pellets for immediate absorption and 50 mg coated pellets for extended release), 50 mg suppositories, and an oral suspension (25 mg/0.5 mL). The usual dose is 75 to 150 mg/d.

In view of its many side effects, indomethacin is not generally recommended for minor aches and fevers.

Ketorolac

Ketorolac is available both for parenteral use and orally as the tromethamine salt. It is available as a racemic mixture, with the S(-) enantiomer responsible for its pharmacologic actions. The parenteral formulation is available as 15 mg/1 mL, 30 mg/1 mL, or 60 mg/2 mL, and the oral formulation is dosed in 10 mg tablets. It is recommended that ketorolac be given only for a maximum period of 5 days. Some guidelines suggest that oral therapy should be used only as a continuation of parenteral therapy (e.g., 2 days parenteral, then 3 days oral). The parenteral formulation contains alcohol and should not be used for spinal administration.

Ibuprofen

Ibuprofen, a propionic acid, is the most commonly used NSAID. Ibuprofen is available over the counter as 200 mg tables and by prescription as 300 mg, 400 mg, 600 mg, and 800 mg tablets, as well as in a 100 mg/5 mL oral suspension form. The usual adult dose is 1200 to 2400 mg/d. Ibuprofen is also available as an intravenous formulation (Caldolor®) (400 mg and 800 mg) that has been approved by the U.S. Food and Drug Administration (FDA) for administration as an intravenous infusion over 30 minutes. However, it can also be administered as an "off-label" intravenous infusion over 5 to 7 minutes.[9]

Meloxicam

Meloxicam is an oxicam derivative and a member of the enolic group of NSAIDs. Although it possesses some COX-2 selectivity (e.g., preferential inhibition of COX-2 over COX-1 is most pronounced at lower doses), meloxicam is not considered as a selective COX-2 inhibitor by the FDA. Meloxicam is available in 7.5 mg tablets. The recommended starting and maintenance dose for osteoarthritis is 7.5 mg orally once a day with a maximal daily dose of 15 mg. Because it is associated with fewer gastrointestinal side effects, unlike most NSAIDs, meloxicam may be given without regard to meals.[10]

COX-2 Inhibitors

Perhaps the most significant difference between tNSAIDs and COX-2 selective inhibitors is noted in clinical situations when the risk of bleeding is high. This is likely due to the fact that there is no COX-2 enzyme in platelets, and therefore COX-2 selective inhibitors tend to have no clinically significant effects on platelets. Although etoricoxib, a more selective COX-2 inhibitor than celecoxib, is widely available throughout Europe, Asia, and Latin America, it is not FDA approved for use in the United States. NSAIDs in combination with proton pump inhibitors or misoprostol are associated with a risk of gastric complications equivalent to that seen with COX-2 inhibitors. However, a theoretical benefit found with COX-2 inhibitors is that unlike tNSAIDs taken in combination with a protective agent, they might reduce the risk of toxicity in the lower gastrointestinal tract.

CELECOXIB

Celecoxib (Celebrex) is the only selective COX-2 inhibitor available for clinical use in the United States. The tablet is reasonably well absorbed after 200 mg is given orally with a high-fat meal. Although absorption is delayed, bioavailability is increased by about 40 percent, resulting in minimal delay in onset. Total protein binding is 97 percent, and it takes about 3 hours to achieve peak plasma concentration. Celecoxib is metabolized extensively in the liver, predominantly via cytochrome P-450 2C9, to three inactive metabolites. The elimination of celecoxib occurs via the kidney (27 percent) and feces (57 percent), with less than 3 percent eliminated as unchanged drug. The half-life is 11 hours. Celecoxib is available as 100 mg and 200 mg tablets and can be given once or twice per day. The usual adult dose is 100 to 400 mg/d, with higher doses generally reserved for acute pain.

Topical NSAIDs

Multiple placebo-controlled studies have demonstrated the efficacy of topical NSAIDs and salicylates for conditions such as tendonitis and other sports injuries, postoperative pain, herpes zoster, and arthritis. Systematic reviews and meta-analyses have estimated that the number needed to treat in order for one patient to experience meaningful benefit ranges from around 3 to 5.5, being slightly higher (i.e., less efficacious) for chronic musculoskeletal pain than for acute pain. There is some evidence that topical NSAIDs might provide relief similar to that obtained through systemic NSAIDs, albeit with considerably fewer side effects. Recent guidelines for osteoarthritis treatment from the National Institute for Health and Clinical Excellence highlight the importance of topical NSAIDs (e.g., diclofenac sodium topical [Voltaren®] gel 1 percent, diclofenac epolamine topical [Flector®] patch 1.3 percent, diclofenac 1 percent topical [Pennsaid] solution 1.5 percent) in the armamentarium of pain management.[11]

ADJUNCTIVE PAIN MEDICATIONS

Adjunctive analgesics (also referred to as adjuvants or co-analgesics) include a wide variety of different agents that all appear to possess antinocipcetive properties. These adjunctive medications include antidepressants (tricyclic antidepressants [TCAs], selective serotonin/norepinephrine reuptake inhibitors [SNRIs]), membrane stabilizers such as calcium channel $\alpha 2$-δ ligands and sodium channel blockers, topical lidocaine and capsaicin, *N*-methyl-D-aspartate (NMDA) receptor antagonists, and α-2 agonists (Table 2.2).

Table 2.2 ADJUNCTIVE PAIN MEDICATIONS

Drug Class	*Agents*	*Indications and Evidence*	*Adverse Effects*
Antidepressants	**TCA** Amitriptyline	• PHN • PDN • Fibromyalgia • Migraine and other headache (e.g., chronic daily headache) prophylaxis	Orthostatic hypotension, constipation, fatigue, dry mouth, tachycardia, weight gain, drowsiness
	TCA Doxepin	• PDN • Acts as an antagonist at H1 and H2 receptors	Sedation, dizziness, drowsiness, nausea
	TCA Nortriptyline	• PDN • PHN • Fibromyalgia • Antagonist at H1, 5-HT1 and 2, α_1-adrenergic, muscarinic, and 5-HT1 Receptors	Sedation, urinary retention, constipation, dry mouth, orthostatic hypotension

(continued)

Table 2.2 (CONTINUED)

Drug Class	*Agents*	*Indications and Evidence*	*Adverse Effects*
Antidepressants	**SNRI** Venlafaxine	• Might be useful for PDN • Fibromyalgia • Migraine prophylaxis	Nausea, somnolence, dry mouth, dizziness, sexual dysfunction, insomnia
	SNRI Duloxetine	• PDN • Fibromyalgia • Chronic musculoskeletal pain	Nausea, vomiting, somnolence, insomnia, dizziness, irritability, dry mouth, headaches
	SNRI Milnacipran	• Fibromyalgia	Nausea, dry mouth, nervousness, palpitations
α2-δ Ligands	Gabapentin	• PHN	Sedation, dizziness, fatigue
	Pregabalin	• PDN • PHN • Fibromyalgia	Dizziness, ataxia, edema, drowsiness, blurred vision

Sodium Channel Blockers	Carbamazepine+	• Drug of choice for trigeminal neuralgia	Nausea, dizziness, drowsiness, visual disturbances, impairment of liver function SIADH-like effects → hyponatremia, aplastic anemia, leucopenia, Stevens-Johnson syndrome, ataxia
	Oxcarbazepine	• Might be effective in certain patients with carbamazepine-unresponsive trigeminal neuralgia • PDN	Somnolence, vomiting, diarrhea, headaches, nausea, dizziness, fatigue, drowsiness, SIADH-like effects, erythema multiform
	Lamotrigine	• Might help central pain • PDN • HIV-related neuropathic pain	Stevens-Johnson syndrome, visual disturbances, toxic epidermal necrolysis, aplastic anemia, dizziness, ataxia, nausea, vomiting, sedation/drowsiness, malaise, headaches; inactivated by hepatic glucuronidation
	Topical lidocaine	• PHN pain	Local site redness, swelling, blisters, changes in skin color, rash, itching

(continued)

Table 2.2 *(CONTINUED)*

Drug Class	*Agents*	*Indications and Evidence*	*Adverse Effects*
Sodium Channel Blockers	Topical capsaicin	• PHN pain	Local site pain/erythema, transient increased arterial pressure
	Tramadol	• PDN • PHN	Drowsiness, nausea, dizziness, dry mouth, constipation, headache, seizure, physical dependence, abuse/addiction
NMDA Receptor Antago-nists	Dextromethorphan	• PDN • Traumatic neuropathic pain	
	Ketamine	• Might be useful for patients with refractory complex regional pain syndrome • PHN	Psychomimetic/dissociative phenomena, delirium, dizziness, hypersalivation, nausea, nystagmus, urinary tract effects sedation, constipation

α-2 Agonists	Clonidine	• Epidural clonidine in combination with epidural opioids for severe pain in cancer patients not adequately relieved by epidural opioids alone	Hypotension; potential rebound effect if abruptly discontinued
	Tizanidine	• Acute intermittent management of increased muscle tone related to spasticity • Certain headaches (e.g., tension-type and chronic daily headache)	Dry mouth, somnolence, dizziness, weakness

PDN, peripheral diabetic neuropathy; PHN, postherpetic neuralgia; HIV, human immunodeficiency virus; SIADH, syndrome of inappropriate antidiuretic hormone secretion.

Antidepressants

Antidepressants are a heterogenous group of drugs that have all demonstrated beneficial activity for patients with major depressive disorder. Antidepressants can be classified in multiple ways; however, one simplistic yet clinically useful categorization divides them into TCAs, SNRIs, selective serotonin reuptake inhibitors (SSRIs), and selective norepinephrine (noradrenalin) reuptake inhibitors (NRIs [NARIs]). Preclinical and clinical studies suggest that both serotonin and norepinephrine reuptake inhibition are necessary in order to effect clinically meaningful analgesia. Thus, drugs that selectively block the reuptake of either serotonin or norepinephrine alone tend to be poor analgesics, though at higher dosages serotonin-specific reuptake inhibitors might result in antinociception as the effects of norepinephrine reuptake become more prominent.

TCAs

The TCAs can be divided into tertiary amines and their de-methylated secondary amine derivatives. The loss of a methyl group (i.e., secondary amine compounds) results in a higher ratio of norepinephrine to serotonin reuptake inhibition, as well as less histamine and α-1 adrenergic (sympathetic) blockade. The tertiary amine TCAs include the following:

- amitriptyline (Evavil)
- imipramine (Tofranil)
- trimipamine (Surmontil)
- clomipramine (Anafranil)
- doxepin (Sinequan)

The secondary amine TCAs include the following:

- nortiptyline (Pamelor)
- desipramine (Norpramin)

- proptriptyline (Vivactil)
- amoxapine (Asendin)

In 1987, Max and colleagues demonstrated that TCAs possess analgesic effects independent of their effects on moods.[12] Later it was found that the analgesic effects of TCAs tend to occur more rapidly (at a week or less after initiating TCA therapy), at lower serum blood levels, and at lower doses than their antidepressive effects.

TCAs have been extensively used in the treatment of different types of neuropathic pain, and multiple randomized controlled trials (RCTs) have demonstrated their efficacy in treating various types of neuropathic pain, excluding HIV pain and chemotherapy-induced peripheral neuropathies.[13] The mechanism of action for TCAs includes both norepinephrine and serotonin reuptake inhibition. Certain TCAs, such as amitriptyline and doxepin, have demonstrated significant sodium channel and α-1 adrenergic blocking ability as well. One of the most commonly used TCAs is nortriptyline, which possesses comparable analgesic efficacy but a more favorable side-effect profile than its cousin, amitriptyline.

TCAs can exhibit a wide range of adverse effects and differ significantly in terms of which TCAs have which effects. Adverse effects include anticholinergic (desipramine has the fewest anticholinergic effects), antihistaminergic (doxepin has the most potent antihistaminergic effects), α-1 adrenergic receptor blockade (e.g., orthostatic hypotension), and cardiac effects (increasing intraventricular conduction, prolonged QT interval [prolonged conduction through the atrioventricular node]).

In addition to orthostatic hypotension, other adverse effects related to anticholinergic activity including urinary retention, constipation, and dry mouth, which in some studies affects a majority of individuals. Cardiac toxicity has been described as a possible side effect of TCAs. Sinus and ventricular arrhythmias have been noted in patients with history of coronary artery disease (CAD) and depression who are taking nortriptyline. A large review demonstrated cardiac complications including myocardial infarction in dosages exceeding 100 mg/d but failed to demonstrate adverse cardiac outcomes in patients on a regimen of less than 100 mg/d. Advantages of using TCAs for analgesic purposes are that they are taken only once daily and are inexpensive relative to other adjuvants. Before committing a patient with neuropathic pain to treatment with TCAs, the lowest effective dose should be used. In patients with a history of arrhythmias and/or CAD, TCAs should be either avoided or used with caution. Obtaining an electrocardiogram prior to starting treatment in patients over 40 years old is recommended.

Multiple reviews evaluating placebo controlled trials have found TCAs to be efficacious for several different types of neuropathic pain.[13–16] In older persons, TCAs, especially tertiary amines such as amitriptyline, might exhibit too many adverse effects to be clinically effective. In fact, amitriptyline consistently appears on the Beers list[17] of medications suggested to be inappropriate for treating older persons. In frail older patients, the SNRI duloxetine might be a reasonable choice. This underscores the distinction between efficacy, which refers to the capacity of a drug to produce a beneficial effect, and effectiveness, which is the capability of producing a beneficial effect in "real-life" circumstances. Clinicians may trial an initial low dose of half a tablet for a week to assess how well the patient tolerates this medication. Duloxetine is also available in 20 mg tablets for old and frail patients. Although the role of SSRIs in providing effective analgesia is uncertain, it appears to be limited at best.[16]

SNRIs

Duloxetine and venlafaxine are antidepressants with both serotonergic and noradrenergic reuptake inhibiting properties. In the treatment of diabetic neuropathy, duloxetine has been demonstrated to be more efficacious than placebo in doses of 60 and 120 mg/d, though the higher dose appears to be associated with similar efficacy but greater side effects.[18,19] The side-effect profile of duloxetine seems to be more favorable than that of TCAs, especially with respect to anticholinergic and cardiac side effects. Nausea is one of the more common side effects, but it can be reduced by lowering the dose.[20] For many patients, nausea is self-limiting and resolves within the first several weeks of usage. Duloxetine has been extensively studied in patients with diabetic neuropathy, fibromyalgia, musculoskeletal back pain, and osteoarthritis and is FDA approved for all four indications. Venlafaxine has been shown to be effective in the treatment of diabetic painful neuropathy and other polyneuropathies, except for postherpetic neuralgia (PHN).[14] A small subset of patients demonstrated cardiac conduction abnormalities; thus, precautions should be taken for patients with a history of cardiac disease. Venlafaxine should be tapered rather than abruptly discontinued because of the potential for a withdrawal syndrome. At doses less than 150 mg/d, venlafaxine behaves more like an SSRI); at doses above 150 mg, it behaves more like an SNRI agent. Therefore, pain relief is more likely to occur with doses of 150 mg/d or greater. Venlafaxine is not currently FDA approved for any pain indication.

Membrane Stabilizers

Calcium Channel α2-δ Ligands

Gabapentin and pregabalin are calcium channel α2-δ ligands. The mechanism of action for each of these is thought to be dependent on their ability, in an excited neuron, to reduce calcium influx into the neuron and consequently inhibit the release of neurotransmitters such as substance-P, glutamate, and norepinephrine. Although calcium channel ligands can lead to dose-dependent somnolence and dizziness, as well as weight gain and peripheral edema, they have few drug–drug interactions. Weight gain might be particularly troublesome in women and individuals with back pain, and it occurs in about 20 percent of patients. The weight gain associated with membrane stabilizers generally tends to be self-limiting and diminishes over time, but many clinicians try to counter-balance this adverse effect through the addition of membrane stabilizers associated with weight loss, such as topiramate and zonisamide. The dose of gabapentinoid drugs must be lowered in patients with renal insufficiency.[14] An additional advantage of gabapentin and pregabalin is that they possess some anxiolytic effects, which can be helpful in alleviating the concurrent anxiety often observed in patients with neuropathic pain. Gabapentin is FDA approved for PHN, whereas pregabalin is approved for PHN, painful diabetic neuropathy (PDN), and fibromyalgia. One randomized controlled study found evidence of supra-additive effects when gabapentin was combined with nortriptyline, relative to either agent administered individually, in patients with PDN or PHN.[21]

Gabapentin exhibits nonlinear pharmacokinetics. This means that as doses are increased, less of the drug is absorbed, and therefore much of it is excreted in the urine rather than being clinically effective. It should ideally be introduced to a patient in a low dose and increased gradually until either analgesia has been achieved or limiting side effects are experienced. The maximum recommended dosage for gabapentin is 3600 mg/d (though physicians sometimes use higher doses), and its effects can be seen as soon as two weeks after treatment is initated, although an adequate therapeutic trial can sometimes take more than a month. Gabapentin is now available in extended-release formulations. Although pregabalin and gabapentin have identical mechanisms of action, pregabalin has improved pharmacokinetics and linear bioavailability, both of which are significant advantages. It is approximately 3 to 6 times more potent than gabapentin. Its onset of analgesia is faster than that of gabapentin secondary to its shorter titration period. The current recommendations for pregabalin dosing are titration up to 300 mg/d for PDN and up to 600 mg/d for PHN and fibromyalgia. For maintenance treatment, it is generally dosed twice per day. However, some elderly patients and/or those patients who are more sensitive to medications might better tolerate a lower dose taken three times per day. The doses for both gabapentin and pregabalin should be reduced in patients with chronic kidney disease.

Sodium Channel Blockers

Multiple sodium channel blockers are used in efforts to ameliorate pain. Antiarrhythmics such as mexilitine are one group, but perhaps the major group comprises anti-epileptic drugs (AEDs). AEDs considered as predominantly sodium channel blockers include phenytoin, carbamazepine, oxcarbazepine, lamotrigine, and zonisamide (the first three are briefly discussed below) (Table 2.3).

CARBAMAZEPINE

Carbamazepine continues to be the drug of choice for the treatment of trigeminal neuralgia. Although carbamazepine has been utilized for PDN and other conditions associated with neuropathic pain, the evidence for such use is not as strong. The drug is predominantly metabolized in the liver (98 percent) via the cytochrome P450 isoenzyme 3A4. During prolonged treatment, carbamazepine induces its own metabolism. The active metabolite of carbamazepine (Carbamazepine-10, 11-epoxide) might partially contribute to carbamazepine intoxication. Excretion is 72 percent renal and 28 percent fecal.

OXCARBAZEPINE

Oxcarbazepine is a keto-analog of carbamazepine metabolized primarily in the liver. Oxcarbazepine is also a reasonable medical option for patients with trigeminal neuralgia and has even

Table 2.3 SELECTED PHARMACOLOGIC DATA OF SODIUM CHANNEL BLOCKERS

Agent	*Bioavailability (%)*	*Protein Binding (%)*	*Elimination Half-life (h)*	*Metabolites*	*Drug Interactions*
Carbamazepine	70–80	76	25–65	Carbamazepine 10, 11-epoxide (active)	Azithromycin, clarithromycin, anti-HIV drugs, valproic acid, phenytonin, topiramte, tramadol, tiagabine, oxcarbazepine, lamotrigine
Oxcarbazepine	Essentially total absorption after oral dose	40–60	Parent:1–25* *Prolonged to 19 hours with CKD IV-V Active metabolite: 9	10-hydroxy carbazepine (active)	Carbamazepine, ethinyl estradiol, evening primrose oil, ginkgo biloba
Lamotrigine	98	56	13–30	2N-glucuronide (inactive)	Oxcarbazepine, carbamazepine, extrogens, ginko biloba, evening primrose oil, valproic acid, phenytoin, ritonavir

been shown to be helpful to certain patients with carbamazepine-unresponsiveness trigeminal neuralgia. As is true of carbamazepine, some clinicians have used oxcarbazepine for PDN and other types of neuropathic pain. In the majority of patients, the effective dose ranged from 600 to 1200 mg/d, although in patients with intractable trigeminal neuralgia doses as high as 2400 mg/d may be used. The main advantage of oxcarbazepine over carbamazepine is its more favorable side-effect profile.

LAMOTRIGINE

Lamotrigine is absorbed rapidly and essentially completely from the gastrointestinal tract. It has a pharmacokinetic profile that appears to be linear, and kinetic parameters after multiple-dose administration are similar to those seen after a single dose. In addition to stabilizing neural membranes by blocking the activation of voltage-sensitive sodium channels (like carbamazepine and oxcarbazepine), it also inhibits the pre-synaptic release of glutamate. Although it is not typically a first- or second-line agent, some clinicians have utilized lamotrigine for intractable neuropathic pain such as PDN, HIV-associated polyneuropathy, central pain (e.g., spinal cord injury, post-stroke pain), and trigeminal neuralgia.

Other Adjuvants

Topical Lidocaine

The lidocaine patch (5 percent) is FDA approved for the treatment of PHN and may be used as part of a multimodal treatment regimen. Several RCTs have established its efficacy over placebo. Its mechanism of action stems from its ability to block sodium channels in peripheral nerves and suppression of ectopic impulses ascending to the dorsal horn. This interferes with peripheral and central sensitization and decreases the likelihood of maladaptive neuroplasticity. In addition, the patch itself is a buffer that decreases the mechanical allodynia associated with damaged nerves. The most common side effect of the patch is mild skin irritation. The patch should not be used in patients sensitive to lidocaine or type 1 antiarrhythmics such as tocainide or mexilitine, nor should it be used in patients with hepatic insufficiency, as lidocaine is metabolized by the liver. Lidocaine crosses the placental barrier and therefore should be avoided by pregnant patients or nursing mothers. The 5 percent lidocaine patch and 5 percent lidocaine-medicated plaster are safe and appear to be effective and well tolerated by patients with PHN and allodynia. Patients with a small focal area of well-localized neuropathic pain associated with stimuli (i.e., evoked pain) might benefit the most from topical lidocaine, though there are anecdotal reports of patients with more generalized conditions such as chronic low back pain experiencing relief. Although topical lidocaine patches are recommended in a 12 hours on, 12 hours off regimen, there are reports of patients using it continuously. Because the drug is not absorbed systemically, there are no systemic adverse effects. Mild local reactions are the most common side effects.

Tramadol

Tramadol is a racemate, with the (+) enantiomer having weak μ-receptor opioid properties that account for about 30 percent of its analgesic activity. The (+) enantiomer also inhibits the reuptake of serotonin, whereas the (–) enantiomer inhibits the reuptake of norepinephrine. Tramadol is available in short-acting and extended-release preparations, with the recommended starting dose for the immediate release tramadol being 50 mg every 6 to 8 hours. Because of the risk of seizures at higher doses, there is a maximum recommended dose of 400 mg/d that needs to be adjusted in patients taking other drugs with pro-convulsive properties (i.e., antidepressants). This regimen should also be adjusted for patients with kidney or liver pathology. Tramadol is not FDA approved for any neuropathic pain indications.

NMDA Receptor Antagonists

Inconsistent outcomes for the use of memantine have been observed; however, it is occasionally tried in patients who have failed other therapies.[14] Dextromethorphan is another NMDA receptor antagonist that has yielded mixed results in clinical trials. It was shown to be effective in a dose-related fashion in selected patients with PDN, but not with PHN.[22] Another controlled study performed in patients with traumatic neuropathic pain found superior pain relief with dextromethorphan relative to placebo.[23]

Ketamine is a potent NMDA receptor antagonist that exerts additional effects on myriad receptor systems, including nicotinic and muscarinic acetylcholine receptors, voltage-gated calcium and sodium channels, D2 dopamine receptors, and γ-amino-butyric acid signaling. In controlled clinical trials, intravenous administration has been shown to be superior to placebo for central pain secondary to spinal cord injury and phantom limb pain, though long-term follow-up in this context is lacking. Controlled studies have also demonstrated short-term benefit in peripheral neuropathic pain. The use of continuous ketamine infusions for refractory complex regional pain syndrome has generated intense interest in the pain management community. Although randomized studies have generally yielded good intermediate-term results, not all studies have been positive. The major limitations of the use of ketamine are the high incidence of psychomimetic side effects and the lack of a readily available oral formulation.[24]

α-2 Adrenoceptor Agonists

There are currently three α-2 adrenoceptor agonists (clonidine, tizanidine, and dexmedetomidine) that have been approved by the FDA for use (not analgesic use) in the United States. The agents all have antinociceptive properties, and they can be especially useful when employed within the context of muscular spasticity/spasms or concomitantly with opioids. The primary use for clonidine is as an antihypertensive agent. It is available in various formulations for multiple routes of administration, including oral, sublingual, transdermal, intravenous, and epidural. Tizandine is primarily used as a muscle relaxant/antispasticity agent in an oral tablet form, but it has also been shown to be effective for headache prophylaxis. In light of their ability to attenuate sympathetic nervous system activity, α-2 adrenoceptor agonists might be especially useful in neuropathic conditions associated with sympathetically maintained pain, such as complex regional pain syndrome. However, their long-term use in this context is based on predominantly anecdotal evidence. Two of the major limiting side effects of α-2 adrenoceptor agonists are sedation and orthostatic hypotension.

Topical Capsaicin

A high-potency (8 percent) capsaicin patch (Qutenza) is FDA approved for the treatment of PHN pain. It is thought to diminish pain sensation via the "defunctionalizaton" of nociceptor fibers in the application area. A single 60-minute application can provide up to 12 weeks of analgesia. Controlled studies have also demonstrated efficacy in HIV-related neuropathy.

The use of topically applied low-concentration (0.075 percent) capsaicin is approved for both nociceptive (arthralgias) and neuropathic pain, having demonstrated efficacy in diabetic neuropathy, PHN, and chronic post-surgical neuropathic pain. Derry and colleagues performed a Cochrane Review in 2009 that included six studies (389 participants) comparing 0.075 percent capsaicin cream with placebo cream and two studies comparing 8 percent capsaicin patch with placebo patch.[25] They concluded that capsaicin, in either repeated applications of a low dose (0.075 percent) cream or a single application of an 8 percent patch, might provide clinically significant pain relief in some patients with neuropathic pain.[25]

SUMMARY

NSAIDs and adjunctive analgesics can be extremely useful agents for alleviating pain and suffering in certain patients with a variety of painful conditions. Whereas NSAIDs have proven efficacy for nociceptive pain (e.g., arthritis and mechanical back pain), the evidence supporting adjuvants is more robust for neuropathic pain. The main limiting side effects of NSAIDs include gastrointestinal toxicity, bleeding, and an increased risk of adverse cardiovascular events in select patients, all of which are most pronounced in the elderly. The most prominent side effects of adjuvants are sedation and cognitive impairment. Clinicians should become familiar with agents in these classes in order to afford their patients optimal care/outcomes.

REFERENCES

1. Argoff CE, Albrecht P, Irving G, Rice F. Multimodal analgesia for chronic pain: rationale and future directions. *Pain Med.* 2009;10(Suppl 2):S53–S66.
2. Smith HS. Potential analgesic mechanisms of acetaminophen. *Pain Physician.* 2009;12(1):269–280.
3. Ferrell B, Argoff CE, Epplin J, et al. Pharmacological management of persistent pain in older persons. *Pain Med.* 2009;10(6):1062–1083.
4. Ing Lorenzini K, Besson M, Daali Y, et al. A randomized, controlled trial validates a peripheral supra-additive antihyperalgesic effect of a paracetamol-ketorolac combination. *Basic Clin Pharmacol Toxicol.* 2011;109(5):357–364.
5. Smith HS. Perioperative intravenous acetaminophen and NSAIDs. *Pain Med.* 2011;12(6):961–981.
6. Simon LS. Nonsteroid anti-inflammatory drugs and cyclooxygenase-2 selective inhibitors. In: Smith HS, ed. *Drugs for Pain.* Philadelphia, PA: Hanley and Belfus; 2003:41–54.

7. Smith HS. Nonsteroidal anti-inflammatory drugs: bedside. In: Smith HS, ed. *Drugs for Pain*. Philadelphia, PA: Hanley and Belfus; 2003:65–82.
8. Argoff CE. Recent developments in the treatment of osteoarthritis with NSAIDs. *Curr Med Res Opin*. 2011;27(7):1315–1327.
9. Smith HS, Voss B. Pharmaockinetics of intravenous ibuprofen: implications of time of infusion in the treatment of pain and fever. *Drugs*. 2012;72(3):327–337.
10. Smith HS, Baird W. Meloxicam and selective COX-2 inhibitors in the management of pain in the palliative care population. *Am J Hosp Palliat Care*. 2003;20(4):297–306.
11. Shah S, Mehta V. Controversies and advances in non-steroidal anti-inflammatory drug (NSAID) analgesia in chronic pain management. *Postgrad Med J*. 2012;88(1036):73–78.
12. Max MB, Culnane M, Schafer SC, et al. Amitriptyline relieves diabetic neuropathy pain in patients with normal or depressed mood. *Neurology*. 1987;37(4):589–596.
13. Sindrup SH, Otto M, Finnerup NB, Jensen TS. Antidepressants in the treatment of neuropathic pain. *Basic Clin Pharmacol Toxicol*. 2005;96(6):339–409.
14. Dworkin RH, O'Connor AB, Backonja M, et al. Pharmacologic management of neuropathic pain: evidence-based recommendations. *Pain*. 2007;132(3):237–251.
15. Finnerup NB, Sindrup SH, Jensen TS. The evidence for pharmacological treatment of neuropathic pain. *Pain*. 2010;150(3):573–581.
16. Saarto T, Wiffen PJ. Antidepressants for neuropathic pain. *Cochrane Database Syst Rev*. 2007;17:CD005454.
17. Beers MH. Explicit criteria for determining potentially inappropriate medication use by the elderly: an update. *Arch Intern Med*. 1997;157(14):1531–1536.
18. Goldstein DJ, Lu Y, Detke MJ, Lee TC, Iyengar S. Duloxetine vs. placebo in patients with painful diabetic neuropathy. *Pain*. 2005;116(1–2):109–118.
19. Wernicke JF, Pritchett YL, D'Souza DN, et al. A randomized controlled trial of duloxetine in diabetic peripheral neuropathic pain. *Neurology*. 2006;67(8):1411–1420.
20. Smith HS, Bracken D, Smith JM. Duloxetine: a review of its safety and efficacy in the management of fibromyalgia syndrome. *J Central Nervous Syst Disease*. 2010:2:57–72.
21. Gilron I, Bailey JM, Tu D, Holden RR, Jackson AC, Houlden RL. Nortriptyline and gabapentin, alone and in combination for neuropathic pain: a double-blind, randomised controlled crossover trial. *Lancet*. 2009;374(9697):1252–1261.
22. Sang CN, Booher S, Gilron I, Parada S, Max MB. Dextromethorphan and memantine in painful diabetic neuropathy and postherpetic neuralgia: efficacy and dose-response trials. *Anesthesiology*. 2002;96(5):1053–1061.

23. Carlsson KC, Hoem NO, Moberg ER, Mathisen LC. Analgesic effect of dextromethorphan in neuropathic pain. *Acta Anesthesiol Scand.* 2004;48(3):328–336.
24. Cohen SP, Liao W, Gupta A, Plunkett A. Ketamine in pain management. *Adv Psychosom Med.* 2011;30:139–161.
25. Derry S, Lloyd R, Moore RA, McQuay HJ. Topical capsaicin for chronic neuropathic pain in adults. *Cochrane Database Syst Rev.* 2009;4:CD007393.

3

Phytomedicines for the Treatment of Pain

JULIA VLACHOJANNIS AND SIGRUN CHRUBASIK

HISTORICAL ASPECTS

Until the end of the 19th century, phytomedicines were the only medicinal option for treating pain. Popular phytomedicines with anti-inflammatory and analgesic properties included willow bark (*Salicis cortex*), goldenrod herb (*Solidaginis herba*), wintergreen herb (*Gaultheriae herba*), aspen bark and leaf (*Populi cortex* and *folium*), and many others. In severe cases of pain, opium, the dried latex or juice of the seed pod of *Papaver somniferum*, was used. For topical treatment, preparations from *Arnica montana* and *Symphytum officinale* were applied. The first medical report on the antipyretic effect of dried and powdered willow bark dates back to 1763.[1] The empirically chosen daily dose (up to 24 g) might have contained up to 1000 mg of salicin, as the crude plant material generally contains about 4 percent salicin.[2] Only after the invention of laboratory facilities was it possible to extract ingredients such as salicin from willow bark, salicylic acid from wintergreen, colchicin from autumn crocus, and morphine from opium and treat patients with isolated single compounds. Shortly thereafter, the compounds could be synthezised, which was a much cheaper means of production than the extraction procedures.

The synthesis of aspirin dates back to 1897. It is generally believed that aspirin originates from *Salix* species. However, willow bark contains only a small amount of salicin, which is the prodrug of various salicylic acid derivatives. A willow bark dose with 240 mg of salicin corresponds to 100 mg of salicylic acid derivatives,[3] an insufficient dose to treat pain. Because the aspirin acetyl group is responsible for inhibiting coagulation, treatment with willow bark preparations does not interfere with blood clotting and can safely be used perioperatively.

Treatment with synthetic drugs (e.g., nonsteroidal anti-inflammatory drugs [NSAIDs]) is associated with adverse events (e.g., gastrointestinal, renal). Therefore, at the end of the 20th century, phytomedicines regained popularity in the treatment of pain. Research shed light on the mechanism of action of the anti-inflammatory-acting phytomedicines, and clinical studies investigated their effectiveness. Unfortunately, phytomedicines were excluded from social healthcare reimbursement in Germany in 2004. As a result of this, research declined in a country that had contributed so much to the field of phyto-analgesia in the past. For example, most of the studies investigating devil's claw preparations were carried out in Germany after Professor Zorn of the University of Jena first described the anti-inflammatory effect of aqueous *Harpagophytum* extract in rats with experimentally induced arthritis.[4]

MECHANISM OF ACTION OF HERBAL ANTI-INFLAMMATORY DRUGS

Phytomedicines contain multiple ingredients with different actions. Their cumulative action is caused by "the active principle" of the particular phytomedicine, reflecting the broader mechanism of action (Table 3.1) relative to synthetic NSAIDs.

Table 3.1 EFFECT MECHANISMS OF PHYTO-ANTI-INFLAMMATORY DRUGS SUGGESTED BY IN VITRO STUDIES[5]

PLEASE: INHIBITION OF COVERS COX-1 UNTIL ENZYMES AND SHOULD BE PLACED IN THE LINE OF ANTIOXIDATIVE

		INHIBITION OF					
		COX-1	*COX-2*	*LOX*	*Cytokines*	*Enzymes*	*Antioxidative Effect*
Persea americana	**Avocado soybean**	Not investigated	Yes	Not investigated	Yes	Hyaluronidase	Yes
+ Glycine max							
***Uncaria* species**	**Cat's claw**	Yes	Yes	Not investigated	Yes	Not Investigated	Yes
Harpagophytum procumbens	**Devil's claw**	No activity	Yes	Yes	Yes	Elastase	Yes
Zingiber officinalis	**Ginger**	Yes	Yes	Yes	Yes	Elastase	Yes
Urtica dioica	**Nettle herb**	Yes	Not investigated	Yes	Yes	Elastase	Yes

Rosa canina	**Rose hip and seed**	Yes	Yes	No activity	Not investigated	Elastase	Yes
Boswellia serrata	**Salai guggal**	Yes	No activity	Yes	Yes	Hyaluronidase	Yes ans pro-oxidative
Curcuma species	**Tumeric root**	Yes	Yes	Yes	Yes	Hyaluronidase	Yes
***Salix* species**	**Willow bark**	Yes	Yes	Yes	Yes	Hyaluronidase	Yes
***Capsicum* species**	**Capsaicin**	Not investigated	Yes	Yes	Not investigated	Elastase	Not investigated
Arnica montana	**Arnica**	Yes	Yes	Yes	Yes	Elastase	Yes
Symphytum officinale	**Comfrey**	Yes	Yes	Not investigated	Not investigated	Not investigated	Yes

COX-1, cyclooxygenase-1; COX-2, cyclooxygenase-2; LOX, lipoxygenase.

NSAIDs mainly interact with the arachidonic acid cascade, inhibiting not only mediators triggering pain but also those important for physiological functions (gut wall, kidney, etc.). As an example from another domain, high blood pressure was usually treated with a single synthetic antihypertensive. In the event of insufficient treatment success, the dose was increased, with a corresponding increase in the incidence of adverse events. Today the state of the art is to treat elevated blood pressure with a combination of up to three or four antihypertensives with different actions. This enables the use of lower doses of single antihypertensives while providing an additive overall effect. This might explain why phytomedicines in general are associated with fewer adverse events than synthetic drugs.

Table 3.1 demonstrates that phytomedicines with anti-inflammatory actions use the same pathways as synthetic NSAIDs or synthetic biologicals (chondroprotective drugs). Although animal studies indicate a chondroprotective effect of some phytomedicines (e.g., avocado and soybean unsaponifiables [ASUs], devil's claw, boswellia), clinical studies so far have not proven a demonstrable chondroprotective effect.[5] This concept has potential clinical importance in specialties such as orthopedics, in which NSAIDs are often stopped so as to avoid poor bone healing, during which time NSAID-responsive patients often complain of worsened pain.

The mechanism of action of topical phytomedicines is less well investigated, except that of capsaicin. This extract from Spanish pepper (*Capsicum* species) acts via the vanilloid receptors (e.g., transient receptor potential cation subfamily V, member 1 [TRPV1]). The binding of capsaicin to this target is accompanied by a decrease in membrane resistance, depolarization, and activation of synaptosomal neurotransmitter release. Following the initial activation (which is often associated with heat sensation and sometimes increased discomfort), the desensitization and depletion of neurotransmitters produce the capsaicin analgesic effect. If capsaicin exposure persists, nerve terminals may degenerate (defunctionalization) and cause prolonged analgesic effects after the treatment's end. For this reason, treatment with capsaicin should be limited to about 3 months so as not to risk irreversible nerve damage. Other capsaicin effects include the inhibition of inducible cyclooxygenase (COX)-2 mRNA expression, lipoxygenase, and free radical scavenging activity.[6] Please be aware that in medicinal plant products, the capsaicinoids are calculated as capsaicin. Preparations containing extracted or synthetic capsaicin (e.g., Zostrix) are no longer considered as phytomedicines.

COMPARISON OF WILLOW BARK EXTRACT AND NSAIDS

In a yeast-induced hyperthermia model in rodents, the antipyretic effect of willow bark extract was weaker than that of acetylsalicylic acid (aspirin) in equipotent doses.[3] But on a dose-by-weight basis, the proprietary aqueous extract STW 33-I (willow bark extract) was at least as effective as aspirin in reducing inflammatory exudates. In rats, willow bark extract (solvent, 30 percent ethanol) inhibited carrageenan-induced paw edema, adjuvant-induced arthritis, heat-induced inflammation, and dextran-induced hind paw edema. The anti-inflammatory effect was dose-dependent; a dose of 120 mg/kg ethanolic extract was equivalent to 600 mg/kg aspirin. Willow bark extract analgesia was also demonstrated in the hot plate test in mice in doses of 60 to 120 mg/kg (equivalent aspirin dose = 600 mg/kg).

The monograph of the European Scientific Cooperative on Phytotherapy (ESCOP)[2] recommends much lower extract doses (a maximum of 240 mg salicin per day) than found in the preparations used to treat fever and pain in the Middle Ages (see above).

With the ESCOP doses, only moderate evidence of effectiveness was demonstrated in the treatment of musculoskeletal pain.[7] One study indicated that ethanolic willow bark extract with 240 mg salicin per day was not inferior to rofecoxib in alleviating acute exacerbations in chronic low back pain sufferers. But in a study comparing this dose to 100 mg diclofenac, the NSAID was superior for pain due to inflammation of the knee joint.[7] According to our observations, higher doses are more effective.

The use of willow bark extract is not restricted to the treatment of musculoskeletal pain. Any pain (including migraine, headache, pain after dental extractions, etc.) might respond to the extract.[2] Because the effect of NSAIDs on blood clotting is a disadvantage in the perioperative period, postoperative pain might also be a promising indication for the use of willow bark preparations.

EVIDENCE OF EFFECTIVENESS OF PHYTOMEDICINES FOR OSTEOARTHRITIS AND LOW BACK PAIN

The interim update of the Cochrane review on osteoarthritis (OA) included 35 studies that investigated 22 phytomedicines.[5] None of the phytomedicines demonstrated good effectiveness based on a meta-analysis of randomized controlled studies. Only 7 of the 35 studies had a confirmatory (fully powered) study design further investigating the trends of effectiveness demonstrated in earlier studies. Four of them investigated a lipophilic fraction of avocado and soybean (ASUs). Although convincing evidence of effectiveness is available for ASU based on three trials, a further confirmatory study over 2 years failed to demonstrate effectiveness, except in a subgroup of people with less severe OA. Joint space loss was significantly reduced in patients with mild OA, possibly indicating that early use of ASU might act preventively. But this suggestion now needs to be confirmed by a study with a confirmatory study design. An increase in dose has not been shown to further improve the ASU effects.

The other three studies with confirmatory study designs investigated ethanolic willow bark extract, a powder from devil's claw, and a tincture made from arnica.

The two studies of willow bark extract included in the interim update of the Cochrane review on OA had contradictory results. The evidence of effectiveness was classified as "conflicting." A review including studies of patients suffering from acute low back pain exacerbations classified the evidence as "moderate."[7] There is no doubt that willow bark preparations are effective in the treatment of musculoskeletal pain;[7] however, individual patients might require higher doses than that recommended by the ESCOP (see above).

Both willow bark extract (solvent, 70 percent ethanol) and aqueous devil's claw extract improved dose-dependently acute exacerbations in chronic low back pain sufferers.[4,7] Available *Harpagophytum* ethanolic extracts are incompletely extracted and contain only around 30 mg harpagoside in the daily dosage, whereas equivalent doses of aqueous extract or powder contain 50 to 60 mg harpagoside. It seems likely that a minimum of 50 mg harpagoside per day is necessary to alleviate OA and low back pain. One survey indicated that with aqueous devil's claw extract, the location of pain (lower back, hip, knee) is not of major importance.[8] Another Cochrane review came to the conclusion that devil's claw, willow bark, and capsaicin seem to reduce low back pain more than placebo.[9]

The definitive study investigating the use of arnica in OA patients was a single study. A number of underpowered studies that investigated the same or other phytomedicines were inconclusive.[5] Further research is necessary to prove the effectiveness of phytomedicines (including Chinese and Ajurvedic herbal mixtures) in the treatment of OA and low back pain.

EVIDENCE OF EFFECTIVENESS OF PHYTOMEDICINES FOR RHEUMATOID ARTHRITIS

The update of the Cochrane review on rheumatoid arthritis (RA) included 20 studies investigating 14 phytomedicines.[10] Meta-analysis was done for studies investigating oils from borage, blackcurrant, and evening primrose, all containing gamma linolenic acid (GLA) as the active principle. GLA doses equal to or higher than 1400 mg/d showed benefit in the alleviation of rheumatic complaints, whereas lower doses of around 500 mg were ineffective.

Three of the 14 studies compared products from *Tripterygium wilfordii* (thunder god vine; Table 3.2) to placebo and returned favorable results, but data could not be pooled because the interventions and measures differed. Serious adverse effects occurred in one study. In a follow-up study, adverse events were mild to moderate and resolved after the intervention ceased. A number of underpowered studies investigating the same or other phytomedicines were inconclusive. Further research is necessary to prove the effectiveness of phytomedicines in the treatment of RA.

EVIDENCE OF EFFECTIVENESS OF PHYTOMEDICINES FOR HEADACHE AND MIGRAINE

The combined anti-spasmodic, anti-inflammatory, and calcium-channel-blocking effects of *Petasites hybridus* provide a rationale for its use in the prophylaxis of migraine.[11] Two trials including 293 patients were included in a systematic review. Both trials investigated the proprietary *Petasites* root extract. The trials were described in a narrative way, taking into consideration methodological quality scores. Pooling of data was not carried out because of the heterogeneity of the results. Treatment with the extract at a higher dose (150 mg) yielded a greater decrease in the frequency of migraine attacks and a greater number of responders (improvement > 50 percent) after treatment over 3 to 4 months than the extract at lower dose (100 mg) and placebo. A study in children also showed favorable results for this proprietary butterbur extract.[12] Definitive studies are now required in order to confirm effectiveness and safety in long-term use before treatment with *Petasites* root extract can generally be recommended for the prophylaxis of migraine.

In folk medicine, feverfew (*Tanacetum parthenium*) is used for the treatment of fevers, migraine headaches, RA, stomachaches, toothaches, and other complaints. A Cochrane review including five randomized, double-blind trials showed insufficient evidence to suggest an effect of feverfew over and above placebo for preventing migraine.[13] Because serotonergic receptors are involved in feverfew's mechanism of action, the concomitant administration of feverfew preparations and serotonin-reuptake inhibitors should be avoided. From time to time, a pause in feverfew treatment is advisable, with a gradual reduction of dosage during the preceding month so as to avoid the occurrence of adverse events. The recently introduced feverfew CO_2 extract seems to have a more potent effect;[13] however, a comprehensive reproductive study is urgently warranted prior to its widespread use.[14] Mixtures of ethanolic extracts of feverfew and *Salix alba* (each 600 mg/d, standardized on 0.2 percent parthenolide and 1.5 percent salicin; drug extract ratio not stated) and of a feverfew and ginger preparation (details not stated; 2 × 2 mL administered sublingually 5 minutes apart and another 2 × 2 mL at between 60 minutes and 24 hours) also show promising results for migraine.[14]

Topical peppermint oil (10 percent) has been studied in two exploratory trials among 73 people with tension headache (n = 328 and n = 419). The oil was superior to placebo and had an effectiveness similar to that of acetaminophen. The onset of pain relief occurred within 15 minutes of administration. Concomitant administration of the peppermint oil in ethanol with acetaminophen resulted in improved relief of pain intensity. In laboratory tests, this preparation was shown to exert a significant analgesic effect, with a reduction in sensitivity to headache, as well as muscle relaxation, a central depressive effect, and an increase in cognitive performance. Allergic reactions might occur following topical peppermint oil use but are very rare.[14]

Perivascular afferent fibers of the superficial temporal artery contain peptides, including Substance P. Recurrent migraineurs reporting pain at pressure (tenderness) on scalp arteries were treated with topical capsaicin (0.1 percent) or Vaseline jelly rubbed over painful arteries. Capsaicin was administered topically in the absence of a migraine attack and, if patients responded with a reduction in palpatory tenderness, also during an acute migraine attack. This exploratory study on 23 migraineurs showed a trend of effectiveness in relieving migraine complaints. Several other studies suggest that the intranasal application of capsaicin might be an alternative treatment in cases of migraine or cluster headache resistant to other drug treatments. Local irritation (heat, pruritus) after topical capsaicin application is common, but it is mostly mild and transient. Systemic adverse events were not observed in any of the clinical trials that investigated topical capsaicin.[14]

Synthetic antidepressants have an established place in the prevention of migraine and tension-type headache treatment. In general, tricyclic antidepressants are more effective that selective serotonin reuptake inhibitors, although they are associated with greater adverse effects. In mild to moderate depression, mood improvement might occur with extracts of St. John's wort. Decreased complaints were associated with fewer adverse events relative to synthetic antidepressants. *Hypericum* extracts containing less that 1 mg of hyperforin (a co-active ingredient) in the daily dosage have so far not been involved in drug interactions, as were St. John's wort extracts with higher hyperforin doses, and they should be preferred over extracts with a higher hyperforin content.[15]

SELF-TREATMENT WITH FOOD SUPPLEMENTS OR PLANT PARTS

In traditional European medicine, preparations from rose hip and seed were used for the treatment of rheumatic complaints,[16] but not until 2004 was the first clinical study showing a trend of effectiveness in a population sample suffering from osteoarthritic pain published. Five studies with exploratory study designs indicate that a powder made from rose hip and seed (Table 3.2) with a dose of up to 10 g/d might alleviate pain in the lower back or due to inflammatory knee pain or RA. The effect size for the different pain locations now needs to be determined in studies with a confirmatory study design.

When comparing the responders according to the OMERACT-OARSI criteria, it seems likely that the rose hip and seed powder (10 g/d initially) is as effective as the aqueous *Harpagophytum* extract with 60 mg harpagoside in the daily dosage (Fig. 3.1).[17] It also seems likely that if the lipophilic compounds are concentrated in a future extract,[18] a more potent rose hip product might be created (which then would no longer be a food supplement). It has to be considered that patients need to drink 300 to 500 mL of any liquid along with the intake of the powder; otherwise, patients might suffer from constipation due to the absorption of gastrointestinal fluid. Patients suffering from irritable bowel syndrome with diarrhea can use the powder to harden their stool by adding only a little additional fluid.

Among the options for self-treatment, a stew from nettle herb (50 to 100 g/d, not heated over 70°C) or a tea from ginger root, blackcurrent leaf, or *Petiveria alliacea* might help one save on synthetic drugs. Freshly squeezed ginger root in a fruit mixture might act as fast as aspirin in alleviating headache. The effectiveness of topical nettle leaf has been known since the Middle Ages, and clinical studies favor its use.[5] Essential oils from peppermint herb (with 10 to 16 percent menthol) and pine needles act as counterirritants and might also help to alleviate pain.[16]

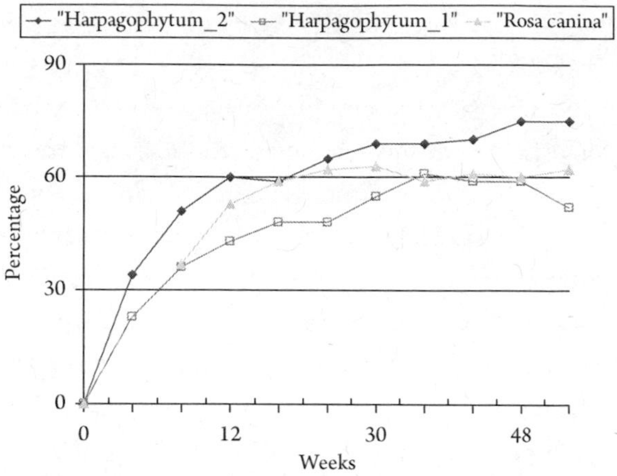

Figure 3.1. The Outcome Measures in Rheumatology and the Osteoarthritis Research Society International (OMERACT-OARSI) response during treatment with *Harpagophytum* extract (60 mg harpagoside per day) in two studies over 1 year and during treatment with a rose hip and seed powder (*Rosa canina*) over 1 year (see Ref. 21).

QUALITY OF PHYTOMEDICINES

Phytomedicines include herbs, herbal materials (fresh juices, gums, fixed oils, essential oils, resins, and dry powders of herbs), herbal preparations (comminuted or powdered herbal materials or extracts, tinctures, and fatty oils of herbal materials produced by extraction, fractionation, purification, concentration, or other physical or biological processes), and finished herbal products (including mixtures). Preparations supplemented by chemically defined active substances, synthetic compounds, and/or isolated constituents from herbal materials are not considered as herbal.[19]

Phytomedicines might be contaminated with other herbs, pesticides, herbicides, heavy metals, or drugs. It is therefore advisable to recommend only products that comply with the principles and guidelines of good manufacturing practice (GMP) for medicinal products and the GMP guideline for starting materials.[20] Collection and/or cultivation, harvest, and primary processing of the starting material all have an impact on the active principle of the phytomedicine. It is therefore impossible for two different brands, or even two batches of one brand, to be identical. There is general agreement that two phytomedicines (or two batches of one brand) are "essentially similar" if they satisfy the criteria of having the same qualitative and quantitative composition in terms of co-active constituents, having the same pharmaceutical form (galenic preparation), and being bioequivalent, also in terms of safety and efficacy. Unless this has not been demonstrated, results of a study with a particular phytomedicine cannot be transferred to another product. For example, for aqueous extract of *Harpagophytum procumbens* with 50 and 100 mg harpagoside in the daily dosage, a dose-dependent effect was demonstrated in a clinical study with a confirmatory study design.[21] In contrast, extract using 60 percent ethanol as an excipient and offering less than 30 mg harpagoside in the daily dosage has not shown any evidence of effectiveness.[4]

The minimum declarations required for phytomedicines in order for studies to be repeatable are (i) the plant part, (ii) the drug extract ratio (how many parts of the starting material were used to prepare one part of extract), (iii) the excipient, (iv) the quantity of native extract per unit (without additives), and (v) the quantity of the marker substance(s) per unit. If possible, the marker should be the active principle. Otherwise, the content of co-active marker substances should be declared, and if they are not known, at least hydrophilic and/or lipophilic marker compounds should be declared. Table 3.2 shows that the declaration of phytomedicines is often insufficient (a complete summary of the products investigated in clinical studies fulfilling the inclusion criteria of the Cochrane group so far will be published in a forthcoming review update).[22] Studies

Table 3.2 CHARACTERISTICS OF SOME PHYTOMEDICINES USED FOR THE TREATMENT OF OA AND RA[5,10]

PLANT					MARKER	
Name	*Part*	*Preparation*	*Drug/Extract Ratio*	*Dose (mg/d)*	*Constituent*	*Dose (mg/d)*
Harpagophytum procumbens	Root	Aqueous extract	1.5–2.5:1	2400	Harpagoside	30
		Ethanolic (60%) extract	4.5–5.5:1	960	Harpagoside	<30
		Cryoground powder		2610	Harpagoside	60
Salix pupurea	Bark	Ethanolic (70%) extract	10–20:1	1360	Salicin	240
Rosa canina	Hip + seed	Powder		5000	Galactolipid	1.5
Curcuma longa	Root	Not stated	Not stated	200	Courcuminoids	20%
Cucuma domestica	Root	Ethanolic extract	Not stated	Not stated	Curcuminoids	500 mg
Zingiber officinale	Root	Acetone extract	20:1	510	Not stated	–
	Root	CO_2 extract	Not stated	1000	Gingerol	40
Zingiber officinale +	Root	Acetone extract	20:1	Not stated	Not stated	–
Alpinia officinale	Root	Not stated	Not stated	Not stated	Not stated	–

Persea gratissima	Oil	Unsaponifiable		300	Not stated	–
Glycine max		Fraction 1/3 P; 2/3 G		600		
Boswellia serrata	Gum resin	Not stated	Not stated	999	Boswellic acid	40%
					Organic acids	65%
	Gum resin	Not stated	Not stated	1200–3600	Boswellic acid	Not stated
Boswellia carteri	Gum resin	Not stated	Not stated	Not stated	Boswellic acid	37.5%
+ *Curcuma longa*	Root	+ Not stated	Not stated	Not stated	Not stated	–
Tripterygium wilfordii	Root	Ethanol/ethyl thereafter	45:1	180	Triptolide	0.09
		Acetate extraction		360	Tripdiolide	0.18
	Root	Chloroform/methanol	Not stated	60	Tripdiolide	0.021
		extract			Tripidiolide	0.041
					Triptonide	0.002

(continued)

Table 3.2 (CONTINUED)

PLANT					MARKER	
Name	*Part*	*Preparation*	*Drug/Extract Ratio*	*Dose (mg/d)*	*Constituent*	*Dose (mg/d)*
Uncaria tomentosa	Bark	Aqueous extract	Not stated	60	Alcaloides*	0.88
Uncaria guianensis	Bark	Aqueous extract	Not stated	100	Not stated	–
Symphytum officinale	Radix	Ethanolic (60%) extract	2:1	3 × 6 cm	Allantoin	0.2–0.5%
Arnica montana	Herb	Tincture, 50% ethanol	20:1	3 × 4 cm	Not stated	–
Petiveria alliacea	Herb	Aqueous extract	9 g/600 mL	600 mL	Not stated	–

[a]Pentacyclic oxindole alcaloide.

Drug extract ratio: parts of crude plant material required to produce one part of extract.

of products that are not comprehensively described are not helpful because their results cannot be transferred to other products of the particular plant part.

SAFETY OF PHYTOMEDICINES

There are no comprehensive safety assessments available for any of the phytomedicines. Safety studies are mandatory if phytomedicines aim to hold a place in pain treatment guidelines. Allergic skin reactions might occur with any medication, but they will subside once the treatment has been stopped. Several reports describe seizures in individuals taking seed oils, particularly in people with a history of seizure disorders, and among individuals taking seed oil in combination with anesthetics or other centrally acting drugs such as chlorpromazine, thioridazine, trifluoperazine, or fluphenazine. Anti-seizure medications might require a dosage increase. People who plan to undergo surgery requiring general anesthesia are advised to stop taking seed oil preparations 2 weeks prior to the operation. Other seed oil adverse events include occasional headache, abdominal pain, nausea, and loose stools.[10]

Willow bark extract contains a gastroprotective principle. In contrast to 100 mg/kg ASA, an ethanolic willow bark extract containing 12 percent salicin in a dose of up to 120 mg/kg did not produce any mucosal lesions in rats, whereas 9 of 10 aspirin-treated rats showed stomach lesions. Acute toxicity studies in rats could not determine the lethal dose of willow bark extract, even in doses 200 times the experimental level. However, data on chronic toxicity are still lacking. Whether a few cytotoxic compounds contained in willow bark extract (e.g., pyrocatechol) might have a clinical impact needs to be elucidated. The studies investigating ethanolic extract with up to 240 mg salicin per day so far have revealed an incidence of adverse events of around 5 percent (mainly mild gastrointestinal complaints). Most adverse events were mild, but life-threatening anaphylactic reactions might occur in patients with a history of allergy to salicylates.[3]

A systematic review of the adverse events during treatment with *Harpagophytum* products included 6892 patients. In none of the double-blind studies was the incidence of adverse events during treatment with *Harpagophytum* higher than that during placebo treatment. The overall adverse event rate was about 3 percent.[23] However, because higher *Harpagophytum* extract doses are more effective, optimum doses and safety have to be studied. The co-active principle (iridoid glycosides) is a bitter principle and is responsible for the gastrointestinal complaints in some patients. Allergies might occur with any phytomedicine. The three studies on preclinical toxicity indicated very low acute toxicity.[24] Data on chronic toxicity including mutagenicity, carcinogenicity, teratogenicity, and embryogenicity were not found.[24]

Among the phytomedicines used for the treatment of pain, the risk/benefit trade-off of *Tripterygium wilfordii* Hook F used in China to treat RA was judged as unfavorable.[25] For all phytomedicines, long-term safety studies are required, given that most pain conditions require long-term treatment.

CONCLUSIONS

The success of treatment with phytomedicines depends on the quality of the medicinal plant product. Product preparation according to the GMP guidelines and a sufficient amount of "active principle" in the daily dosage help to optimize treatment outcomes. Phytomedicines have a broader mechanism of action than NSAIDs and are associated with a lower risk of adverse events. The most potent all-round phytomedicine for pain is willow bark extract, provided the dose is high enough. In many cases the recommended extract doses, with a maximum of 240 mg salicin per day, are insufficient to achieve acceptable pain relief. Likewise, preparations from devil's claw should contain at least 50 mg of harpagoside in the daily dosage. The indication for medicinal products from *Harpagophytum procumbens* and ASU is OA, whereas GLA-containing seed oils and preparations from thunder god vine are preferred for RA. Many phytomedicines have a promising action for OA and RA because they use the same molecular pathways as synthetic medications, but the quality of the clinical trials that have investigated the products are, unfortunately, too low to allow a definitive conclusion. Dose-finding studies are required. Preparations from butterbur and feverfew, St. John's wort, peppermint oil, and capsaicin are treatment options for migraine and headache patients. For self-treatment of painful conditions, a powder from rose hip and seed, a stew of nettle herb, or a tea from blackcurrent or *Petiveria alliacea* might allow a patient to reduce his or her intake of synthetic pain medications. Alternatively, topical nettle administration or the use of peppermint or pine needle oil as a counterirritant might be helpful.

REFERENCES

1. Stone E. An account of the success of the bark of the willow in the cure of agues. *Philos Trans R Soc Lond.* 1763;53:195–200.
2. ESCOP. Salicis cortex. In: European Scientific Cooperative on Phytotherapy, ed. *ESCOP Monographs.* 2nd ed. Exeter, UK: ESCOP; 2003:445–451.
3. Vlachojannis J, Magora F, Chrubasik S. Willow species and aspirin: different mechanism of actions. *Phytother Res.* 2011;25:1102–1104.
4. Chrubasik S, Conradt C, Black A. The quality of clinical trials with *Harpagophytum procumbens. Phytomedicine.* 2003;10:613–623.
5. Cameron M, Blumle A, Gagnier JJ, Little CV, Parsons T, Chrubasik S. Evidence of effectiveness of herbal medicinal products in the treatment of arthritis. Part 1: osteoarthritis. *Phytotherapy Res.* 2009;23:1497–1515.
6. Weiser T, Roufogalis B, Chrubasik S. Comparison of the effects of pelargonic acid vanillylamide and capsaicin on human vanilloid receptors. *Phytotherapy Res.* 2012. doi: 10.1002/ptr.4817.

7. Vlachojannis JE, Cameron M, Chrubasik S. A systematic review on the effectiveness of willow bark for musculoskeletal pain. *Phytother Res.* 2009 23:897–900.
8. Chrubasik S, Thanner J, Kuünzel O, Conradt C, Black A, Pollak S. Comparison of outcome measures during treatment with the proprietary *Harpagophytum* extract Doloteffin in patients with pain in the lower back, knee or hip. *Phytomedicine.* 2002;9:181–194.
9. Gagnier JJ, van Tulder M, Berman B, Bombardier C. Herbal medicine for low back pain. *Cochrane Database Syst Rev.* 2006;(2):CD004504.
10. Cameron M, Gagnier JJ, Chrubasik S. Herbal therapy for treating rheumatoid arthritis. *Cochrane Database Syst Rev.* 2011;(2):CD002948.
11. Agosti R, Duke RK, Chrubasik JE, Chrubasik S. Effectiveness of Petasites hybridus preparations in the prophylaxis of migraine: a systematic review. *Phytomedicine.* 2006;13(9–10):743–746.
12. Sun-Edelstein C, Mauskop A. Alternative headache treatments: nutraceuticals, behavioral and physical treatments. *Headache.* 2011;51(3):469–483.
13. Pittler MH, Ernst E. Feverfew for preventing migraine. *Cochrane Database Syst Rev.* 2004;(1):CD002286.
14. Vlachojannis J, Cameron M, Chrubasik S. Herbal medicinal treatment options for headache and migraine. *Headache.* 2011;51:1350–1351.
15. Vlachojannis J, Cameron M, Chrubasik S. Addendum to the interactions with St. John's wort products. *Pharmacology Res.* 2011;63:254–256.
16. Blumenthal M. The Complete German Commission E Monographs. Austin, TX: American Botanical Council; 1998.
17. Chrubasik C, Wiesner L, Black A, Muüller-Ladner U, Chrubasik S. A one-year survey on the use of a powder from *Rosa canina lito* in acute exacerbations of chronic pain. *Phytother Res.* 2008;22:1141–1148.
18. Wenzig EM, Widowitz U, Chrubasik S, Bucar F, Knauder E, Bauer R. Phytochemical and in vitro pharmacological comparison of two rose hip preparations. *Phytomedicine.* 2007;15:826–835.
19. World Health Organization. Traditional medicine: definitions. World Health Organization Web site. http://www.who.int/medicines/areas/traditional/definitions/en/index.html.
20. Schmidt O. FDA and EMEA presentation on hot GMP and regulatory topics. Active Pharmaceutical Ingredients Committee Website. www.api-conference.org/pa4.cgi?src=eca_news_data.htm&nr=488&show=daten/news/GMP_News_488.htm&id=S11510781142". Access April 2012.
21. Chrubasik S, Junck H, Breitschwerdt H, Conradt C, Zappe H. Effectiveness of *Harpagophytum* extract WS 1531 in the treatment of exacerbation of low back pain: a randomized, placebo-controlled, double-blind study. *Eur J Anaesthesiol.* 1999;16:118–129.
22. Cameron M, Chrubasik S. Herbal therapy for treating osteoarthritis. *Cochrane Database Syst Rev.* Unpublished data.

23. VlachojannisJ, Roufogalis BD, Chrubasik S. Systematic review on the safety of Harpagophytum preparations for osteoarthritic and low back pain. *Phytother Res.* 2008;22:149–152.
24. ESCOP. Harpagophyti radix. In: European Scientific Cooperative on Phytotherapy, ed. *ESCOP Monographs*. 2nd ed. Exeter, UK: ESCOP; 2003:233–240.
25. Canter PH, Lee HS, Ernst E. A systematic review of randomised clinical trials of *Tripterygium wilfordii* for rheumatoid arthritis. *Phytomedicine.* 2006;13:371–377.

PART II

NON-PHARMACOLOGIC PAIN THERAPIES

4

Behavioral Interventions for Chronic Pain: Exercise and Cognitive-Behavioral Therapy

DAVID A. WILLIAMS AND AFTON L. HASSETT

The field of pain medicine has demonstrated a reasonably good ability to reduce acute pain, but it remains challenged in providing anything more than modest effects when addressing chronic pain.[1] The ability to treat one form of pain successfully but not the other stems from the fact that chronic pain is not a simple extension of acute pain; rather, their mechanisms differ, and so must their treatments. Melzack and Wall[2] first proposed that in order for pain to be perceived by humans there needed to be an integration of sensory, affective, and cognitive inputs. Current neuroimaging studies support this early theory by demonstrating separate neural pathways corresponding to sensation, affect, and cognition, with pain perception being an integrated balance of the three.[3] In the case of chronic pain, affective and cognitive pathways play more prominent roles than that for acute pain.[4] Thus, the application of sensory-based acute pain treatments in the context of chronic pain are likely to fail, given that two-thirds of the problem (i.e., cognition and affect) will remain under-addressed.

Interventions for chronic pain that focus on cognitive and affective components of pain have been developed largely within the disciplines of health psychology and behavioral medicine. Such interventions tend to focus directly upon pain relief, relief from comorbid symptoms (e.g., fatigue, sleep problems, difficulty thinking), and improvements of functional status. Behavioral medicine does not attempt to "cure" chronic pain; instead it uses a "management" model, much as would be done with other chronic conditions such as diabetes and asthma. Three decades' worth of research on chronic pain management outcomes has consistently documented the superiority of addressing all components of chronic pain using a multidisciplinary approach,[5,6] even though such practice is not currently the norm because of numerous economic and systemic barriers.[7,8] As the number of individuals with pain increases, the cost of retaining outdated and insufficient treatments will have more staggering economic consequences. We will need to revisit interventions that address all components of pain.

Non-pharmacologic interventions such as cognitive-behavioral therapy (CBT) and exercise have substantial efficacy in the management of chronic pain conditions including low back pain,[9] arthritis (e.g., osteoarthritis, rheumatoid arthritis), complex regional pain syndrome,[10] chronic pelvic pain,[11] and conditions such as fibromyalgia and chronic widespread pain.[12] Both exercise and, especially, CBT have also demonstrated efficacy in the treatment of depression and anxiety, but these conditions are not the focus of this chapter. Instead, we focus on specifically what CBT and exercise can do specifically for pain, even though depression and anxiety are often concomitant targets of care in the case of chronic pain. Currently, exercise and CBT interventions for pain come in many varieties, despite their more general label. In this chapter we help to clarify the types of exercise and CBT interventions for which there are the best evidence of efficacy in the treatment of chronic pain conditions.

COGNITIVE-BEHAVIORAL THERAPY (CBT)

The strong evidence base supporting the use of CBT for the management of pain[9,13,14] has evolved over the past 30 years. CBT is actually a hybrid of two efficacious forms of therapy: behavioral therapy and cognitive therapy. Behavioral therapy for chronic pain is grounded in the work of Fordyce's operant model,[15] as well as in classical conditioning and social learning theory. Fordyce's model (behavioral therapy) focuses upon how aspects of patients' environments lead to the development or maintenance of pain through reinforcement (e.g., guarding, grimacing, absenteeism, avoidance, or modeling others with pain). Cognitive therapy has its roots in the psychological treatment for depression.[16] Cognitive therapy focuses on thoughts, beliefs, expectations, and attributions that can lead to overwhelming emotions, suffering, and additional pain intensity and/or diminished functional status. First, maladaptive thoughts and emotions need to be identified, after which skills are taught for altering these thoughts and beliefs in a manner that is better aligned with the management of pain. CBT is a hybrid of both, and for any given patient, behavioral or cognitive elements may be differentially emphasized. In practice, CBT for pain typically involves three components: (1) *education,* in which patients are introduced to a model for understanding their pain and the role that individuals can play in the management of the condition; (2) *symptom management skills acquisition,* in which patients learn skills for directly reducing symptoms; and (3) *lifestyle adaption skills,* in which patients learn more general skills for obtaining and improved quality of life and integrating symptom management into daily practice (Fig. 4.1). The next sections describe some of the specific skills that are used in CBT, along with representative studies supporting the use of these skills for the management of pain.

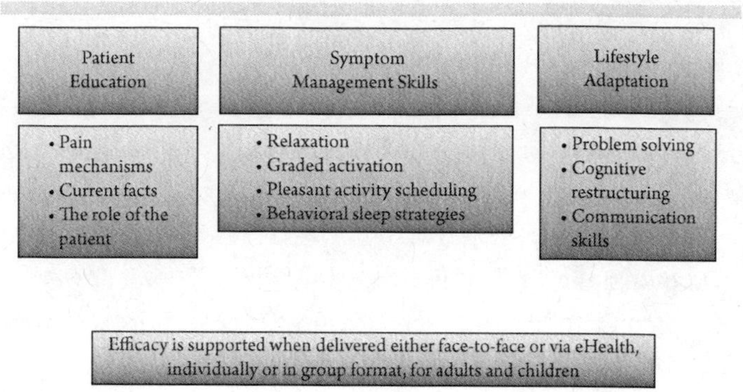

Figure 4.1. Components of cognitive behavioral therapy for pain.

Education

The purpose of education is to establish rapport with the patient and help ensure that the patient and the clinician are thinking about pain and their respective responsibilities for the management of pain from a common perspective. Education typically involves providing the patient with current facts concerning the type of pain he or she is experiencing, the latest approaches to treatment, and a theoretical framework for understanding the role of the patient in pain management. Education by itself is not considered sufficiently robust or adequate as a standalone treatment, given that knowing what needs to change does not ensure that behavioral action will actually occur.

Symptom Management Skills

The *relaxation response* is one of the most commonly applied behavioral approaches to pain management.[17] It can be taught using a variety of methods (e.g., progressive muscle relaxation, visual imagery, hypnosis, biofeedback), with each method relying upon repeated practice, behavioral principles of reinforcement, and training the body to alter its physiological state in response to a conscious desire for relaxation and quiescence.

A second skill often applied in CBT for pain is termed "*graded activation*" or "*time-based pacing*."[18] Performing tasks can enhance one's self-esteem and improve affect. Thus, on "good days," patients often unwittingly engage in more activity than personal limitations allow and consequently suffer several "bad days" of symptom flares, lost productivity, and lowered self-esteem. Graded activation is a method of pacing that can improve physical functioning while minimizing the likelihood of pain flare-ups. Key to this strategy is pacing activities based upon time (which is subjectively neutral) rather than upon pain or the completion of tasks given (which can be affectively charged). Functional time based upon pain level tends to diminish over time, whereas functional time based upon a time interval tends to increase over time because there are fewer flare-ups. For this to work, the patient and therapist must work together to develop a plan for steadily increasing the amount of time spent on specified targeted behaviors. Time-based pacing can be used as a complementary skill to help ensure the long-term adoption of exercise regimens, work-related activities, and pleasant activities such as social outings and sporting activities.

A skill complementary to graded activation is *pleasant activity scheduling*. When pain is chronic, people often eliminate enjoyable activities and reserve time only for essential tasks. Although cutting back on pleasurable activities might make sense in the short term, this is exactly the wrong strategy for managing chronic pain. Engaging in pleasant activities is a natural way to elevate mood[19] and promotes confidence in one's body that might allow it to function at a higher level. As emotions represent a prominent component of chronic pain, activities that enhance mood can directly impact the processing of the affective component of pain. Scheduling pleasant activities into one's day helps to ensure that such events will happen. They should be given the same priority as a meeting, a doctor's appointment, or a deadline.[20] Combining graded activation with the scheduling of pleasant activities helps to reinforce the use of each skill and allows patients to engage in pleasant activities longer and with diminished risk of a flare-up.

Individuals with chronic pain have a number of problems related to getting a good night's sleep, including difficulty falling asleep, being awakened by pain or discomfort, or, after being sleep, awakening with feelings of being unrefreshed and unrestored. *Behavioral sleep strategies*, if used regularly, can help individuals get needed restorative sleep with additional benefits in improved mood, better management of pain, less fatigue, and improved mental clarity.[21] Some of these skills focus on timing strategies (e.g., having regular sleep routines), sleep behaviors (e.g., attempting to sleep only when in need of sleep), and behavioral avoidance of stimulating activities (e.g., watching action movies or consuming nicotine or caffeine).

Lifestyle Adaptation Skills

Individuals with chronic pain face interpersonal and functional challenges that rarely affect healthy individuals. Thus, in order to reduce negative affect associated with dealing with such complex problems and to overcome challenges associated with integrating new behavioral skills into one's daily routine, *problem-solving skills* are provided to patients. Problem-solving skills are systematic processes for breaking large problems down into smaller, more solvable pieces.[22] What is taught in therapy is a strategy for solving problems in general, rather than for determining specific solutions; in this way patients learn a strategy that can be carried into the future as new problems arise.

Beliefs held about the nature of a problem often influence the types of solutions one is able to generate so as to deal with the problem.

For example, strong convictions of one's helplessness, the futility of trying to control illness, or the inability to contribute meaningfully in life tasks are examples of learned automatic thinking patterns that can impede creative problem solving and successful adaptation to living with chronic pain. *Cognitive restructuring*[16] is a cognitive skill that is used to challenge the rationality of negative automatic thoughts and which seeks to instill alternative thinking capable of promoting greater functioning and well-being. Cognitive restructuring invites individuals to explore the origin of learned automatic thinking patterns that contribute to maladaptive behavioral responses. With practice, one can replace old thinking patterns with new ones that are more consistent with well-being and pain control.

Individuals with chronic pain often experience challenges in their dealings with other people. For example, a patient's spouse might become frustrated with that patient's limitations. Employers might become less sympathetic over time, and busy physicians might not have sufficient time to hear the many important details that patients wish to communicate. Assertiveness training and *communications skills training* can help one more effectively garner the support of others in managing pain[23] and are essential skills for managing pain over the long term.

Methods of CBT Service Delivery

CBT can be delivered in either a one-to-one format between a trained therapist and a single patient or with a therapist in a group setting. The duration of therapy is typically brief, involving between 6 and 12 sessions, with booster sessions being used to reinforce change over the longer term. Some communities do not have trained therapists, and in such cases receiving such care would impose a severe travel burden on patients attempting to receive long-distance care. However, there are e-Health alternatives for more rural areas.

For example, the delivery of coping skills training can be accomplished over the telephone,[24] CBT skills can be taught and supported by lay coaches,[25] and Web sites that do not employ therapists can provide patients with the content of cognitive and behavioral approaches, all of which can have a significant effect on symptoms.[14,26]

Literature reviews of CBT for the management of pain typically support the efficacy of CBT, with effects being comparable or in some cases superior to the effects of medications on pain.[9,13,14] Integrating this relatively low-cost pain treatment modality into more routine pain care should be a priority for practitioners who want to offer a broader spectrum of evidence-based care to their patients with chronic pain.

EXERCISE

There is little doubt that exercise is an effective treatment for patients with chronic pain. Moreover, exercise might be particularly essential for improving health and functioning in patients with chronic pain, given that deconditioning and obesity are ubiquitous. However, simply prescribing exercise might not result in the desired improvements. Exercise can take many forms, and there is evidence of the benefits of some forms of exercise and little to support the practice of others. Exercise can be aerobic or geared toward increasing strength and flexibility. It can be of high intensity and frequency or involve only adding a few more steps each day. A good exercise program can be land-based or water-based, range from whole-body exercise to cycling, or involve structured approaches such as Pilates, Qigong, or Tai Chi. In the first subsection below we provide an overview of the different types of exercise and the evidence base for each with regard to the treatment of patients with chronic pain. We also offer practical suggestions to promote the successful implementation of an exercise program, given the challenges a healthcare practitioner is bound to encounter when working with this population.

Anaerobic Exercise

As recently as 20 years ago, the etiology of chronic pain was presumed to be muscle pathology; thus, exercise interventions aimed to build muscle strength or address deconditioning. However, there is little evidence supporting a prominent role of muscle pathology in chronic pain conditions, and instead central nervous system dysregulation figures prominently.[27] Therefore, despite support for the benefits of muscle strength training in terms of pain reduction, evidence that strength training actually addresses the underlying pathology is lacking. Nonetheless, gentle and regular strength training, as opposed to moderate- or heavy-intensity strength training, is considered best.[28]

Most patients with chronic pain also experience muscle stiffness and reduced range of motion. *Flexibility training* includes stretching and bending with the aims of decreasing stiffness, increasing range of motion, and minimizing the risk of injury. Although few studies have evaluated flexibility training (stretching) for chronic pain, the most effective aerobic exercise programs include a flexibility-training component. However, when flexibility training is tested head-to-head with aerobic training, the latter almost always results in better outcomes, including reductions in pain and increased fitness and function. Although yoga does not fit into one discrete category, some consider it as flexibility training. The evidence for yoga is quite good; it has been shown to have multiple benefits for patients with chronic pain.[29]

Aerobic Exercise

Aerobic exercise for chronic pain can be *land based* or *water based* and consists of physical activity performed at least at a moderate intensity over an extended period of time. Pool-based aerobic exercise programs are particularly attractive to individuals with pain because of the added benefits of lower impact, increased resistance, and relief from immersion in warm water. Exercise of moderate intensity (i.e., with the individual working at 60 to 70 percent of his or her age-adjusted maximum heart rate, or about 110 beats per minute for a 40-year-old) is associated with improved fitness and fat burning.

There is an excellent evidence base supporting the efficacy of aerobic exercise in improving pain and functioning in individuals with chronic pain. Hauser and colleagues reported in a recent meta-analysis evaluating 35 randomized controlled trials (RCTs) that land-based and water-based aerobic exercise significantly reduced pain in patients with fibromyalgia.[30] Evidence suggests that exercise might also result in improvements in fatigue, sleep, cognitive complaints, and depression.

Intensity and Frequency

An evidence-based review of the exercise literature was published recently and concluded that there was robust evidence in favor of light to moderate aerobic exercise as a treatment for pain.[30] The authors suggested that aerobic exercise training start very slowly at the initiation of a program, at activity levels just below capacity. Then the activity should be increased in duration and intensity gradually until patients are exercising at low to moderate intensity (e.g., 50 to 70 percent of the age-adjusted maximum heart rate) for 20 to 30 minutes per session at least two to three times per week. Training programs should last for at least 4 weeks, and education is particularly helpful during the early stages of a new exercise program. Ideally, the training program will fit into a patient's lifestyle and thus become a more permanent aspect of his or her life. To enhance success, patients should be cautioned that experiencing increased symptoms is normal, and if this occurs they should decrease, but not stop, exercise until symptoms improve. Lastly, if there is concern about adverse effects, patients should always consult with their physicians. These recommendations are consistent with published guidelines.[31]

Attrition, Persistence, and Motivation

What might be the best way to engage patients who are obese, apathetic, sedentary, depressed, fatigued, and experiencing pain during regular exercise? This problem has plagued RCTs evaluating exercise in chronic pain conditions; studies typically report attrition rates ranging from 30 to 90 percent. Moreover, in this patient population, initial improvements in fitness are not always associated with symptomatic improvement—often patients get worse before they get much better. Thus, tailoring the exercise treatment program to the particular needs, preferences, and interests of each patient is the key to deriving benefit from and improving adherence to a new exercise program. *Exercise should be fun, and goals need to be easily attainable.* To truly enhance the chances for success, a combination of exercise and CBT aimed at modifying dysfunctional thoughts and beliefs is the optimal non-pharmacological therapeutic approach to chronic pain.

CONCLUDING REMARKS

It is likely that clinicians will continue to utilize pharmacological agents as frontline approaches to chronic pain management; however, clinicians need to be aware that reliance on medications and procedural interventions alone is unlikely to meaningfully impact the growing number of cases of chronic pain.[1] Non-pharmacological interventions that actively involve the patient in pain management, such as exercise and CBT, need to be used more routinely in chronic pain care. The challenge in using these interventions has been not a lack of efficacy but limited access to providers, a lack of reimbursement for services, and a lack of knowledge on the part of providers regarding the benefits of these interventions. Unlike pharmacological agents, exercise and CBT do not have large marketing forces behind them. Nonetheless, optimal pain management appears to involve combined pharmacological and non-pharmacological approaches to care.

REFERENCES

1. Institute of Medicine. *Relieving Pain in America: A Blueprint for Transforming Prevention, Care Education, and Reserach.* Washington, DC: The National Academies Press; 2011.
2. Melzack R, Wall PD. Pain mechanisms: a new theory. *Science.* 1965;150(699): 971–979.
3. Tracey I, Mantyh PW. The cerebral signature for pain perception and its modulation. *Neuron.* 2007;55(3):377–391.
4. Apkarian AV, Bushnell MC, Treede RD, Zubieta JK. Human brain mechanisms of pain perception and regulation in health and disease. *Eur J Pain.* 2005;9(4):463–484.
5. Chou R, Loeser JD, Owens DK, et al. Interventional therapies, surgery, and interdisciplinary rehabilitation for low back pain: an evidence-based clinical practice guideline from the American Pain Society. *Spine.* 2009;34(10):1066–1077.
6. Turk DC. Clinical effectiveness and cost-effectiveness of treatments for patients with chronic pain. *Clin J Pain.* 2002;18(6):355–365.
7. Schatman ME. The role of the health insurance industry in perpetuating suboptimal pain management. *Pain Med.* 2011;12(3):415–426.
8. Richeimer SH. Are we lemmings going off a cliff? The case against the "interventional" pain medicine label. *Pain Med.* 2010;11(1):3–5.
9. Hoffman BM, Papas RK, Chatkoff DK, Kerns RD. Meta-analysis of psychological interventions for chronic low back pain. *Health Psychol.* 2007;26(1):1–9.
10. Bruehl S, Chung OY. Psychological and behavioral aspects of complex regional pain syndrome management. *Clin J Pain.* 2006;22(5):430–437.
11. Reiter RC. Evidence-based management of chronic pelvic pain. *Clin Obstet Gynecol.* 1998;41(2):422–435.
12. Carville SF, Arendt-Nielsen S, Bliddal H, et al. Eular evidence-based recommendations for the management of fibromyalgia syndrome. *Ann Rheum Dis.* 2008;67(4):536–541.

13. Glombiewski JA, Sawyer AT, Gutermann J, Koenig K, Rief W, Hofmann SG. Psychological treatments for fibromyalgia: a meta-analysis. *Pain.* 2010;151(2):280–295.
14. Macea DD, Gajos K, Daglia Calil YA, Fregni F. The efficacy of Web-based cognitive behavioral interventions for chronic pain: a systematic review and meta-analysis. *J Pain.* 2010;11(10):917–929.
15. Fordyce WE. *Behavioral Methods for Chronic Pain and Illness.* St. Louis, MO: Mosby; 1976.
16. Beck AT, Rush AJ, Shaw BF, Emery G. *Cognitive Therapy for Depression.* New York: Guilford Press; 1979.
17. Integration of behavioral and relaxation approaches into the treatment of chronic pain and insomnia. NIH Technology Assessment Panel on Integration of Behavioral and Relaxation Approaches into the Treatment of Chronic Pain and Insomnia. *JAMA.* 1996;276(4):313–318.
18. Gil KM, Ross SL, Keefe FJ. Behavioral treatment of chronic pain: four pain management protocols. In: France R, Krishnan K, eds. *Chronic Pain.* New York: American Psychiatric Press; 1988:376–413.
19. Lewinsohn PM. The behavioral study and treatment of depression. In: *Progress in Behavior Modification.* Hersen, M., Eisler RM, Miller, PM, editors. Vol 1. New York: Academic Press; 1975, pp. 19–64.
20. Williams DA, Cary MA, Groner KH, et al. Improving physical functional status in patients with fibromyalgia: a brief cognitive behavioral intervention. *J Rheumatol.* 2002;29(6):1280–1286.
21. Morin CM, Culbert JP, Schwartz SM. Nonpharmacological interventions for insomnia: a meta-analysis of treatment efficacy. *Am J Psychiatry.* 1994;151(8):1172–1180.
22. D'zurilla TJ, Goldfried MR. Problem solving and behavior modification. *J Abnorm Psychol.* 1971;78(1):107–126.
23. Talen MR, Muller-Held CF, Eshleman KG, Stephens L. Patients' communication with doctors: a randomized control study of a brief patient communication intervention. *Fam Syst Health.* 2011;29(3):171–183.
24. Naylor MR, Keefe FJ, Brigidi B, Naud S, Helzer JE. Therapeutic interactive voice response for chronic pain reduction and relapse prevention. *Pain.* 2008;134(3):335–345.
25. Lorig K, Feigenbaum P, Regan C, Ung E, Chastain RL, Holman HR. A comparison of lay-taught and professional-taught arthritis self-management courses. *J Rheumatol.* 1986;13(4):763–767.
26. Williams DA, Kuper D, Segar M, Mohan N, Sheth M, Clauw DJ. Internet-enhanced management of fibromyalgia: a randomized controlled trial. *Pain.* 2010;151(3):694–702.
27. Phillips K, Clauw DJ. Central pain mechanisms in chronic pain states—maybe it is all in their head. *Best Pract Res Clin Rheumatol.* 2011;25(2):141–154.

28. Brosseau L, Wells GA, Tugwell P, et al. Ottawa Panel evidence-based clinical practice guidelines for strengthening exercises in the management of fibromyalgia: part 2. *Phys Ther*. 2008;88(7):873–886.
29. Langhorst J, Klose P, Dobos GJ, Bernardy K, Hauser W. Efficacy and safety of meditative movement therapies in fibromyalgia syndrome: a systematic review and meta-analysis of randomized controlled trials. *Rheumatol Int*. 2012.
30. Hauser W, Klose P, Langhorst J, et al. Efficacy of different types of aerobic exercise in fibromyalgia syndrome: a systematic review and meta-analysis of randomised controlled trials. *Arthritis Res Ther*. 2010;12(3):R79.
31. Brosseau L, Wells GA, Tugwell P, et al. Ottawa Panel evidence-based clinical practice guidelines for aerobic fitness exercises in the management of fibromyalgia: part 1. *Phys Ther*. 2008;88(7):857–871.

5

Complementary and Alternative Medical Therapies for Pain

RICHARD E. HARRIS AND SUZANNA M. ZICK

Complementary and alternative medicines (CAM) are a heterogeneous group of therapies delivered by providers such as acupuncturists and chiropractors; self-care modalities such as yoga and Tai Chi; and dietary supplements such as herbs, vitamins, and minerals. These treatments are generally not covered by insurance, taught at medical schools, or available at hospitals or clinics. One recent national survey done in 2007 found that over 38 percent of adults had used at least one of 36 types of CAM therapies in the past 12 months. That survey revealed that the top 10 diseases for which CAM was most commonly utilized included six pain disorders, with the top four being back pain (17.1 percent), neck pain (5.9 percent), joint pain (5.2 percent), and arthritis (3.5 percent).[1] Similarly, in a telephone survey of over 1000 people aged 50 years and older, 47 percent of responders reported using CAM in the past 12 months, and 73 percent of those indicated that they used CAM "to reduce pain or treat painful conditions."[2] People's reasons for using CAM to treat pain—in particular chronic pain—are not entirely understood. However, the limited and/or mixed effectiveness and the high incidence of side effects associated with conventional treatments might be the primary drivers for high CAM utilization in these populations.

Because of the heterogeneous nature of CAM therapies and the variety of pain disorders for which they are utilized, it is outside of the scope of this chapter to cover all CAM treatments for every pain condition. Consequently, we chose to highlight three CAM treatments—acupuncture, massage, and chiropractic—that, according to the 2007 National Health Interview Survey, are the among the most prevalent modalities used for treating chronic pain.[1–3] We also chose to focus on three of the most prevalent chronic pain disorders: chronic non-specific low back pain, knee osteoarthritis (OA), and fibromyalgia (FM) in adults. Herbal therapies are described in Chapter 3 ("Phytomedicines for the Treatment of Pain"). This chapter is organized into three sections on, respectively, massage, acupuncture, and chiropractic. Within each section, the efficacy, effectiveness, safety, and cost-effectiveness (as appropriate) of each of these therapies are described for chronic non-specific low back pain, knee OA, and FM.

MASSAGE AND CHRONIC PAIN

Massage is a heterogeneous therapy in which both superficial and deeper layers of muscle and connective tissue are rubbed, kneaded, or stretched to bring about relaxation, break muscle spasms, and enhance function. Massage is most often applied by a therapist, although caregivers such as spouses can also deliver massage treatments, and some types of self-administered massage are practiced.

Massage and OA of the Knee

Only one published pilot study has examined the effect of massage on improving pain and function in OA of the knee. Eight weeks of Swedish massage (twice per week for 4 weeks and then once weekly in weeks 5 to 8) was compared to a wait-list control in 68 adults.

Patients randomized to massage experienced significant improvements in pain, physical functioning, stiffness, and Western Ontario and McMaster Osteoarthritis Index (WOMAC) global scores. Although this was a pilot study, effect sizes at the 8-week assessments were large, ranging from 0.64 to 0.86—greater than a large acupuncture study performed for OA of the knee.[4] Larger studies of Swedish massage for OA of the knee are currently underway.

Massage and Chronic Low Back Pain

Eleven randomized clinical trials conducted to date have investigated the efficacy of massage for non-specific chronic low back pain.[5–10] We did not include studies that examined acupressure or foot reflexology, as both of these techniques more closely approximate the application of the traditional Chinese medicine (TCM) practice of acupuncture than other forms of bodywork. Those articles on acupressure are included in the section on acupuncture. The massage studies in general were of moderate to good quality. These trials tended to have larger sample sizes, with five having over 100 participants, and they included both short- and long-term assessments (see Table 5.1).

The types of massage investigated in the 11 studies were heterogeneous and included Thai massage, which is conducted on a mat on the floor and involves stretching and deep muscle massage whereby the therapist uses his or her hands, knees, legs, and feet to move the patient into a series of yoga-like stretches; Swedish massage, which uses five styles of long, flowing strokes (effleurage [sliding or gliding], petrissage [kneading], tapotement [rhythmic tapping], friction [cross fiber], and vibration/shaking); structural massage or integration, which focuses on decreasing muscular strain throughout the body using slow, deep manipulation of fascia and muscle; neuromuscular/trigger point massage, which is a deep tissue technique that helps to release trigger points (trigger points are knots of tense

Table 5.1 CHARACTERISTICS OF CLINICAL MASSAGE STUDIES FOR FIBROMYALGIA, OSTEOARTHRITIS OF THE KNEE AND CHRONIC LOW BACK PAIN

Author(s), Year	*Type of Massage*	*Control Group(s)*	*N*	*Length of Treatment*	*Any Significant Effect on Pain vs. Control Group(s)?*		*Any Significant Effect on Pain vs. No Treatment?*	*Any Significant Effect on Other Outcomes vs. Control Group(s)?*	*Study Quality*
					Short Term (End of Treatment)	*Long Term (Longer Follow-up > 1 month)*			
	KNEE OSTEOARTHRITIS								
Perlmen et al., 2006	Swedish	No treatment	68	8 weeks	Yes	Yes	Yes	Yes: improved stiffness, physical functioning, and time to walk 15 m	High

Buttagat et al., 2009	Thai	Bed rest	36	1 session	Yes	Not assessed	Yes	Yes: improved anxiety, flexibility, and muscle tension	Moderate
Chatchawan et al., 2005[a]	Thai	Swedish	180	3 to 4 weeks	No	No	Yes	No	Moderate
Cherkin et al., 2001[a]	Combination Swedish, deep-tissue, trigger point, and neuromuscular	Acupuncture and self-care education	262	10 weeks	Yes (massage superior to both control groups)	Yes (massage superior to acupuncture but not self-care)	Yes	Yes, Roland Disability Scale	Moderate

(continued)

Table 5.1 (CONTINUED)

Author(s), Year	*Type of Massage*	*Control Group(s)*	*N*	*Length of Treatment*	*Any Significant Effect on Pain vs. Control Group(s)?*		*Any Significant Effect on Pain vs. No Treatment?*	*Any Significant Effect on Other Outcomes vs. Control Group(s)?*	*Study Quality*
					Short Term (End of Treatment)	*Long Term (Longer Follow-up > 1 month)*			
Cherkin et al., 2011	Structural massage	Relaxation massage and usual care	401	10 weeks	Yes (either massage type superior to usual care)	No	Yes	Yes, Roland Disability Scale	Good
Field et al., 2007[a]	Swedish	PMR	30	5 weeks	No	Not assessed	Yes	Yes: sleep disturbance	Very low

Franke et al., 2000[a]	Swedish plus either group or individual exercise	Acupressure plus individual exercise or group exercise	109	1 month	No (acupressure superior)	No (acupressure superior)	Yes	No	Low
Hernandez-Reif, 2011[a]	Swedish	Relaxation	24	5 weeks	Yes	Not assessed	Yes	Yes: depression, anxiety, and sleep	Low
Kumnerddee, 2009	Thai	Acupuncture	18	10 days	No (acupressure superior on the McGill Pain Questionnaire)	Not assessed	Yes	No	Low

(continued)

Table 5.1 (CONTINUED)

Author(s), Year	*Type of Massage*	*Control Group(s)*	*N*	*Length of Treatment*	*Any Significant Effect on Pain vs. Control Group(s)?*		*Any Significant Effect on Pain vs. No Treatment?*	*Any Significant Effect on Other Outcomes vs. Control Group(s)?*	*Study Quality*
					Short Term (End of Treatment)	*Long Term (Longer Follow-up > 1 month)*			
Little et al., 2011	Swedish, neuromuscular work, and trigger point release[b]	Alexander technique,[b] usual care,[c] or exercise counseling	579	3 months	Yes (superior to exercise alone only)	No (six lessons of Alexander technique plus exercise were superior to other approaches)	Yes	Yes: quality of life, enablement, health transition, and fearing physical activity (superior to exercise	Moderate

Mackawan et al., 2005[a]	Thai	Joint mobilization	67	1 session	Yes	None	Yes	No	Moderate
Preyde, 2000[a]	Comprehensive massage therapy includes soft tissue work, trigger point and neuromuscular work, and exercise and posture education	Soft tissue work, exercise and posture education, or sham laser therapy	98	1 month	Yes (superior to all other groups)	Yes (superior to all other groups)	Yes	Yes: anxiety (superior to all other groups)	Moderate
	FIBROMYALGIA								
Alnigenis et al., 2001[d]	Swedish	SC/SCPC	37	24 weeks	Not assessed	Not assessed	Yes	Not assessed	Very low

(continued)

Table 5.1 (CONTINUED)

Author(s), Year	*Type of Massage*	*Control Group(s)*	*N*	*Length of Treatment*	*Any Significant Effect on Pain vs. Control Group(s)?*		*Any Significant Effect on Pain vs. No Treatment?*	*Any Significant Effect on Other Outcomes vs. Control Group(s)?*	*Study Quality*
					Short Term (End of Treatment)	*Long Term (Longer Follow-up > 1 month)*			
Asplund, 2003[e]	MLD	None	17	4 weeks	Yes; improvement of 35 mm	Yes; improvement of 17 mm	Yes	Yes: stiffness, sleep, well-being	Very low
Brattberg, 1999[d]	CTM	No treatment	48	10 weeks	Yes	No	Yes	Yes: depression, FIQ	Low
Castro-Sanchez et al., 2011	MRT	Sham (disconnected magnotherapy	64	20 weeks	Yes on both measures	Yes on VAS	Yes	Yes: trait anxiety	Low

Ekici et al., 2008[e]	MLD	CTM	50	3 weeks	No	Not assessed	Yes	Yes; FIQ	Low
Field et al., 2002[d]	Swedish and shiatsu	PMR	24	5 weeks	Yes	Not assessed	Yes	Yes: sleep, stiffness, fatigue	Very low
Gordon et al., 2006[e]	Mechanical (Cellu M6)	None	10	15 weeks	Yes: improvement of 16.5 mm, decrease of 8 tender points	Not assessed	Yes	Yes; FIQ	Very low
Lund et al., 2006[e]	Swedish	GR	19	6 weeks	No	Not assessed	Yes	Yes; NHP for pain and emotional reaction	Very low

(continued)

Table 5.1 (CONTINUED)

Author(s), Year	*Type of Massage*	*Control Group(s)*	*N*	*Length of Treatment*	*Any Significant Effect on Pain vs. Control Group(s)?*		*Any Significant Effect on Pain vs. No Treatment?*	*Any Significant Effect on Other Outcomes vs. Control Group(s)?*	*Study Quality*
					Short Term (End of Treatment)	*Long Term (Longer Follow-up > 1 month)*			
Sunshine et al., 1996[d]	Swedish	Sham (TENS) and TENS	30	5 weeks	Not assessed	Not assessed	Yes	Not assessed	Low

WOMAC = Western Ontario and McMaster Universities Osteoarthritis Index; TENS = transcutaneous electrical nerve stimulation; FIQ = Fibromyalgia Impact Questionnaire; SC = standard of care; SCPC = standard of care followed by a phone follow-up; MLD = manual lymph drainage; CTM = connective tissue massage; PMR = progressive muscle relaxation; GR = guided relaxation; NHP = Nottingham Health Profile; MRT = myofacial release therapy; PPT = pressure pain threshold; VAS = Visual Analog Scale; FRCT = factorial randomized clinical trial.

[a]Referenced and reviewed in Furlan AD, Imamura M, Dryden T, Irvin E. Massage for low back pain: an updated review within the framework of the Cochrane Back Review Group. *Spine (Phila Pa 1976)*. 2009;34(16):1669–1684.

[b]Participants were randomized to two study arms of Alexander technique: 6 sessions or 24 sessions.

[c]Half of all participants in each study arm (Alexander, massage, usual care) were randomized to receive exercise counseling.

[d]Referenced and reviewed in Porter NS, Jason LA, Boulton A, Bothne N, Coleman B. Alternative medical interventions used in the treatment and management of myalgic encephalomyelitis/chronic fatigue syndrome and fibromyalgia. *J Altern Complement Med*. 2010;16(3):235–249.

[e]Referenced and reviewed in Kalichman L. Massage therapy for fibromyalgia symptoms. *Rheumatol Int*. 2010;30(9):1151–1157.

or spasmodic muscles, which can "refer" pain to other parts of the body); and comprehensive massage therapy, which comprises various soft-tissue techniques such as friction and neuromuscular massage.

Massage techniques were compared to numerous other therapies, including sham laser, exercise, joint mobilization, acupuncture, usual care, self-care, and relaxation. Seven of the 11 studies found massage to be beneficial for relieving pain at the short-term assessments relative to a variety of control groups including exercise and usual care, with the lower quality studies more likely to find no benefit of massage (3 of 4). However, only two of six studies found long-term (>6 months) benefits that persisted after treatment was stopped.

Massage for FM

There have been 10 studies—2 open label and 8 randomized clinical trials—examining the effect of various types of massage on FM (see Table 5.1).[5–7] All of the studies were small (between 1 and 64 participants) and of poor quality. They used a wide variety of outcomes measures, many of which have not been validated in the FM population. Similar to studies evaluating massage for chronic low back pain, those performed for FM included a heterogeneous array of treatments, control groups, and inclusion criteria. Although five of the studies[5–8] reported significantly improved pain either immediately after or for as long as 6 months post-intervention, the heterogeneity and low quality of the studies make these results difficult to interpret. As a result, better quality studies are needed before any clear clinical recommendations can be made for FM patients.

ACUPUNCTURE AND CHRONIC PAIN

Acupuncture as a component of East Asian medicine and TCM is based largely on the philosophy that the placement and stimulation of very fine needles into specific points on the body (acupoints) can treat pain and other symptoms.[9] TCM has been practiced in China for over 5000 years and until fairly recently was the primary form of healthcare in China. The methods for the stimulation of acupoints are quite diverse and involve manual manipulation, pressure with fingers or other devices (termed acupressure), thermal stimulation, electrical stimulation, or even chemical injection of specific compounds. Typically these diverse manipulations all fall under the rubric of what is clinically termed "acupuncture." A typical treatment session involves intake of symptoms, pulse and tongue diagnosis, and needle insertion/manipulation. Usually this is performed by a trained acupuncturist, and treatments may extend to multiple sessions over weeks to months, depending on patient response. One obstacle encountered in acupuncture research is the development of a non-invasive control procedure that would effectively work as a placebo. Acupuncture controls include (1) insertion of needles into non-acupoints, (2) insertion of needles superficially either on or off acupoints (termed minimal acupuncture), (3) pricking the skin without skin penetration, and (4) using a sham needle that retracts into the needle handle. A common control used for electrical acupuncture involves attaching wires to the needles but not actually running electricity through them. Often one or more of these control procedures are used in acupuncture clinical trials to control for the "placebo effect" or "non-specific effects" of the intervention that are not involved with needle insertion.

Acupuncture and OA of the Knee

We identified nine randomized clinical trials and one open label study of acupuncture treatment of chronic knee OA (see Table 5.2).[10] Five studies used manual manipulation of the needle for the active treatment, and the other five investigated the effects of electrical

Table 5.2 CHARACTERISTICS OF ACUPUNCTURE CLINICAL STUDIES FOR FIBROMYALGIA, OSTEOARTHRITIS OF THE KNEE, AND CHRONIC LOW BACK PAIN

Author, Year	*Type of Acupuncture*	*Control Group(s)*	*N*	*Length of Treatment*	*Any Significant Effect on Pain vs. Control Group(s)?*		*Any Significant Effect on Pain vs. No Treatment?*	*Any Significant Effect on Other Outcomes vs. Control Group(s)?*	*Study Quality*
					Short Term (End of Treatment)	*Long Term (Longer Follow-up; >1 Month)*			
	KNEE OSTEOARTHRITIS								
Christensen et al., 1992[a]	TCM; manual	Wait list	32	3 weeks	Yes; acupuncture superior to wait list	Not assessed	Yes	Yes; acupuncture improves mobility	Low
Berman et al., 1999[a]	TCM; e-stim	Standard care	73	8 weeks	Yes; acupuncture superior to standard care	Yes; acupuncture superior to standard care	Yes	Yes; acupuncture improves disability	Very good

(continued)

Table 5.2 *(CONTINUED)*

Author, Year	*Type of Acupuncture*	*Control Group(s)*	*N*	*Length of Treatment*	*Any Significant Effect on Pain vs. Control Group(s)?*		*Any Significant Effect on Pain vs. No Treatment?*	*Any Significant Effect on Other Outcomes vs. Control Group(s)?*	*Study Quality*
					Short Term (End of Treatment)	*Long Term (Longer Follow-up; >1 Month)*			
Sangdee et al., 2002[a]	E-stim	diclofenac	193	4 weeks	Yes; acupuncture superior to drug	Not assessed	Yes	Yes; acupuncture increases function	Very low
Berman et al., 2004[a]	TCM; e-stim	Sham or education control	570	26 weeks	N.S.	Yes; acupuncture superior to sham and education	Yes	Yes; acupuncture increases function	Very good

Tukmachi et al., 2004[a]	TCM; e-stim	Medication alone	35	5 weeks	Yes; acupuncture superior to medication	Not assessed	Yes	Yes; acupuncture improves stiffness	Low
Camila et al., 2004[a]	TCM; e-stim + diclofenac	Sham acupuncture + diclofenac	97	12 weeks	Yes; acupuncture superior to sham	Overview of	Yes	Yes; acupuncture improves function	Moderate
Witt et al., 2006[a]	Acupuncture with individualized formula	Standard care	532	3 months	Yes; acupuncture superior to control	Not assessed	Yes	Yes; acupuncture improves physical function	Good
Scharf et al., 2006[a]	TCM; with individualized formula	Minimal acupuncture or wait list	1007	6 weeks	Mixed; acupuncture favors no treatment but not minimal acupuncture	Mixed; acupuncture favors no treatment but not minimal acupuncture	Yes	Not assessed	Good

(continued)

Table 5.2 *(CONTINUED)*

Author, Year	*Type of Acupuncture*	*Control Group(s)*	*N*	*Length of Treatment*	*Any Significant Effect on Pain vs. Control Group(s)?*		*Any Significant Effect on Pain vs. No Treatment?*	*Any Significant Effect on Other Outcomes vs. Control Group(s)?*	*Study Quality*
					Short Term (End of Treatment)	*Long Term (Longer Follow-up; >1 Month)*			
Foster et al., 2007[a]	TCM; manual individualized formula	Sham acupuncture or exercise	352	3 weeks; 6 treatments	N.S.	N.S.	Yes	N.S.	Moderate
Williamson et al., 2007[a]	TCM; manual	Physical therapy or education	181	6 weeks	Yes (knee score); no VAS	N.S.	Yes	Not assessed	Good
	NON-SPECIFIC CHRONIC LOW BACK PAIN								
Mendelson et al., 1983[b]	TCM; manual	2 percent lidocaine + superficial needling	77	4 weeks per period	N.S.	N.S.	Yes	N.S.	Low

Carlsson et al., 2001[c]	TCM; manual and e-stim	Sham TENS	50	8 weeks + taper of 4 months	Yes: acupuncture superior to control	Yes: acupuncture superior to control	Yes	Yes; acupuncture improves work activity	Good
Leibing et al., 2002[c]	TCM; body and ear	Physiological therapy + superficial needling	131	12 weeks	N.S.	N.S.	Yes	Yes; acupuncture improves distress	Good
Meng et al., 2003[c]	TCM; e-stim	Standard care	55	5 weeks	Yes; acupuncture superior to standard care	Not assessed	Yes	Yes; acupuncture improves disability	Moderate
Yeung et al., 2003[c]	E-stim + exercise	Exercise alone	52	4 weeks	Yes; favors acupunctrue + exercise	Yes; favors acuupncture + exercise	Yes	Yes; acupuncture improves disability	Good

(continued)

Table 5.2 (CONTINUED)

Author, Year	*Type of Acupuncture*	*Control Group(s)*	*N*	*Length of Treatment*	*Any Significant Effect on Pain vs. Control Group(s)?*		*Any Significant Effect on Pain vs. No Treatment?*	*Any Significant Effect on Other Outcomes vs. Control Group(s)?*	*Study Quality*
					Short Term (End of Treatment)	*Long Term (Longer Follow-up; >1 Month)*			
Hsieh et al., 2004	Acupressure	Physical therapy	146	4 weeks	Yes; acupuncture superior to physical therapy	Yes; acupuncture superior to physical therapy	Yes	Not assessed	Moderate
Sator-Katzenschlager et al., 2003[c]	Ear acupuncture + e-stim	Ear acupuncture alone	61	6 weeks	Yes; favors acupuncture + e-stim	Yes; favors acupuncture + e-stim	Yes	Yes; improved activity	Low

2006[b]	with semistandard formula	puncture or wait-list control			puncture favors no treatment but not minimal acupuncture	puncture favors no treatment but not minimal acupuncture		puncture improves disability	
Hsieh et al., 2006	Acupressure	Physical therapy	129	4 weeks	Yes; acupressure superior to physical therapy	Yes; acupressure superior to physical therapy	Yes	Yes; acupressure improves disability and function	Low
Itoh et al., 2006[c]	Trigger point acupuncture; manual	Non-penetrating acupuncture	19	3 weeks per period	Yes; acupuncture superior to sham	Not assessed	Yes	Yes; acupuncture improves disability	Low

(continued)

Table 5.2 (CONTINUED)

Author, Year	*Type of Acupuncture*	*Control Group(s)*	*N*	*Length of Treatment*	*Any Significant Effect on Pain vs. Control Group(s)?*		*Any Significant Effect on Pain vs. No Treatment?*	*Any Significant Effect on Other Outcomes vs. Control Group(s)?*	*Study Quality*
					Short Term (End of Treatment)	*Long Term (Longer Follow-up; >1 Month)*			
Thomas et al., 2006[b]	TCM; with individualized formula	Standard care	239	3 months	N.S.	Yes; acupuncture superior to standard care	Yes	No effect on disability	Good
Witt et al., 2006[b]	Acupuncture; individualized	Standard care	2931	3 months	Trend for acupuncture superior to standard care	Not assessed	Yes	Yes; acupuncture improves function and is cost-effective	Good

Haake et al., 2007[b]	TCM; manual	Minimal acupuncture or standard care	1162	6 weeks	Not assessed	Mixed; acupuncture favors no treatment but not minimal acupuncture	Yes	Yes; acupuncture improves disability	Good
	FIBROMYALGIA								
Deluze et al., 1992[d]	TCM; e-stim	Minmal acupuncture with e-stim	70	3 wks	Yes; acupuncture superior to control	Not assessed	Yes	Not assessed	Moderate
Assefi et al., 2005[d]	TCM; manual	Unrelated acupuncture, minimal acupuncture, or non-insertion	96	12 weeks	N.S.; acupuncture not superior to control	N.S.; acupuncture not superior to control	Yes	Not assessed	Good

(continued)

Table 5.2 (CONTINUED)

Author, Year	*Type of Acupuncture*	*Control Group(s)*	*N*	*Length of Treatment*	*Any Significant Effect on Pain vs. Control Group(s)?*		*Any Significant Effect on Pain vs. No Treatment?*	*Any Significant Effect on Other Outcomes vs. Control Group(s)?*	*Study Quality*
					Short Term (End of Treatment)	*Long Term (Longer Follow-up; >1 Month)*			
Harris et al., 2005[d]	TCM; manual	Minimal acupuncture + stimulation, minimal acupuncture with no stimulation, or acupuncture with no stimulation	114	9 weeks	N.S.; acupuncture not superior to any control	Not assessed	Yes	No	Good

Martin et al., 2006[d]	TCM; e-stim	Sham acupuncture; non-insertive	50	2 to 3 weeks	Yes; acupuncture superior to control	N.S.	Yes	Yes; acupuncture improves fatigue and anxiety	Moderate

N.S. = not significant; TCM = traditional Chinese medicine; e-stim = electrical stimulation; TENS = transcutaneous electrical nerve stimulation; VAS = Visual Analog Scale; NRS = Numerical Rating Scale; SF-MPQ = Short Form of the McGill Pain Questionnaire; WOMAC = Western Ontario and McMaster Universities Osteoarthritis Index; MPI = Multidisciplinary Pain Inventory; FIQ = Fibromyalgia Impact Questionnaire; SC = standard of care.

[a]Referenced and reviewed in Manheimer E, Cheng K, Linde K, et al. Acupuncture for peripheral joint asteoarthritis. *Cochrane Database Systemic Reviews.* 2010 Jan 20;(1):CD001977

[b]Referenced and reviewed in Yuan J, Purepong N, Kerr DP, Park J, Bradbury I, McDonough S. Effectiveness of acupuncture for low back pain: a systematic review. *Spine (Phila Pa 1976)*. 2008;33(23):E887–E900.

[c]Referenced and reviewed in Rubinstein SM, van Middelkoop M, Kuijpers T, et al. A systematic review on the effectiveness of complementary and alternative medicine for chronic non-specific low-back pain. *Eur Spine J.* 2010;19(8):1213–1228.

[d]Referenced and reviewed in Langhorst J, Klose P, Musial F, Irnich D, Hauser W. Efficacy of acupuncture in fibromyalgia syndrome—a systematic review with a meta-analysis of controlled clinical trials. *Rheumatology (Oxford)*. 2010;49(4):778–788.

stimulation. Controls used in these studies were quite diverse and included minimal needling, education, exercise, physical therapy, wait-listing, and even medications such as diclofenac. The quality of the studies ranged from low to very good, with the majority of trials (seven of the nine) having moderate to good scores.

In all studies examined, acupuncture significantly reduced pain outcomes when analyzed in isolation (i.e., pre- versus post-acupuncture alone). Relative to trials that had a wait-list or standard-of-care control arm, acupuncture was effective in the short term for reducing pain (four of four trials). Modest evidence also existed of acupuncture being superior to no treatment or standard of care for long-term effects (two of two trials). Three studies reported that acupuncture had been more effective than medications such as diclofenac for knee OA in the short term.

These trials largely suggest that acupuncture might be better than either no treatment or standard of care; however, when compared to sham or placebo acupuncture, two large well-designed trials (n = 1007 and n = 352) failed to show the superiority of acupuncture over sham acupuncture. This result might mean acupuncture is simply a placebo for this disorder or that sham treatment is not an inert intervention. Very few adverse events were reported with these trials, and some studies also suggest that acupuncture might be cost-effective for knee OA.[11]

Acupuncture and Chronic Low Back Pain

We identified 13 clinical trials investigating the efficacy of acupuncture in the treatment of chronic low back pain (see Table 5.2).[12–15] The majority of these studies (9 of 13) were of moderate to good quality. Acupuncture methods were diverse and included TCM, ear stimulation, trigger point acupuncture, and acupressure. Needle stimulation involved either manual manipulation or electrical stimulation.

Control groups were also quite diverse and included wait-list controls, standard of care, exercise, physical therapy, sham transcutaneous electrical nerve stimulation, minimal acupuncture, and lidocaine injection. Given the diversity of acupuncture methods and the control interventions, it might be premature at this point to infer findings across studies. Regardless, there was strong evidence (13 of 13 trials) that acupuncture reduced pain in the short term when examined in isolation (i.e., pre- versus post-acupuncture). Similar findings were also reported when acupuncture was compared to wait list (one trial) or standard of care (three trials). In these trials, acupuncture was superior in the short term and the long term for reducing pain.

However, similar to the studies of acupuncture for knee OA, all studies that involved a sham or placebo acupuncture control that were of good quality (three of three trials; total $n = 1591$) failed to show superiority of acupuncture over sham controls. It is important to note that the only studies involving a sham control that reported acupuncture as being superior to sham were of low methodological quality and involved few participants (two trials; $n = 19$ and 61). Adverse events were rare and included pain upon needle insertion and minor bleeding. Modest evidence also exists of acupuncture's being cost-effective for chronic low back pain with respect to accepted national thresholds for quality adjusted life years.[16] These data indicate that acupuncture is safe, cost-effective, and superior to no treatment and standard of care, but not superior to sham controls.

Acupuncture and FM

We identified four clinical trials investigating the efficacy of acupuncture for the treatment of FM (see Table 5.2).[17] All of these studies were of moderate to good quality. Acupuncture methods across these trials were more uniform than for the OA and chronic low back pain studies. All trials included TCM theory and used either manual manipulation (two trials) or electrical stimulation (two trials). Control groups for these studies were non-insertion sham, minimal insertion, or sham electrical stimulation. Similar to the findings for chronic low back pain and knee OA, there was moderate evidence (four of four trials) that acupuncture reduced pain when examined in isolation (i.e., pre- versus post-acupuncture). However, findings were mixed when comparing efficacy using sham controls. The two studies that used minimal acupuncture as a control failed to show the superiority of acupuncture in the short term. These trials were of good quality and had the largest sample sizes ($n = 96$ and 114). The two studies that reported significant differences between acupuncture and sham acupuncture were of lower quality and were somewhat smaller studies ($n = 50$ and 70).

Similar to findings for chronic low back pain and knee OA, acupuncture is superior to no treatment for FM; however, manual acupuncture does not appear to be superior to sham controls. As the methodology of acupuncture research is diverse, future studies are needed to explore the efficacy of these diverse practices in a controlled setting. We recommend that researchers and clinicians utilize standardized reporting methods for acupuncture clinical trials (please see http://www.stricta.info/).

CHIROPRACTIC CARE AND CHRONIC PAIN

Chiropractic treatment is a "hands on" therapy wherein the practitioner uses manual therapy, including manipulation of the spine, other joints, and soft tissues, in order to reduce pain. Although the treatment is largely manual, chiropractic care may also include exercises, as well as health and lifestyle counseling. Traditionally chiropractic care proposes that vertebral subluxation interferes with the body's innate healing system and that manual manipulation of the spine can correct these deficiencies. Typical sessions involve mobilization (low velocity combined with small- or large-amplitude movement techniques) or manipulation (high-velocity impulse or thrust) of joints. The latter of these two methods may be accompanied by an audible "crack" of the manipulated joint. As with other CAM interventions, there are multiple diagnostic techniques and philosophies utilized by chiropractic care givers; however, the components of manipulation and mobilization are commonly utilized.

Chiropractic Care and OA of the Knee

We identified only two randomized clinical trials using chiropractic treatment of chronic knee OA (see Table 5.3).[18,19] Although both trials used mobilization of the joint, one study used sham ultrasound combined with an inert gel as a control, and the other trial compared chiropractic care to manual contact or no-contact controls. These two studies were of moderate to good quality and enrolled a total of 178 participants (n = 140 and 38).

Limited evidence exists that chiropractic care is beneficial when studied in isolation (i.e., pre- versus post-therapy); only one of these two trials reported beneficial effects of chiropractic in the short term for knee OA. Furthermore, when compared to sham controls or manual contact, neither trial reported significant effects of chiropractic care in the short term for reducing pain. The one study that examined chiropractic care for long-term effects on knee pain did not find any significant benefit over control. One trial did find improvement in knee function and a reduction in pressure pain tenderness at the knee following treatment. There is a need for more studies with larger sample sizes to assess the effects of chiropractic care for knee OA. There is insufficient evidence at present to conclude whether chiropractic care is effective in treating knee OA.

Table 5.3 CHARACTERISTICS OF CHIROPRACTIC CLINICAL STUDIES FOR FIBROMYALGIA, OSTEOARTHRITIS OF THE KNEE, AND CHRONIC LOW BACK PAIN

Author, Year	*Type of Chiropractic Care*	*Control Group(s)*	*N*	*Length of Treatment*	*Any Significant Effect on Pain vs. Control Group(s)?*		*Any Significant Effect on Pain vs. No Treatment or Over Time?*	*Any Significant Effect on Other Outcomes vs. Control Group(s)?*	*Study Quality*
					Short Term (End of Treatment)	*Long Term (Longer Follow-up; >1 Month)*			
	KNEE OSTEOARTHRITIS								
Bennell et al., 2005	Mobilization	Sham ultrasound + inert gel	140	12 weeks	N.S.	N.S.	Yes	N.S.	Moderate
Moss et al., 2007	Mobilization	Manual contact or no contact	38	1 treatment	Mixed; improvement in PPT but not VAS or WOMAC	Not assessed	No	Yes; improvement in function	Good

	NON-SPECIFIC CHRONIC LOW BACK PAIN								
Evans et al., 1978[a]	SM	Wait list	32	3 weeks	Could not be estimated	Not assessed	Yes	Not assessed	Very low
Koes et al., 1992[a]	SM	Physical therapy	131	3 months	N.S.	Yes; favors SM	Yes	Not assessed	Very low
Hemmila et al., 1997[a]	Bone setting; SM	Physical therapy or exercise	114	6 weeks	N.S.	Yes; favors bone setting	Yes	Not assessed	Low
Licciardone et al., 2003[a]	SM	Sham or no treatment	199	5 months (seven treatments)	Mixed; SM favors no treatment but not sham	Mixed; SM favors no treatment but not sham	Yes	N.S.	Very low
Giles et al., 2003[a]	SM	Acupuncture or medication	109	9 weeks	no direct comparisons	no direct comparisons	Yes	N.S.	Very low

(continued)

Table 5.3 (CONTINUED)

Author, Year	*Type of Chiropractic Care*	*Control Group(s)*	*N*	*Length of Treatment*	*Any Significant Effect on Pain vs. Control Group(s)?*		*Any Significant Effect on Pain vs. No Treatment or Over Time?*	*Any Significant Effect on Other Outcomes vs. Control Group(s)?*	*Study Quality*
					Short Term (End of Treatment)	*Long Term (Longer Follow-up; >1 Month)*			
Rasmussen-Barr et al., 2003[a]	Manual treatment; mobilization	Stabilizing training	47	6 weeks	N.S.	N.S.	Yes	No; no improvement in disability	Low
Cambron et al., 2006[a]	Flexion distraction	Exercise	235	4 weeks	N.S.	N.S.	Yes	Yes; flexion distraction improves disability	Low
Ferreira et al., 2007[a]	SM	Motor exercise or general exercise	240	8 weeks	N.S.	N.S.	Yes	Yes; SM improves disability	Good

Skillgate et al., 2007[a]	SM; naprapathy	Education support	409	8 weeks	N.S.	Yes; SM superior to control	Yes	Yes; SM improves disability	Good
Paatelma et al., 2008[a]	SM	McKenzie Method or education	134	6 treatments	N.S.; SM not superior to education or McKenzie	N.S.; SM not superior to education or McKenzie	Yes	N.S.	Moderate
Hondras et al., 2009[a]	SM; HVLA or LVVA	Conservative medical care	240	6 weeks	N.S.	Not assessed	Yes	Yes; both SM groups improve disability	Good
Rasmussen et al., 2008[a]	SM: HVLA	Exercise	72	4 weeks	N.S.	N.S.	Yes	Not assessed	Low
Wilkey et al., 2008[a]	SM; individualized	Pain clinic	30	8 weeks	SM superior to control	Not assessed	Yes	Yes; SM improves disability	Very low

(continued)

Table 5.3 (CONTINUED)

Author, Year	*Type of Chiropractic Care*	*Control Group(s)*	*N*	*Length of Treatment*	*Any Significant Effect on Pain vs. Control Group(s)?*		*Any Significant Effect on Pain vs. No Treatment or Over Time?*	*Any Significant Effect on Other Outcomes vs. Control Group(s)?*	*Study Quality*
					Short Term (End of Treatment)	*Long Term (Longer Follow-up; >1 Month)*			
	FIBROMYALGIA								
Blunt et al., 1997	SM	Wait list	21	4 weeks	Yes; SM superior to control	Not assessed	Yes	Yes; SM improves range of motion	Low

N.S. = not significant; SM = spinal manipulation; HVLA = high velocity low amplitude; LVVA = low velocity variable amplitude; VAS = Visual Analog Scale; NRS = Numerical Rating Scale; PPT = pressure pain threshold; SF-MPQ = Short Form of the McGill Pain Questionnaire; CPQ = Chronic Pain Questionnaire; WOMAC = Western Ontario and McMaster Universities Osteoarthritis Index; MPI = Multidisciplinary Pain Inventory; FIQ = Fibromyalgia Impact Questionnaire; SC = standard of care.

[a]Referenced and reviewed in Rubinstein SM, van Middelkoop M, Assendelft WJ, de Boer MR, van Tulder MW. Spinal manipulative therapy for chronic low-back pain: an update of a Cochrane review. *Spine (Phila Pa 1976)*. 2011;36(13):E825–E846.

Chiropractic Care for Chronic Low Back Pain

We identified 13 clinical trials investigating the efficacy of chiropractic care for the treatment of chronic low back pain (see Table 5.3).[20] Unfortunately, the majority of these studies (9 of 13) were of low to very low quality. Chiropractic methods were diverse and included spinal manipulation, bone setting, manual treatment, naprapathy, and flexion distraction. Control or comparison groups were also diverse and included wait-list controls, exercise, education, physical therapy, sham manipulation, McKenzie method, conservative medical care, and standard of care. Given the diversity of methods and the control interventions used, it might be premature at this point to infer findings across studies. Regardless, there was strong evidence (13 of 13 trials) that chiropractic care reduces pain when examined in isolation (i.e., pre- versus post-treatment).

When compared to control treatments, chiropractic care was not found to be superior in the short term for treating chronic low back pain (8 of 13 trials). The results for long-term effects on pain were similar, with five of nine trials failing to show the superiority of chiropractic care for low back pain. In analyses of only the trials that were of moderate to good quality (four trials), there was no evidence of the clinical benefit of chiropractic care for back pain in the short term immediately following treatment, and only one study showing long-term benefit. As with acupuncture, adverse events were rare. These trials suggest that chiropractic care, although safe, might be better than no treatment but not superior to controls such as physical therapy and education.

Chiropractic Care for FM

We were able to find only one study examining the effect of chiropractic care on FM pain.[21] This study compared spinal manipulation to a wait-list control in 21 participants. Similar to knee OA and low back pain, chiropractic treatment was associated with less pain when comparing before- and after-treatment pain scores. Spinal manipulation was also superior to the wait-list control group when assessed in the short term. This study did not examine the long-term benefits of chiropractic care. Of note, chiropractic treatment did improve patients' range of motion. More studies of chiropractic treatment are needed to confirm or refute these initial findings.

CONCLUSION

Multiple CAM clinical trials have been published about chronic low back pain, knee OA, and FM. Because significant heterogeneity exists within CAM modalities and their matching controls, definitive conclusions might be premature at this point. Inert control or sham procedures have yet to be developed for many CAM interventions. That said, acupuncture, massage, and, to a lesser extent, chiropractic care appear to be beneficial relative to no treatment. Moreover, in some cases these CAM treatments are superior to the current standard of care. Whereas CAM may induce analgesic benefits in the short term, requiring ongoing treatment similar to conventional pain medications, acupuncture has the added benefit of long-term analgesia without continued sessions. Overall, these CAM treatments are largely safe, and in some cases they are even cost-effective, making them important tools our clinical armamentarium. More rigorous clinical trials are needed.

REFERENCES

1. Barnes P, Bloom B, Nahin R. *Complementary and Alternative Medicine Use among Adults and Children: United States,* Natural Health Statistics Report. 2008 Dec 10;12:1–23.

2. American Association of Retired Persons, National Center for Complementary and Alternative Medicine. *Complementary and Alternative Medicine: What People Aged 50 and Older Discuss with Their Health Care Providers.* 2011; http://nccam.nih.gov/sites/nccam.nih.gov/files/news/camstats/2010/NCCAM_aarp_survey.pdf, accessed on November 30th, 2012.
3. TerhorstL, Schneider MJ, Kim KH, Goozdich LM, Stilley CS. Complementary and alternative medicine in the treatment of pain in fibromyalgia: a systematic review of randomized controlled trials. *J Manipulative Physiol Ther.* 2011;34(7):483–496.
4. Perlman AI, Sabina A, Williams AL, Njike VY, Katz DL. Massage therapy for osteoarthritis of the knee: a randomized controlled trial. *Arch Intern Med.* 2006;166(22):2533–2538.
5. Kalichman L. Massage therapy for fibromyalgia symptoms. *Rheumatol Int.* 2010;30(9):1151–1157.
6. Porter NS, Jason LA, Boulton A, Bothne N, Coleman B. Alternative medical interventions used in the treatment and management of myalgic encephalomyelitis/chronic fatigue syndrome and fibromyalgia. *J Altern Complement Med.* 2010;16(3):235–249.
7. Furlan AD, Imamura M, Dryden T, Irvin E. Massage for low back pain: an updated systematic review within the framework of the Cochrane Back Review Group. *Spine (Phila Pa 1976).* 2009;34(16):1669–1684.
8. Castro-Sanchez AM, Mataran-Penarrocha GA, Granero-Molina J, Aguilera-Manrique G, Quesada-Rubio JM, Moreno-Lorenzo C. Benefits of massage-myofascial release therapy on pain, anxiety, quality of sleep, depression, and quality of life in patients with fibromyalgia. *Evid Based Complement Alternat Med.* 2011;2011:561753.
9. Xinnong C. *Chinese Acupuncture and Moxibustion.* Vol 1. Bejing: Foreign Languages Press; 1999.
10. Manheimer E, Cheng K, Linde K, et al. Acupuncture for peripheral joint osteoarthritis. *Cochrane Database Systemic Reviews.* 2010 Jan 20;(1):CD001977.
11. Reinhold T, Witt CM, Jena S, Brinkhaus B, Willich SN. Quality of life and cost-effectiveness of acupuncture treatment in patients with osteoarthritis pain. *Eur J Health Econ.* 2008;9(3):209–219.
12. Yuan J, Purepong N, Kerr DP, Park J, Bradbury I, McDonough S. Effectiveness of acupuncture for low back pain: a systematic review. *Spine (Phila Pa 1976).* 2008;33(23):E887–E900.
13. Rubinstein SM, van Middelkoop M, Kuijpers T, et al. A systematic review on the effectiveness of complementary and alternative medicine for chronic non-specific low-back pain. *Eur Spine J.* 2010;19(8):1213–1228.
14. Hsieh LL, Kuo CH, Lee LH, Yen AM, Chien KL, Chen TH. Treatment of low back pain by acupressure and physical therapy: randomised controlled trial. *BMJ.* 2006;332(7543):696–700.

15. Hsieh LL, Kuo CH, Yen MF, Chen TH. A randomized controlled clinical trial for low back pain treated by acupressure and physical therapy. *Prev Med.* 2004;39(1):168–176.
16. Ratcliffe J, Thomas KJ, MacPherson H, Brazier J. A randomised controlled trial of acupuncture care for persistent low back pain: cost effectiveness analysis. *BMJ.* 2006;333(7569):626.
17. Langhorst J, Klose P, Musial F, Irnich D, Hauser W. Efficacy of acupuncture in fibromyalgia syndrome—a systematic review with a meta-analysis of controlled clinical trials. *Rheumatology (Oxford).* 2010;49(4):778–788.
18. Bennell KL, Hinman RS, Metcalf BR, et al. Efficacy of physiotherapy management of knee joint osteoarthritis: a randomised, double blind, placebo controlled trial. *Ann Rheum Dis.* 2005;64(6):906–912.
19. Moss P, Sluka K, Wright A. The initial effects of knee joint mobilization on osteoarthritic hyperalgesia. *Man Ther.* 2007;12(2):109–118.
20. Rubinstein SM, van Middelkoop M, Assendelft WJ, de Boer MR, van Tulder MW. Spinal manipulative therapy for chronic low-back pain: an update of a Cochrane review. *Spine (Phila Pa 1976).* 2011;36(13):E825–E846.
21. Blunt KL, Rajwani MH, Guerriero RC. The effectiveness of chiropractic management of fibromyalgia patients: a pilot study. *J Manipulative Physiol Ther.* 1997;20(6):389–399.

PART III

ADDITIONAL CONSIDERATIONS IN THE PAIN PATIENT

6

Management of Addiction in the Pain Patient

CALEB KROLL AND GLENN TREISMAN

Case Presentation

Mr. Smith is a 51-year-old electrician with a past medical history significant for hypertension, obesity, cigarette dependency, prior marijuana use, and chronic low back pain who presents to your office with worsening low back pain over the past 6 months. You have been treating his mechanical low back pain for several years with non-steroidal anti-inflammatory drugs (NSAIDs), muscle relaxants, and referrals to physical therapy. You have also given him some short courses of opioids in the past when pain exacerbations have interfered with his ability to work. Unfortunately, his back pain now occurs every day and is not relieved by NSAIDs. A recent MRI revealed nonspecific degenerative changes but no disc herniations.

Mr. Smith is now requesting chronic opioids for his persistent pain because these are the only medications that have provided relief in the past. He does have a brother who has undergone rehabilitation for illicit drug abuse.

Is Mr. Smith a candidate for chronic opioid therapy (COT)? What risk factors does he have for addiction? How would you risk-stratify him before initiating treatment? What are the challenges of COT in this patient?

Addiction to prescribed opioids has reached epidemic proportions in the United States. The appropriate use of opioid analgesic medications for a short duration is seldom associated with addiction, but chronic opioid treatment for ongoing pain is more controversial. The recognition several decades ago that many patients with terminal medical conditions were not receiving adequate opioid doses resulted in the much more liberal use of opioids in palliative care settings. Postoperative pain was also found to be under-treated, and this resulted in a major effort in organized medical settings to monitor patients more aggressively for pain. Partly as a result of the development of universal pain rating scales, the description of pain as a "vital sign," and efforts by the Joint Commission on Hospital Accreditation, the identification of pain in medical settings has increased, and therefore clinicians have been more aggressive about pain treatment. Opioids are clearly effective for reducing pain acutely, but their efficacy is less clear in the treatment of chronic pain. Given the increased risk of addiction in chronic treatment, the best approach to patients with chronic pain is more ambiguous than it is for acute pain.

Chronic pain has been distinguished from acute pain by its duration, but it can also be distinguished mechanistically. Briefly, chronic pain is the result of an adaptation by the nervous system such that pain continues after an injury has healed. Opioids can clearly produce a temporary reduction in this type of pain, but their ongoing use is frequently marked by the reemergence of pain.

Defining addiction is equally problematic. Although a variety of criteria exist, addiction is an evolving process in which patients develop maladaptive patterns of use of drugs that worsen over time. In simplistic behavioral terms, the addicted person increases his or her use of a drug despite increasing consequences and decreasing benefits.

Finally, the goals of interventions for pain need to be better elucidated. The relief of all types of pain is not always possible. One definable goal for treatment is improved function, quality of life, and longevity. In terminal patients, we often see pain relief as the best contribution we can make toward a better quality of life. These patients must balance their desire to be alert and interactive with their discomfort. In patients with chronic pain, the goal must include aspects of life beyond just physical comfort. What do opioids allow patients to accomplish that they cannot accomplish without opioids? How do opioids improve function and quality of life, and is there a cost in terms of longevity? Although these are complex questions, they are answerable; unfortunately, they often get lost in the pursuit of providing pain relief as a primary goal.

PREVALENCE OF CHRONIC PAIN

Chronic pain is a substantial economic and public health concern. Studies indicate that more than 25 percent of the general population experience pain lasting longer than 3 months, with an annual economic burden exceeding $100 billion, over half of which is due to lost productivity in the workforce.[1] The World Health Organization estimates that 20 percent of individuals worldwide have some degree of chronic pain.[2] For many, chronic pain can become an all-consuming and debilitating disease, taxing personal, social, and financial resources. Furthermore, the presence of chronic pain is known to be associated with higher rates of psychiatric illnesses such as depression and substance abuse.[3] This combination of factors increases the risk of opioid abuse and addiction in chronic pain patients. Further complicating this risk is the dramatic increase in prescribed opioids over the past 20 years. From 1997 to 2002, prescriptions for the most common opioids for medical use greatly increased—morphine by 73 percent, hydromorphone by 96 percent, fentanyl by 226 percent, and oxycodone by 403 percent.[4] Between 1997 and 2006, opioids were the most frequently prescribed drug class in the United States, with retail sales increasing by 176 percent.[2] Thus, patients with chronic pain who are on opioids are likely to be encountered in any medical practice.

DEFINITION OF CHRONIC PAIN

Surprisingly, there is no consensus definition of chronic pain, though many experts define it as pain lasting longer than 3 months beyond the expected period of ongoing tissue damage.[5] It is also important to note that there are chronic conditions that are typically associated with acute pain, such as rheumatoid arthritis, which has a chronic time course but causes ongoing acute tissue destruction. Over time, many pain syndromes last beyond the expected time of tissue healing, thus evolving from acute pain to chronic. The distinction is important because chronic pain as defined as "pain in the absence of ongoing tissue destruction" is an independent risk factor for accelerating disability and the development of substance use disorders. Furthermore, chronic pain defined this way is less responsive to opioids.

SUBSTANCE ABUSE AND CHRONIC PAIN

It is well known that the prevalence of substance use disorders in patients with chronic pain is higher than in the general population. In one study of patients at a primary care clinic who received at least 6 months of opioid prescriptions over 1 year, 25 percent were found to exhibit behaviors consistent with opioid abuse.[6] In another review, the prevalence ranged from 3 percent to 19 percent.[7]

Patients are at the highest risk of developing substance use disorders in the first few years after the development of chronic pain symptoms.[8] This risk is greatest among patients with a history of drug abuse or comorbid psychiatric conditions such as depression or anxiety. These patients are more often started and continued on opioids for chronic pain than others, and they tend to receive higher doses.[9] In a large review examining abuse/addiction rates and aberrant drug-related behaviors (ADRB), Fishbain and colleagues estimated an abuse/addiction rate of 3.27 percent in patients with a history of alcohol or illicit drug use.[10] In those with no history of abuse, the rate was 0.19 percent.[10] The biggest challenge facing physicians caring for chronic pain patients is avoiding the iatrogenic dysfunction associated with opiate abuse abuse. The accurate assessment of addictive behaviors in chronic pain patients is further compounded by disagreements over the definitions of addiction, physical dependence, and even chronic pain.

ADDICTION, DEPENDENCE, AND PSEUDOADDICTION

Central to the issue of chronic pain and addiction risk is the confusion surrounding the terms "misuse," "abuse," "dependence," "addiction," and "pseudoaddiction." Addiction is a chronic neurobiological disorder produced by repeated behavior associated with exposure to a substance that activates the brain reward circuitry, with increasing exposure over time producing a loss of control over the use of the substance.[11] A simplified definition favored by some experts is *escalating drug-taking behavior despite increasing adverse consequences of the behavior and diminishing benefits.*

A consensus panel convened in 2001 determined that the "four C's" of addiction are critical in differentiating patients legitimately using opioids from those who are addicted.[11] These include adverse *consequences* from continued drug use, loss of *control* over use of the drug, intense *craving,* and *compulsivity.*[11] It is important to recognize that this definition does not necessitate the development of physical dependence or tolerance in order for a diagnosis of addiction to be made (see Fig. 6.1). Experimental and clinical experience demonstrates that patients on COT can be both tolerant and dependent

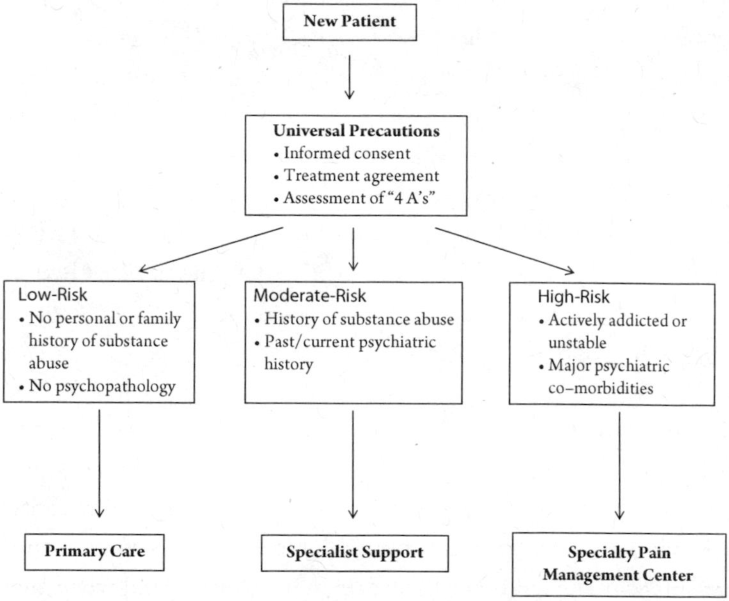

Figure 6.1. Abuse risk algorithm.

without exhibiting any of the destructive and consequence-producing behaviors characteristic of addiction. The panel defined physical dependence as a drug-class-specific withdrawal symptom that can be produced by abrupt cessation, rapid dose reduction, or decreasing blood levels of the drug.[11] Therefore, physical dependence can occur concurrently with addiction, but it is not required. In fact, many highly addictive stimulants, such as cocaine, produce relatively little physical dependence. There are also many classes of drugs not associated with addiction, such as antidepressants, beta-blockers, and corticosteroids, that produce physical withdrawal symptoms if abruptly stopped.

Tolerance is defined as a reduction in a substance's physiologic effects over time due to changes induced by repeated exposure.[11] This is commonly seen in opioid-tolerant patients who are receiving COT and require increasing doses in order to achieve the same level of pain relief. Patients who are opioid tolerant usually display a pattern of gradual increase in dosage; in contrast, addicted patients will often require a rapid increase in dose, which will be followed by a plateau, followed by a subsequent escalation.[5] Tolerance, like physical dependence, can be present in both patients suffering from addiction and those requiring COT for legitimate reasons.

Pseudoaddiction involves a pattern of addictive behaviors that can be attributed to inadequately treated pain. These behaviors include drug seeking, the use of deception to obtain opioids, "clock watching," and illicit drug use. Critical to distinguishing pseudoaddiction from true addiction is that these ADRB will resolve if the patient's pain is adequately treated.[11] In other words, if the patient is truly addicted, simply increasing the dose of opioids to treat the patient's pain will not stop the drug-seeking behavior, whereas a sufficient increase will stop the aberrant behavior(s) in the case of pseudoaddiction. There are some problems with the concept of psuedoaddiction, as some patients will only consider their pain adequately treated when they are intoxicated. Despite the problems, there are patients who improve

Table 6.1 COMPARISON OF PHYSICAL DEPENDENCE, TOLERANCE, AND ADDICTION

	Dependence	*Tolerance*	*Addiction*
Behavior characterized by "4 C's"	N	N	Y
Drug-class-specific withdrawal symptoms	Y	N	Sometimes
Reduction in drug effects over time due to repeated exposure	N	Y	Sometimes
Observed only in addictive substances	N	N	Y

their function when given opiates and who are impaired when their access to opiates in disrupted.

An understanding of the behavioral elements and clinical signs of addiction are essential for any physician treating chronic pain patients receiving COT. It is important to recognize that most patients, because of the normal physiologic effects of opioids, will experience physical dependence and tolerance. These patients are at an increased risk of becoming addicted, and so evidence of behaviors involving the "four C's" should prompt the provider to heighten monitoring or possibly consider altering the treatment course (see table 6.1).

ADDICTION AND THE BRAIN REWARD CIRCUITRY

A key feature of addictive drugs is their ability to produce reward or pleasure. Interestingly, of the approximately 30,000,000 known chemical compounds, only 100 are addictive.[12] There are few similarities among these compounds aside from their ability to activate the reward circuitry of the brain. This reward circuitry, first discovered in the 1950s, is located primarily in the medial forebrain bundle.[13] Over time it was realized that there were an assortment of brain loci and tracts forming an "in-series" circuit linking the ventral tegmental area, nucleus accumbens, and ventral pallidum via the medial forebrain bundle.[14] Addictive drugs of different classes act on this circuit at different points to produce a behavioral "reward," which can be defined as an increase in the behavior that occurred immediately before the drug was administered. Opioids act on synapses located in the ventral tegmental area.

The crucial neurotransmitter activated by addictive drugs is dopamine. Some addictive drugs are direct dopamine agonists, others are indirect agonists, and some work transsynaptically. This functional dopamine agonism is one of the few features shared among all addictive compounds.

Blum et al. proposed in the mid-1990s that many behaviors associated with addiction are driven by a deficiency in the brain reward system.[15] The thought was that some patients who develop addiction are born with or acquire a deficiency in the dopaminergic substrates of the reward circuitry and become addicted while trying to correct this deficiency.[15] Blum's hypothesis is supported by animal research that shows that atrophy of the transport system for the dopamine-synthesizing enzymes in the medial forebrain bundle is associated with drug-seeking behavior.[16] This behavioral phenotype can be reproduced by genetic modification, supporting a genetic model of vulnerability for addiction.

In humans, twin studies support the idea of a genetic influence in drug addiction, with the inherited risk ranging between 40 and 60 percent.[17] Although the exact roles of individual genes have not yet been characterized, it is thought that addiction is likely polygenic.

Whereas genetics clearly play a role in some patients with addiction, many patients with addiction have no appreciable genetic risk. Moreover, even in the best models, genetics account for only about half the risk.

The concept of multiple vulnerabilities is useful clinically, as it allows the identification of characteristics that predict vulnerability to drug addiction. Many of these factors have been successfully modeled at the animal level, and some are conceptually congruent with Blum's formulation of reward deficiency. These include psychiatric conditions that disable the reward circuitry, such as major depression and bipolar disorder. Included as well are personality traits that increase reward sensitivity or decrease impulse control, such as novelty-seeking traits, impulsivity, sociopathy, and behavior disorders. The clinician caring for chronic pain patients should screen for these conditions before initiating COT. Those patients felt to be at higher risk might warrant specialist evaluation as part of a multimodal approach to care.

PAIN AND DEPRESSION

Patients with chronic pain often suffer from co-morbid psychiatric conditions, making it difficult to treat their pain. Depression in particular is a known risk factor for the development of chronic pain. In one study, 33 to 50 percent of patients presenting to chronic pain clinics were found to have a concurrent diagnosis of major depression.[18] As mentioned previously, depression is also a known risk factor for the development of alcohol or substance abuse, with some studies placing depressed patients at a 6-fold increased risk of addiction.[10] Depression interferes with treatment management, aggravates other medical illnesses, and amplifies the symptoms of pain that patients report to their physician.

In patients suffering from chronic pain, depression is also associated with an increased rate of aberrant drug-taking behavior and opioid use.[3] A study by Braden et al. found that rates of long-term opioid use were three times higher in patients with a history of depression.[19] There have been several hypotheses concerning the trend of patients with depression misusing opioids, including inappropriate self-medication to treat a depressed mood and being overly focused on pain symptoms.[3] Regardless, it is crucial that patients in chronic pain be screened for depression and appropriately treated, as it is a known risk factor for the development of worsening or refractory pain symptoms.

SCREENING FOR ABUSE RISK

Given the increasing number of patients being treated with COT, it is essential for the practitioner to incorporate a method of screening for abuse risk. All patients are at some risk for addiction, and therefore a "universal precautions" model would recommend preventive measures for each patient including initial assessment, an opioid treatment agreement, informed consent, regular urine drug screens (UDS), periodic review of the pain diagnosis and the development of co-morbid conditions, appropriate documentation, and a feasible exit strategy.[20] Additionally, all treatment should be directed at specific functions that will ideally improve with opioid therapy. Patients should also be evaluated for the presence of opioid-related risk factors, including genetic predisposition, personal or family history of substance use disorders, history of sexual abuse, a poor social support system, and cigarette dependency.[20] A large systematic literature review aimed at predicting opioid misuse in chronic pain patients found that the strongest predictor was a personal history of alcohol or illicit drug use.[21] This approach allows the clinician to stratify the patient into one of three risk categories (low, moderate, and high) based on his or her past history of substance use disorder and past or current history of psychiatric comorbidities.[5] Low-risk patients can usually be followed in the primary care setting, those at moderate risk might require some specialist support, and high-risk patients should be referred to a specialty pain center[5] (see Fig. 6.1).

There are multiple tools available for screening patients at risk for opioid misuse before beginning COT. Three of these tools are recommended in guidelines for the treatment of chronic non-cancer pain.[20] The Screener and Opioid Assessment for Patients with Pain is a 14-item self-report questionnaire measured on a 5-point scale, with a total score of 8 or greater suggesting a high risk of abuse. The Opioid Risk Tool (ORT) is composed of five self-report items that provide a gender-specific score. A total ORT score below 3 denotes a low risk of opioid misuse, a score of 4–7 signifies moderate risk, and a score greater than 8 suggests high risk. Both of these tools examine risk factors such as a personal or family history of substance abuse, history of sexual abuse, and comorbid psychiatric disorders. The third tool, named Diagnosis, Intractability, Risk, Efficacy (DIRE), includes characteristics of the patient's pain in addition to risk factors for substance misuse. The "risk" category is further subdivided into four subcategories including psychological co-morbidities, chemical health, reliability, and social support. The DIRE is a clinician-rated scale scored out of 21 points. Patients with scores above 14 are considered to be at low risk for abuse. Although there are weaknesses associated with each of these screening tools, research has shown that they can be very effective when combined with other assessment methods such as UDS and psychological evaluations.

UDS are becomingly an increasingly popular component of the universal precautions risk assessment for patients on COT.

The purpose of UDS is to assess compliance with the prescribed treatment regimen. When used in conjunction with other monitoring measures, UDS can help to elucidate whether the patient is taking illicit or unauthorized prescriptions. An abnormal UDS, however, cannot be used to definitively diagnose addiction or predict future ADRB. In fact, some studies have shown that up to 45 percent of patients on COT will have an aberrant UDS result.[22] If an aberrant result is detected, the clinician should document it and consider either tightening the monitoring measures or altering the treatment plan. Examples of additional measures might include more frequent clinic visits, additional UDS, and limiting the amount or types of opioids prescribed. It is important to use clinical judgment in this situation, however, because either the absence or presence of additional opioids could also indicate pseudoaddiction due to a change in the patient's pain.

It is critical to have an effective monitoring policy in any clinic that prescribes COT to patients. The choice of which screening tools to use will vary from clinic to clinic depending on the patient mix and time available for assessment. At each visit the patient should be reassessed for the 4 A's: analgesia, activities of daily living, adverse effects, and ADRB.[20] Once patients are risk-stratified, appropriate monitoring and treatment can be tailored for each patient. For example, a low-risk patient with no ADRB can likely be seen in clinic less often and perhaps be given more medication per visit than a moderate- or high-risk patient. Reassessment is crucial, though, and one cannot assume that a low-risk patient will never misuse opioids or that a high-risk patient always will. Furthermore, it is not uncommon for a patient's risk categorization to change as life stressors or medical co-morbidities fluctuate in intensity. In such situations, the frequency of surveillance might need to be adjusted until the aggravating factors improve or stabilize.

CHALLENGES OF COT

The use of opioids for pain relief in patients suffering from chronic pain can dramatically improve their comfort, which might in turn enhance their quality of life. The benefits of COT, however, must be weighed against the risks of decreased function and quality of life that are produced by misuse or addiction, endocrine deficiencies, and other associated medical co-morbidities such as sleep-disordered breathing and opioid-induced hyperalgesia (OIH). Moreover, the efficacy of COT has been questioned by several studies suggesting little benefit for long-term pain relief.[5]

A large Cochrane review evaluating the efficacy of COT with a sample size of 4893 individuals showed that a considerable percentage of those patients stopped taking the opioids because of adverse effects (22.9 percent) or inadequate pain relief (10.3 percent).[23] Another systematic review evaluating the efficacy of opioids relative to non-opioid or placebo treatment in chronic low back pain patients failed to find a significant advantage of opioid treatment.[24] These studies illustrate a persistent problem with COT in that many patients are unable to tolerate the side effects or are being treated with opioids for a chronic pain condition (e.g., diabetic peripheral neuropathy) that might respond better to other medications. Although COT can be an effective treatment for chronic pain, this is likely true only in a carefully selected and closely monitored subset of patients.

In addition to the questionable efficacy of COT, there are several other potentially problematic adverse effects. A number of studies have revealed that opioids decrease testosterone, gonadotropin, estrogen, luteinizing hormone, and adrenocorticotrophin levels.[5] Symptoms can include decreased libido and muscle mass, infertility, depression, fatigue, and osteoporosis. Patients on COT should be closely monitored for symptoms of endocrine deficiency, and if such symptoms are detected, the patients should have their opioid regimen rotated or reduced. If this is unsuccessful, hormone replacement therapy can be considered.

There is some research to suggest that patients on COT are at increased risk for sleep-related breathing disorders. One study showed that 75 percent of patients on COT for at least 6 months exhibited evidence of obstructive or central sleep apneas on overnight polysomnograms.[25] Another study found that 30 percent of patients on chronic methadone therapy showed signs of central sleep apnea on polysomnograms, which is considerably higher than the rate observed in the general population.[20] Sleep apnea can interfere with restorative sleep and place the patient at increased risk for respiratory depression. Because sleep-related breathing disorders appear to be correlated with COT, early detection and interventions are needed in order to minimize the risks.

One of the most controversial and poorly understood conditions associated with COT is OIH. This phenomenon occurs when a patient on COT develops increased sensitivity to painful stimuli as a result of maladaptive neuroplasticity. Studies performed in humans have shown that this enhanced sensitivity can occur within hours of initiating opioid therapy. OIH can be difficult to differentiate from tolerance clinically because both are associated with increased pain in the face of a constant opioid dose and both are temporarily improved by an increase in opioid dose. A diagnosis of OIH is suggested by a pattern in which opioid dose increases produce relatively smaller and shorter improvements in pain. A prolonged drug holiday is the optimal means to distinguish true tolerance from OIH. Reducing the opioid dose will result in a temporary worsening of pain with both conditions, but with OIH the increased pain should ideally diminish to below baseline within 6 weeks. Other possible causes for opioid-treatment failure should also be considered, such as disease progression, withdrawal, and addiction.

Patients receiving COT for the treatment of chronic pain might display a variety of ADRB. It is important to realize that the presence of ADRB does not necessarily imply addiction and, as mentioned earlier, could be secondary to inadequate pain control (pseudoaddiction) stemming from tolerance or disease progression. A study of 904 patients receiving COT reported that patients with four or more ADRB were at greater risk for a concurrent substance use disorder.[5] ADRB more closely associated with substance misuse include frequently changing doctors, current abuse of alcohol or illicit drugs, stealing or borrowing drugs, frequently losing opioid prescriptions, or refusal to change to non-opioid therapy in spite of adverse side effects.[5] If ADRB do appear, the clinician should heighten monitoring and conduct additional assessments to determine the underlying origin of the behavior. If the evidence points to opioid addiction, the patient should be referred to a supervised detoxification program.

The risks of continuing patients on COT must be weighed against the risk of inadequately treating a patient's pain. Although the efficacy of COT in chronic pain patients has been questioned, there is likely a subset of patients who will benefit and enjoy an improved quality of life. Given the potential side effects of COT, clinicians should continually monitor these patients and be prepared to initiate opioid rotation or start adjunctive therapies as indicated. These patients should also always be monitored for ADRB, and if such behaviors are discovered, they should be further investigated. For those patients who do not attain appropriate benefit or who suffer from the aforementioned adverse effects, it would be prudent to taper opioids and seek out alternative pain therapies.

CONCLUSION

Chronic pain is a worldwide public health problem that afflicts patients in every medical setting. It is well-established that patients with chronic pain are at increased risk for substance use disorders relative to the general population. This risk is increased by co-morbid psychiatric conditions such as depression. Every clinician caring for patients with chronic pain should have a means of evaluating the addiction risk of this population in order to provide the most appropriate treatment. Once the patient is risk-stratified, an appropriate level of monitoring can be initiated. If the patient is felt to be a candidate for COT, it becomes necessary to have a thorough understanding of the potential risks involved in this treatment so they can be weighed against the therapeutic benefit. Some patients on COT will display ADRB, and the presence of these behaviors should prompt further monitoring, alternative therapies, and possibly referral to a specialist. Further research into the factors that predispose patients to addiction and into alternative therapies for chronic pain conditions is needed to help combat the growing trend of opioid misuse and addiction.

CASE RESOLUTION

Mr. Smith might be a candidate for COT if opioids would improve his quality of life and provide functional improvement, as demonstrated by his ability to continue working full time and/or exercising to help with weight loss. Mr. Smith would score a 3 on the ORT because of his family history of substance abuse. This would place him in the low-risk category, although his history of cigarette dependency would slightly heighten his risk. It would be reasonable to initiate COT in the primary care setting after having him sign an opioid contract, undergo initial UDS, and agree on the goals of therapy. As is the case for any patient on COT, he would need to be monitored for ADRB at every follow-up clinic visit.

REFERENCES

1. Pleis JR, Lucas JW, Ward BW. Summary health statistics for US adults: National Health Interview Survey, 2008. *Vital Health Stat.* 2009;10:1–157.
2. Turk D, Wilson H, Cahana A. Treatment of chronic non-cancer pain. *Lancet.* 2011;377:2226–2235.
3. Clark MR, Treisman GJ. Optimizing treatment with opioids and beyond. *Adv Psychosom Med.* 2011;30:92–112.
4. Gilson AM, Ryan KM, Joranson DE, Dahl JL. A reassessment of trends in the medical use and abuse of opioid analgesics and implications for diversion control: 1997–2002. *J Pain Symptom Manage.* 2004;28:176–188.
5. Cheatle MD, O'Brien CP. Opioid therapy in patients with chronic noncancer pain: diagnostic and clinical challenges. *Adv Psychosom Med.* 2011;30:61–91.
6. Reid MC, Engles-Horton LL, Weber MB, et al. Use of opioid medications for chronic noncancer pain syndromes in primary care. *J Gen Intern Med.* 2002;43:238–240.
7. Manchikanti L, Cash K, Damron K, et al. Controlled substance abuse and illicit drug use in chronic pain patients. An evaluation of multiple variables. *Pain Physician.* 2006;9:215–226.
8. Brown RL, Patterson JJ, Rounds LA, Papasouliotis O. Substance abuse among patients with chronic back pain. *J Fam Pract.* 1996;43:152–160.
9. Galati SA, Clark MR. Substance use disorders and detoxification. In: Benzon HR, Raja SN, Liu SS, Fishman SM, Cohen SP, eds. *Essentials of Pain Medicine.* 3rd ed. Philadelphia, PA: Elsevier Saunders; 2011:184–191.
10. Carinci AJ, Mao J. Pain and opioid addiction: what is the connection? *Curr Pain Headache Rep.* 2010;14:17–21.
11. American Pain Society. *Definitions Related to the Use of Opioids for the Treatment of Pain. A Consensus Document from the American Academy of Pain Medicine, the American Pain Society, and the American Society of Addiction Medicine.* Glenview, IL: American Academy of Pain Medicine; 2001.
12. Gardner EL. Brain reward mechanisms. In: Lowinson JH, Ruiz P, Millman RB, Langrod JG, eds. *Substance Abuse. A Comprehensive Textbook.* 4th ed. Philadelphia: Lippincott Williams & Wilkins; 2005:48–97.
13. Olds J. Pleasure centers in the brain. *Sci Am.* 1956;95:105–116.
14. Wise RA, Bozarth MA. Brain reward circuitry: four circuit elements "wired" in apparent series. *Brain Res Bull.* 1984;12:203–208.
15. Blum K, Cull JG, Braverman ER, Comings DE. Reward deficiency syndrome. *Am Sci.* 1996;84:132–145.
16. Beitner-Johnson D, Guitart X, Nestler EJ. Dopaminergic brain reward regions of Lewis and Fischer rats display different levels of tyrosine hydroxylase and other morphine- and cocaine-regulated phosphoproteins. *Brain Res.* 1991;561:147–150.

17. Uhl GR, Drgan T, Johnson C, et al. "Higher order" addiction molecular genetics: convergent data from genome-wide association in humans and mice. *Biochem Pharmacol.* 2008;75:98–111.
18. Clark MR, Treisman GJ. Perspectives on pain and depression. *Adv Psychosom Med.* 2004;25:1–27.
19. Braden JB, Sullivan MD, Ray GT, et al. Trends in long-term opioid therapy for noncancer pain among persons with a history of depression. *Gen Hosp Psychiatry.* 2009;31:564–570.
20. Webster LR, Dove B. Risk stratification and management of opioids. In: Benzon HR, Raja SN, Liu SS, Fishman SM, Cohen SP, eds. *Essentials of Pain Medicine.* 3rd ed. Philadelphia, PA: Elsevier Saunders; 2011:101–106.
21. Turk DC, Swanson KS, Gatchel RJ. Predicting opioid misuse by chronic pain patients: a systematic review and literature synthesis. *Clin J Pain.* 2008;24:497–508.
22. Michna E, Jamison RN, Pham LD, et al. Urine toxicology screening among chronic pain patients on opioid therapy: frequency and predictability of abnormal findings. *Clin J Pain.* 2007;23:173–179.
23. Noble M, Treadwell JR, Tregear SJ, et al. Long-term opioid management for chronic noncancer pain. *Cochrane Database Syst Rev.* 2010;1:CD006605.
24. Martell BA, O'Connor PG, Kerns RD, et al. Systematic review—opioid treatment for chronic back pain: prevalence, efficacy, and association with addiction. *Ann Intern Med.* 2007;146:116–127.
25. Webster LR, Choi Y, Desai H, et al. Sleep-disordered breathing and chronic opioid therapy. *Pain Med.* 2008;9:425–432.

7

A Circular Conundrum: Sleep Disruption Worsens Pain and Pain Medications Disrupt Sleep

MICHAEL STERNBERG, HELEN A. BAGHDOYAN, AND RALPH LYDIC

The relevance of disordered sleep to health is clear from the foundation in 1993 of the National Center on Sleep Disorders Research within the National Heart, Lung, and Blood Institute. The 2011 statistics from the National Institutes of Health (NIH) indicate that 25 to 30 percent of the general population has sleep disorders that are "proven contributors to disability, morbidity, and mortality." The ability of disordered sleep to enhance pain is noted repeatedly in the 2011 NIH Sleep Disorders Research Plan (http://www.nhlbi.nih.gov/health/prof/sleep/sleep_splan.htm). A major, unwanted side effect of pain medications is sleep disruption.[1,2] Thus, care providers and pain patients must contend with an unfavorable, circular problem: sleep disruption promotes pain, and pain medications disrupt sleep. Related issues include the underappreciated concepts of devaluing sleep and failing to distinguish sleep traits from sleep states. Drug-induced obtundation of wakefulness is commonly misperceived as sleep. A frequently occurring example is misdiagnosing as a state of sleep what is actually a dissociated state of consciousness caused by drugs that produce anti-nociception. The drug-induced state may include some sleep-like traits such as immobility with eyes closed, as well as slow and regular breathing. A polysomnographic recording of this same patient, however, would make clear that the presence of such traits should not be confused with the state of sleep. The goal of this chapter is to highlight evidence that pain disrupts the experience of normal, restorative sleep and that all currently available drugs prescribed for managing pain also disrupt sleep. Editorial mandates limit citations, and interested readers are referred elsewhere for systematic reviews.[3–6]

STATES OF PAIN AND SLEEP SHARE OVERLAPPING CONTROL SYSTEMS

The reciprocal relationship between sleep and pain arises from the overlap between brain regions and neurotransmitter systems that regulate sleep and nociception. The expression of sleep and wakefulness has a circadian (about 24 h) rhythm. Embedded in the circadian rhythm of sleep is the ultradian (about 90 min) oscillation between the rapid eye movement (REM) and the non-rapid eye movement (NREM) phases of sleep. At a gross behavioral level, REM and NREM sleep might be misperceived as similar states. Electrographic recordings, however, demonstrate that these two sleep states have more differences than similarities. NREM sleep is characterized by the persistence of somatic muscle tone; slow-wave cortical electroencephalogram (EEG) activity; slow, rolling eye movements; and regular breathing and heart rate. REM sleep is distinguished by autonomic dysregulation including, but not limited to, skeletal muscle atonia, rapid eye movements, poor temperature regulation, fast and irregular breathing, and heart rate and blood pressure surges that can reach levels associated with maximal exertion during exercise. Cerebral blood flow and metabolism during REM sleep are as active as observed during wakefulness, and this cortical activation is accompanied by the experience of dreaming.[3]

Maintaining a normal temporal organization of the NREM and REM phases of the sleep cycle is critical to the experience of restorative sleep. Sleep onset begins with the initiation of NREM sleep, which comprises several distinct stages. As sleep stages progress, one's arousal threshold increases (see Roehrs cited in Ref. 7). The greatest percentage of time asleep is spent in NREM stage 2. Periods of REM sleep occur approximately every 90 min, and epochs of REM sleep increase in duration and frequency over the course of the night. The ratio of REM sleep to NREM sleep decreases with age, amplifying the potential for sleep-disrupting effects of pain medications in the elderly. Figure 7.1 illustrates the dynamic changes in the human brain that occur during the normal oscillation among states of wakefulness, NREM sleep, and REM sleep.

Sleep fragmentation, like sleep deprivation, decreases daytime neurocognitive function and impairs affect. Deficits in reaction time, productivity, mood, and learning are all observed following a night without satisfactory sleep. There is a dose-dependent relationship between the degree of impairment and the number of nights of poor sleep. Directly relevant to this chapter, inadequate sleep also depresses immune responses and increases sensitivity to painful stimuli.[1,7] The negative health consequences of sleep loss and sleep fragmentation include increased risk of death.[8] The negative effects of sleep disruption are so widespread in part because sleep is actively generated by a diffuse neural network that contributes to multiple, overlapping control systems. Similarly, painful stimuli are processed in multiple brain regions and neural networks. The details of these overlapping neuronal networks are beyond the scope of this chapter and can be visualized by comparing established pain networks[9] with multiple neural systems[5] and neurotransmitters[4] contributing to the regulation of sleep and wakefulness.

The subjective experience of pain is influenced by emotional and cognitive factors, as well as the specific context in which one thinks about the pain. These numerous influences enable painful stimuli to access a broad array of neural networks, also illustrated by Fig. 7.2 from Tracey.[9] Comparison of the sleep-dependent changes in brain activity (Fig. 7.1) with brain regions activated by pain (Fig. 7.2) helps one to visualize the key points of this chapter. First, just as no single brain region regulates pain, there is no "sleep center" or "anesthesia center." A second key feature illustrated by a comparison of Figs. 7.1 and 7.2 is the significant overlap between brain regions that changes during states of pain and states of sleep. This overlap illustrates many of the brain substrates mediating the bidirectional interaction between pain and sleep. Finally, Figs. 7.1 and 7.2 emphasize that when medications are administered systemically, they are distributed to all areas of the brain, and thus act on receptors throughout the nervous system. In contrast, regional anesthesia for the management of chronic pain offers the advantage of site-directed pain relief that does not alter multiple brain regions. An exciting, ongoing research effort is specifying the brain regions and neurochemical mechanisms by which pain medications alter pain and states of sleep.[2,10]

Chronic pain, defined as pain that persists or recurs for more than 3 months, further complicates attempts to identify a concrete "pain matrix." Over time, chronic pain can modulate the brain's detection of salient events by prioritizing the experience of pain and activating brain regions that are not part of the pain matrix of a healthy adult.[11] Imaging techniques illustrate the broad, unique cerebral signature induced by chronic pain states. The activation of multiple brain regions by chronic pain recruits the hypothalamic–pituitary–adrenal axis and activates the brain's stress response system. The stress response can also disrupt sleep by elevating levels of corticotrophin-releasing hormone and hyperactivating the locus coeruleus–norepinephrine systems (see Roehrs cited in Ref. 7).

Approximately 116 million Americans are affected by chronic pain, and two-thirds of these patients report unsatisfactory sleep.[1,12] Chronic pain patients taking analgesic drugs might be the most vulnerable to the adverse consequences of drug-induced sleep disruption because of the long-term nature of the pain. Their need for pain medication propagates the aforementioned cyclical pain–sleep relationship by simultaneously increasing pain sensitivity and the effective dose of medication. The higher prevalence of chronic pain in the elderly, who already experience more disrupted sleep relative to their younger counterparts, adds additional complexity to this problem.[3]

PAIN MEDICATIONS DISRUPT SLEEP

All drugs prescribed to treat pain that also have been studied using electrographic recordings have been shown to disrupt sleep. The following subsections highlight the effects on sleep, where studied, of the four classes of drugs commonly used on and off label to treat pain. These drug groups include opioids, tricyclic antidepressants (TCAs), membrane stabilizers, and serotonin-norepinephrine reuptake inhibitors (SNRIs).

Opioids: Morphine and Fentanyl

Morphine and fentanyl promote analgesia through activation of μ-opioid receptors in the central nervous system. Opioids obtund wakefulness and suppress REM sleep, in part via effects on the transmission of choline and γ-aminobutyric acid (GABA) in multiple brain regions.[2,5] Cholinergic mechanisms in the pontine reticular formation contribute to the initiation of REM sleep, and endogenous acetylcholine levels are highest in the pontine reticular formation during REM sleep. Morphine and fentanyl inhibit REM sleep, in part by decreasing cholinergic tone in the pontine reticular formation.[1] GABAergic transmission in the pontine reticular formation promotes wakefulness,[2] and morphine decreases GABAergic transmission in the pontine reticular formation.[4] Thus, altering GABAergic transmission in the pontine reticular formation might be another mechanism by which morphine disrupts sleep and wakefulness.

Acetylcholine release in the prefrontal cortex is greatest during wakefulness and REM sleep. Cholinergic input to prefrontal cortex arises from neurons in the basal forebrain.[5] Systemic morphine administration or microdialysis delivery of morphine to the basal forebrain reduces wakefulness and disrupts REM sleep by decreasing acetylcholine release in the prefrontal cortex. Morphine activates μ-opioid receptors in the basal forebrain, causing a decrease in acetylcholine release in the prefrontal cortex and a decrease in arousal (see Osman cited in Ref. 10).

Buprenorphine is a partial μ-opioid agonist and a κ-opioid antagonist that provides effective pain management. When buprenorphine was administered intravenously or via microdialysis to the pontine reticular formation or to the basal forebrain of rat, the temporal organization of sleep was disrupted.[10] Buprenorphine caused increased time awake, decreased REM sleep, and delayed onset of NREM and REM sleep. Interestingly, coadministration of the sedative-hypnotic eszopiclone countered the buprenorphine-induced inhibition of sleep.[10] This suggests the potential for increasing the efficacy of opioids in treating pain by means of pretreatment with sedative-hypnotic drugs that enhance sleep.

Buprenorphine also decreases adenosine levels in basal forebrain regions known to modulate sleep and nociception. Endogenous adenosine promotes sleep and decreases nociception. Thus, the buprenorphine-induced decrease in basal forebrain adenosine suggests one possible mechanism by which buprenorphine disrupts sleep architecture.[10]

TCAs: Amitriptyline, Nortriptyline, Desipramine, and Imipramine

TCAs have been utilized for several decades to treat chronic pain. TCAs have widespread effects on the central nervous system due to binding to multiple neurotransmitter receptors including serotonin, norepinephrine, histamine, and acetylcholine. TCAs also bind to voltage gated sodium channels. All TCAs antagonize serotonin and norepinephrine reuptake transporters, thereby increasing serotonergic and noradrenergic tone in the central nervous system. The extent to which a TCA antagonizes various reuptake transporters depends on the specific binding affinity of the drug. Clearly, the overall effect on sleep and nociception of TCAs is the result of a complex interaction of their specific binding affinities and dose, the length of use, and the type of patient taking the medication. All TCAs share a cyclic structure but differ from one another in side-chain structure and amine classification (secondary, tertiary, etc.). Side-chain variation contributes to receptor binding selectivity and differential effects on sedation and REM sleep suppression observed among TCAs.[13]

Tertiary TCAs, such as amitriptyline and imipramine, are often subjectively classified as the most sedating of the TCAs because they produce the most consistent disruptions of sleep architecture. The sedating effects of amitriptyline and imipramine might be due to their stronger serotonergic effects relative to secondary amine tricyclics.[3]

Amitriptyline suppresses REM sleep and latency to sleep onset, but it increases total sleep time and periodic limb movements during the sleep phase. Difficulty waking and drowsiness contribute to the hangover effect often described after a patient is prescribed amitriptyline. Imipramine also decreases REM sleep, but it shows differential effects on sleep latency and total sleep time.[3,13]

Secondary TCAs, such as nortriptyline and desipramine, are less sedating than tertiary TCAs and show less sleep disruption, likely due in part to their stronger adrenergic activity and weaker serotonergic activity.[3] Rarely tested outside of depressed patient populations, these medications decrease REM sleep and total sleep time while increasing waking after sleep onset and periodic limb movements.[13]

The sedating effects of TCAs are limited to subjective patient reports of improved sleep continuity and quality. A comprehensive search of the available literature suggests that the only patients reported to show objective improvements in sleep while taking TCAs are depressed patients or patients with other co-morbid conditions. Depressed patients, especially those concurrently suffering from a chronic pain condition, are more likely to be prescribed TCAs. Given that TCAs disrupt sleep architecture, patient reports of improved sleep quality are thought to arise from the TCA-induced lessening of depression. A PubMed search for studies conducted in the past 10 years documenting beneficial effects of the aforementioned TCAs on the sleep of healthy individuals produced no results.

Membrane Stabilizers: Gabapentin, Pregabalin, and Carbamazepine

Membrane stabilizers, also known as anti-epileptics, are a useful tool for managing chronic pain conditions such as fibromyalgia and neuropathic pain due to diabetic neuropathy or postherpetic neuralgia. Gabapentin, originally created as an anticonvulsant analogue of GABA, began to be recognized as an effective analgesic agent for treating neuropathic pain in the mid-1990s.[14] Pregabalin is another GABA analogue that has a structure similar to that of gabapentin. Pregabalin was synthesized as a more potent successor to gabapentin. These medications desensitize neurons following tissue damage but have insignificant effects on pain transmission in the absence of tissue damage.[14]

Carbamazepine is one of the classic, older anti-epileptic drugs still available today. It has been used less frequently since the advent of gabapentin and pregabalin because it causes greater cognitive impairment.[3] Carbamazepine binds to voltage gated sodium channels, stabilizing the inactivated, open conformation and blocking the passage of sodium ions.[15] Carbamazepine, like all anti-epileptic drugs and TCAs, makes it more difficult for a neuron to fire an action potential. There is evidence that carbamazepine and tertiary TCAs such as imipramine actually share a binding site in the sodium channel.[15]

Gabapentin, pregabalin, and carbamazepine all produce significant increases in total sleep time and the percentage of slow wave sleep in healthy adult volunteers.[16–18] However, their effects on REM sleep vary. Some studies indicate that gabapentin increases REM sleep; other studies indicate that gabapentin slightly reduces REM sleep and produces sleep fragmentation.[16]

Pregabalin is a newer medication, and a PubMed search for studies of its effects on the sleep of healthy individuals located only one paper.[18] This double-blind study involved polysomnographic analysis of sleep in healthy volunteers prescribed pregabalin. In addition to an increase in total sleep time and the percentage of NREM sleep characteristic of all anti-epileptics, pregabalin also significantly reduced latency to sleep onset and improved sleep efficiency by decreasing the number of awakenings after sleep onset relative to placebo. Pregabalin treatment produced no statistically significant changes in the REM sleep composition of these healthy volunteers.[18]

Carbamazepine has been used for several decades, and recent studies of its effect on the sleep of healthy volunteers also are rare. Individuals treated with a 10-day course of carbamazepine showed a 209 percent increase in slow wave sleep relative to baseline measurements.[17] There were no statistically significant findings concerning changes in REM sleep, but this study did note a tendency toward shortened REM periods.[17]

SNRIs

Duloxetine and venlafaxine are two prominent, yet relatively new, SNRIs that are indicated for the treatment of chronic pain conditions. These drugs bind to monoamine reuptake transporters, inhibiting the removal of serotonin and norepinephrine from the synapse. Increased serotonergic and noradrenergic tone is associated with antidepressant and anti-nociceptive effects. Although patients who are prescribed SNRIs report equal rates of insomnia and somnolence, increased monoaminergic tone is known to disrupt sleep architecture. The majority of studies investigating the sleep-disrupting effects of SNRIs have involved patients with coexisting disorders such as depression, anxiety, or fibromyalgia. A PubMed search for studies testing the effects of venlafaxine or duloxetine on the sleep of healthy individuals located only one study for each of these drugs. The lack of information concerning the effects of SNRIs on healthy individuals highlights an important area of future research if these medications are to be used to treat chronic pain conditions in otherwise healthy patients.

A 4-day regimen of venlafaxine administered to healthy volunteers caused an increase in time spent awake and decreased NREM sleep. Venlafaxine also caused an immediate and severe suppression of REM sleep, and REM sleep was completely abolished on the fourth night.[19] Venlafaxine significantly increased periodic limb movements during sleep.

Duloxetine, the most recent SNRI available, causes sleep disruptions that are similar in many ways to the disruptions caused by other SNRIs and antidepressants. Duloxetine has been reported to cause an increase in the onset to REM latency, a decrease in the percentage of REM sleep, and an increase in NREM stage 2 sleep time.[20] This study also reported dose-dependent REM sleep suppression. SNRIs increase monoaminergic activity and have REM-suppressing activity, but it is clear that these effects vary by medication, dose, and time at which the drugs are administered. The variable data and lack of studies in this area present exciting opportunities for future clinical studies. Given the data available, SNRIs with once daily dosing may cause less sleep disturbance when administered in the morning.

There are also data suggesting that SNRIs such as duloxetine might decrease postoperative opioid requirements. The combination of duloxetine and morphine produced no adverse drug-related effects and reduced the morphine requirement necessary to regulate tolerable pain levels.[21] These findings are promising because previous studies testing combinations of gabapentin and pregabalin to reduce postoperative opioid requirements reported increased sedation and dizziness.[21] Reducing a patient's opioid requirement by coadministering SNRIs might be particularly useful for treating pain in elderly patients in whom opioids commonly cause delirium. These data suggest novel research opportunities to determine whether similar polypharmacy focused on reducing opioid requirements could attenuate the sleep-disrupting effects of higher doses of opioids. Future research on the concomitant administration of SNRIs and opioids is needed in order to determine safety and efficacy for chronic pain patients.

SLEEP: A UNIQUE OPPORTUNITY FOR PAIN MEDICINE

Sleep is a cross-cutting biological process that significantly impacts neurocognitive function, autonomic physiology, immune response, metabolism, and pain.[3] Achieving adequate and restorative sleep is a health requirement for each of the 7 billion humans on Earth, making sleep research the ultimate in translational science. Sleep is disrupted by pain and by the pharmacological management of pain. An as-yet unexploited opportunity for pain medicine is to facilitate research that successfully links sleep neurobiology and clinical care. Asking patients how they slept has apparent, but poor, validity. Questionnaire data regarding sleep are not validated by objective, electrographic measures of sleep in normal individuals[22] or insomnia patients (see Carskadon et al., 1976, cited in Ref. 22). This is of particular relevance to the present chapter because many current misconceptions about the effects of pain medications on sleep are inferred from patient questionnaire data. The scarcity of objective data provides an opportunity to confirm or refute these subjective evaluations with electrographic studies quantifying the effects of pain medications on sleep. For the clinician, it would be useful to have a table rating the objective effects of pain medications on the sleep of pain patients without co-morbid disease. Such tables exist evaluating sleep medications for the treatment of sleep disorders,[3] but no electrographic data are presently available for use in evaluating the relative efficacy of different sleeping medications in pain patients. The design of such studies will need to incorporate the complexities of pharmacogenetics, types of pain, and patient variables such as age, sex, and race. Studies designed to collect such data represent an exciting research opportunity. There is also an opportunity to extend to the study of sleep the pioneering investigations clarifying the action of opioids on respiratory control in children (see Brown cited in Ref. 6). A comparison of the 1990 and 2005 editions of *Brain Control of Wakefulness and Sleep*[5] makes clear the enormous progress that has been achieved in understanding the neurobiology of sleep. The recency of this progress is illustrated by fact that in 2012, the eighth edition of *Basic Neurochemistry* included the first chapter devoted to sleep.[2] The measurement of neurotransmitters and putative biomarkers in pain studies will be translational only if linked to objective measures of sleep.[23] Finally, evidence that healthcare providers receive inadequate training about sleep[24,25] illustrates another area in which pain medicine can take a leadership role. The Institute of Medicine advocates that promoting sleep education will benefit patients and care givers alike (see Colten and Altevogt, 2006, cited in Ref. 2).

CONCLUSIONS

Pain and all available pharmacologic therapies for pain can adversely affect sleep. Despite subjective patient reports of improved sleep with some medications, the limited available objective testing (EEG) demonstrates abnormal sleep architecture. Of the medications commonly used for pain, gabapentinoids have the least adverse effects on sleep. TCAs have sedating properties thus should be dosed in the nighttime, and secondary TCAs (nortriptyline) do not disturb sleep as much as the older TCAs. The increased monoaminergic tone from SNRIs disrupts sleep architecture and may provide a rationale for morning dosing of this class of medications. The sleep-disrupting effects of opioids have been well-documented and are unambiguous.

Additional studies can determine whether sedative hypnotics attenuate opioid-induced sleep disturbance. Proper sleep is a key component to health, and future research is needed on the complex interrelationships between sleep, pain, and response to medications for pain.

ACKNOWLEDGMENTS

This work was supported by National Institutes of Health Grant Nos. HL40881 (RL), HL65272 (RL), and MH45361 (HAB) and by the Department of Anesthesiology. This work was not an industry-supported study, and the authors have no financial conflicts of interest.

REFERENCES

1. Lydic R, Baghdoyan HA. Neurochemical mechanisms mediating opioid-induced REM sleep disruption. In: Lavigne G, Sessle BJ, Choinière M, Soja PJ, eds. *Sleep and Pain.* Seattle, WA: International Association for the Study of Pain (IASP) Press; 2007:99–122.
2. Baghdoyan HA, Lydic R. The neurochemistry of sleep and wakefulness. In: Brady ST, Albers RW, Price DL, Siegel GJ, eds. *Basic Neurochemistry*. New York: Elsevier; 2012:982–999.
3. Kryger MH, Roth T, Dement WC, eds. *Principles and Practice of Sleep Medicine.* 5th ed. New York: Elsevier; 2011.
4. Watson CJ, Baghdoyan HA, Lydic R. Neuropharmacology of sleep and wakefulness. *Sleep Med Clinics*. 2010;5:513–528.
5. Steriade M, McCarley RW. *Brain Control of Wakefulness and Sleep*. 2nd ed. New York: Plenum Press; 2005.
6. Lydic R, Baghdoyan HA. Sleep, anesthesiology, and the neurobiology of arousal state control. *Anesthesiology*. 2005;103:1268–1295.
7. Chhangani BS, Roehrs TA, Harris EJ, et al. Pain sensitivity in sleepy pain-free normals. *Sleep*. 2009;32:1011–1017.
8. Cappuccio FP, D'Ellia L, Strazzullo P, Miller MA. Sleep duration and all-cause mortality: a systematic review and meta-analysis of prospective studies. *Sleep*. 2010;33:585–592.

9. Tracey I. Imaging pain. *Br J Anaesth.* 2008;101:32–39.
10. Gauthier EA, Guzick SE, Brummett CM, Baghdoyan HA, Lydic R. Buprenorphine disrupts sleep and decreases adenosine concentrations in sleep-regulating brain regions of Sprague Dawley rat. *Anesthesiology.* 2011;115:743–753.
11. Legrain V. The pain matrix reloaded. A salience detection system for the body. *Prog Neurobiol.* 2011;93:111–124.
12. Institute of Medicine. *Relieving Pain in America: A Blueprint for Transforming Prevention, Care, Education, and Research.* Washington, DC: The National Academies Press; 2011.
13. Mayers A, Baldwin D. Antidepressants and their effect on sleep. *Hum Psychopharmacol.* 2005;20:533–559.
14. Gilron I. Gabapentin and pregabalin for chronic neuropathic and early post-surgical pain: current evidence and future directions. *Curr Opin Anaesthesiol.* 2007;20:456–472.
15. Yang Y-C, Huang C-S, Kuo C-C. Lidocaine, carbamazepine, and imipramine have partially overlapping binding sites and additive inhibitory effect on neuronal Na+ channels. *Anesthesiology.* 2010;113:160–174.
16. Foldvary-Schaefer N, Sancez De leon I, Karafa M, Mascha E, Dinner D, Morris HH. Gabapentin increases slow-wave sleep in normal adults. *Epilepsia.* 2002;43:1493–1497.
17. Yang JD, Elphick M, Sharpley AL, Cowen PJ. Effects of carbamazepine on sleep in healthy volunteers. *Biol Psychiatry.* 1989;26:324–328.
18. Hindmarch I, Dawson J, Stanley N. A double-blind study in healthy volunteers to assess the effects on sleep of pregabalin compared with alprazolam and placebo. *Sleep.* 2005;28:187–193.
19. Salin-Pascual RJ, Galicia-Polo L, Drucker-Colin R. Sleep changes after four consecutive days of venlafaxine administration in normal volunteers. *J Clin Psychiatry.* 1997;58:348–350.
20. Chalon S, Pereira A, Lainey E, et al. Comparative effects of duloxetine and desipramine on sleep EEG in healthy subjects. *Psychopharmacology.* 2005;177:357–365.
21. Ho K-Y, Tay W, Yeo M-C, et al. Duloxetine reduces morphine requirements after knee surgery. *Br J Anaesth.* 2010;105:371–376.
22. Baker FC, Maloney S, Driver HS. A comparison of subjective estimates of sleep with objective polysomnographic data in healthy men and women. *J Psychosom Res.* 1999;47:335–341.
23. Phillipson EA. If it's not integrative, it may not be translational. *Clin Invest Med.* 2002;25:94–96.

24. Strohl KP, Veasey S, Harding S, et al. Competency-based goals for sleep and chronobiology in undergraduate medical education. *Sleep*. 2003;26:333–336.
25. Gamaldo CE, Salas RE. Sleep medicine education: are medical schools and residency programs napping on the job? *Nat Clin Pract Neurol*. 2008;4:344–346.
26. Braun AR, Balkin TJ, Wesenten NJ, et al. Regional cerebral blood flow throughout the sleep-wake cycle: an $H_2{}^{15}O$ PET study. *Brain*. 1997;120:1173–1197.

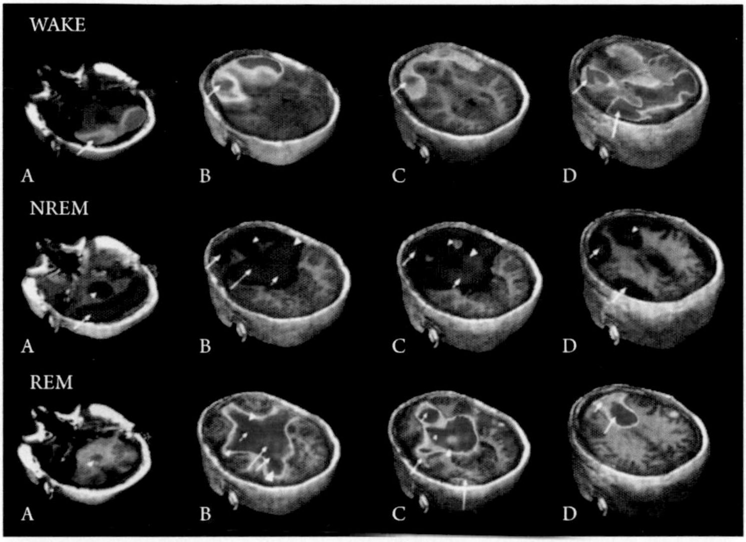

Figure 7.1. Regional human brain activity varies as a function of sleep and wakefulness. These PET images were among the first to illustrate brain-region-dependent changes (arrows) in regional cerebral blood flow (rCBF) during states of wakefulness (WAKE), non-rapid eye movement sleep (NREM), and rapid eye movement sleep (REM). In WAKE states there are increases (red color) in rCBF. During the NREM phase of sleep there are significant decreases (purple color) in rCBF. REM sleep is an activated brain state and is characterized by increases (red color) in rCBF. For each of the three states, the horizontal plane illustrated progresses from ventral (A) to dorsal (D). The original images from Braun et al. (Braun AR, Balkin TJ, Wesenten NJ, et al. Regional cerebral blood flow throughout the sleep-wake cycle: an $H_2{}^{15}O$ PET study. *Brain*. 1997;120:1173–1197) were reorganized and relabeled to facilitate comparison with Fig. 7.2.

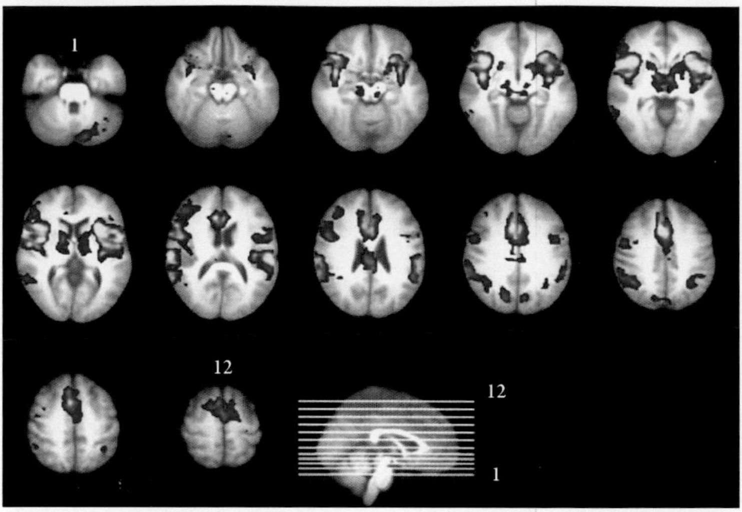

Figure 7.2. Neural networks activated by pain (red and yellow) when visualized by means of blood-oxygen-level-dependent functional magnetic resonance imaging signals. The horizontal brain scans have been organized from most ventral (1, at top left) to most dorsal (12, in the third row of scans). The image at the bottom right illustrates the horizontal level of each brain scan. These images are from Tracey, who describes this constellation of brain activation as a cerebral signature of pain. From Tracey I. Imaging pain. *Br J Anaesth*. 2008;101:32–39.

PART IV

CASE-BASED PAIN CHAPTERS

8

Low Back Pain

STEVEN P. COHEN, ARTEMUS FLAGG, AND JULIE H. Y. HUANG

CASE PRESENTATION

A 43-year-old male presents with a 7-month history of low back pain (LBP) extending into his posterolateral thigh. His pain began after he was rear-ended in a motor vehicle accident. Neurological exam is non-focal except for abnormal gait biomechanics. After failed trials with epidural steroids and duloxetine, the patient obtained short-term relief with a sacroiliac (SI) joint injection. Subsequent SI joint radiofrequency denervation, in combination with physical therapy and rehabilitation, provided him with excellent long-term relief.

EPIDEMIOLOGY

LBP is commonly encountered in the primary care setting, and it is the fifth most common reason for all physician visits in the United States.[1] Americans spend an estimated minimum of $50 billion per year on back pain. Back pain is the most frequent cause of disability in people younger than 45 years old, with 2 percent of the work force submitting worker's compensation claims each year. Approximately one-half of all working Americans admit to having had back pain symptoms in the past year, and 8 percent had at least one episode of severe LBP. Yet these costs are not spread out equally: approximately 5 percent of people with back pain account for 75 percent of the costs.[2]

Males and females are at roughly equal risk for LBP, though younger individuals tend to be disproportionately male, and women are at higher risk after the age of 60. Genetics appears to play a role in LBP. Patients with first-degree relatives who have a history of discogenic LBP are more likely to develop back pain themselves than relatives of "control" patients, and they are more likely to require spine surgery.[3] A genetic predisposition might play a role in facet arthropathy, in addition to discogenic LBP.

COURSE OF LBP

Many patients do not seek medical care for back pain. Among those who do seek care (and undoubtedly many who do not), symptoms and the ability to work typically improve rapidly in the first month. However, up to one-third of patients report persistent back pain of at least moderate intensity 1 year after an acute episode, and one in five continue to experience substantial limitations in activity.[4]

PREDICTORS OF ACUTE EPISODES AND CHRONICITY

Factors influencing persistence can be divided into genetics, anatomical-biomechanical, occupational, lifestyle, and psychosocial. In general, LBP risk factors are better at predicting the persistence of LBP than acute episodes. Studies have shown that first-degree relatives of individuals with LBP are at greater risk of developing the condition, with the risk being six times higher in identical twins.[5] Biomechanical disorders, such as altered gait mechanics, true and apparent leg length discrepancies, and structural or functional scoliosis, can all predispose a person to acute or persistent LBP. Occupations that require heavy physical activity, expose the patient to whole-body vibration, or entail static work posture are associated with back pain. Satisfaction with work and secondary gain issues (e.g., litigation or compensation claims) also seem to affect recovery from back pain episodes. Lifestyle risk factors for back pain disability include emotional distress, sleep disturbances, excessive or low baseline activity levels, and educational level. Psychosocial factors are perhaps the most studied and important risk factors associated with persistent LBP and include depression, anxiety, poor coping skills, somatization, and catastrophization.

CATEGORIZATION

Acute vs. Chronic

LBP is commonly categorized into acute, sub-acute, and chronic symptoms. Acute back pain is usually defined by a period of complaint of 6 weeks or shorter, sub-acute as a period between 6 and 12 weeks, and chronic LBP as longer than 12 weeks. Longer durations of LBP and other pain conditions have been shown to be associated with poorer treatment outcomes (see Table 8.1).[6]

Mechanical vs. Neuropathic

Distinctions among the different etiologies are perhaps the most important ones to make when categorizing back pain, as they inform

Table 8.1 RISK FACTORS FOR THE DEVELOPMENT AND PERSISTENCE OF LOW BACK PAIN

Physical	*Psychological/ Emotional*	*Behavioral*	*Social*
Previous LBP episode	Depression	Fear-avoidance behavior	Low levels of education
Physically demanding job	High levels of job stress	Low levels of physical activity (i.e., sedentary lifestyle)	Poor job satisfaction
Obesity	Somatization	Poor coping skills	Smoking
Greater baseline disease burden	High anxiety levels	Negative attitude	Not having the ability to return to work in limited capacity
Sleep disturbance	Catastrophization		

Note: Relationship between these factors and LBP is generally greater for the persistence of pain than the development of an acute episode.

treatment at every level. LBP can be classified as mechanical, neuropathic, or secondary to another cause. Mechanical LBP refers to pain caused by an abnormal stress placed on the vertebral column or

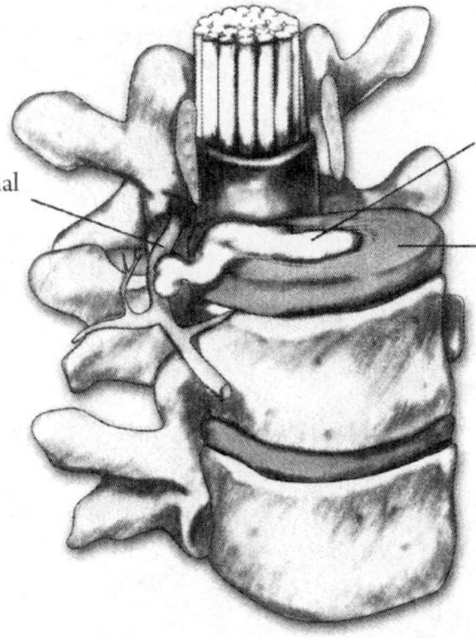

Figure 8.1. Herniated nucleus pulposus causing nerve root impingement. Radicular symptoms may result from either chemical mediators released from degenerated discs or mechanical irritation. From Cohen SP, Argoff CE, Carragee EJ. Management of low back pain. *BMJ*. 2008;337:a2718.

supporting structures. Common causes of mechanical pain can include the facet or SI joints, muscles, ligaments, and discs. Osteoporosis frequently results in back pain from vertebral fractures, though there is some evidence that osteoporosis in and of itself may cause pain. The International Association for the Study of Pain defines neuropathic pain as "pain initiated or caused by a primary lesion or dysfunction of the nervous system."[7] The most common cause of neuropathic back pain (i.e., radiculopathy) in younger people is a herniated disc, with the peak prevalence occurring in patients between 35 and 55 years of age. In people over 60, the principal cause of radicular symptoms is spinal stenosis (see Figs. 8.1 and 8.2).

Many patients present with a combination of mechanical and neuropathic pain. Degenerative discs can cause pain because of endplate fractures, annular fissures, and an increased load burden borne by the annulus fibrosus. These tears in the annulus can also

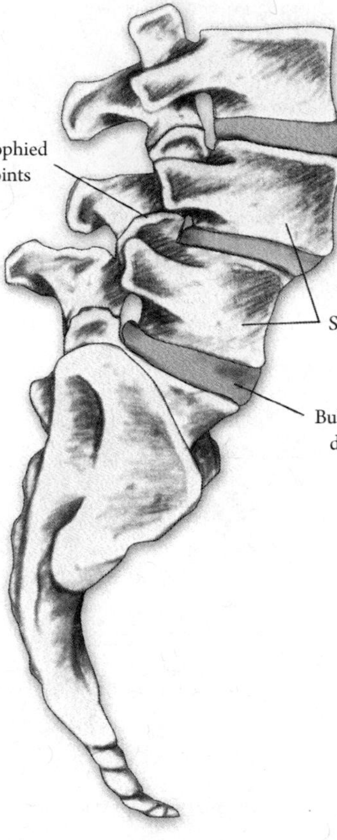

Figure 8.2. Sagittal view of a lumbar spine demonstrating central and foraminal spinal stenosis at L4–5 and L5–1. From Cohen SP, Argoff CE,Carragee EJ. Management of low back pain. *BMJ*. 2008;337:a2718.

result in the leakage of inflammatory cytokines that irritate adjacent nerve roots and decrease the amount of stress required in order to "herniate" the nucleus pulposus. Both of these scenarios can result in radicular symptoms. Hypertrophied facet joints frequently result in foraminal stenosis, which can also cause radiculopathy. Another frequent cause of "mixed" mechanical and neuropathic LBP is failed back surgery syndrome. Recent studies examining the breakdown

Table 8.2 DISTINGUISHING FEATURES OF NEUROPATHIC AND NOCICEPTIVE LOW BACK PAIN

Clinical Characteristic	*Neuropathic Spinal Pain*	*Nociceptive Spinal Pain*
Etiology	Mechanical compression of nerve root or, less commonly, chemical irritation or nerve root ischemia	Tissue damage (e.g., muscle tear or spasm, degenerative spondylosis)
Inciting event	Common in younger patients with herniated disc	Very common with acute myofascial pain, fairly common (40 percent to 50 percent) with SI joint pain, uncommon with discogenic or facetogenic pain
Descriptors	Lancinating, shooting, electrical-like, stabbing	Throbbing, aching, pressure-like
Sensory deficits	Frequent (e.g., numbness, tingling)	Infrequent and, if present, in non-dermatomal distribution
Motor deficits/ reflexes	Neurological weakness might be present if motor fibers affected Diminution in reflexes might be present	Might have pain-induced weakness; reflexes generally normal

(continued)

Table 8.2 (CONTINUED)

Clinical Characteristic	*Neuropathic Spinal Pain*	*Nociceptive Spinal Pain*
Physical exam signs	Straight leg raising test has high sensitivity but only moderate specificity	Numerous, generally non-specific
Hypersensitivity	Allodynia or hyperalgesia sometimes present	Not present
Referral pattern	Distal radiation common	Distal radiation less common; proximal radiation frequent, but in non-dermatomal distribution
Paroxysms	Exacerbations common and unpredictable; neurogenic claudication exacerbated by activity	Severe exacerbations less common and associated with activity
Autonomic signs	Sometimes present	Not present

Adapted from Wilkinson IM, Cohen SP. Epidural steroid injections. Curr Pain Headache Rep. 2011;16:50–59.

of chronic LBP using validated instruments have determined that "neuropathic" pain accounts for between 37 percent and 59 percent of cases.[8] Among the various instruments used to distinguish neuropathic from non-neuropathic pain, the painDETECT screening questionnaire is specifically designed for LBP. Relative to mechanical pain, neuropathic pain is typically associated with greater disability and a poorer quality of life (see Table 8.2).

History

A comprehensive medical history can provide important clues as to etiology. Patients with neuropathic pain often describe their symptoms with terms such as "sharp," "burning," and "stabbing," whereas those presenting with mechanical pain are more likely to characterize their pain as throbbing or aching. Because over 90 percent of radicular pain involves the L4–S1 nerve roots, neuropathic pain generally extends to below the knee, often in a dermatomal distribution (though multiple dermatomes may be affected). Patients generally experience some sensory deficits, which can consist of numbness, paresthesias, and/or dysesthesias (painful abnormal sensations). Unlike patients with spinal stenosis, which tends to have a more insidious onset, people with a herniated disc can sometimes identify a specific event that led to their symptoms, such as lifting a heavy object. Neuropathic pain is likely to have more unpredictable, greater "exacerbations" than mechanical pain, which is clasically worsened by activity.

Mechanical pain results from pain sensed by the "nociceptor" sensory fibers after an injury to muscle, soft tissue (ligaments, tendons), bones, joints, discs, or skin (or other organs). Most cases of mechanical pain resolve within weeks, with or without interventions, and are assumed to be due to muscle or soft-tissue injury. Muscle tears and spasms can develop following an innocuous event such as a cough, sneeze, or change in position. Mechanical pain frequently extends into the leg, including below the knee in a non-dermatomal distribution on occasion. Pain arising from degenerative conditions such as facet arthropathy and disc disease usually develops gradually, whereas vertebral fractures generally follow a traumatic inciting event. In contrast to facet and disc pathology, SI joint pain is more likely to be unilateral, with between 40 percent and 50 percent of individuals being able to cite a specific precipitating event. The most common of these are motor vehicle accidents, falls, and sports injuries or repetitive training.

PHYSICAL EXAMINATION

Physical examination can almost never provide a definitive diagnosis, but it is generally used to identify individuals who might benefit from diagnostic imaging or referrals for surgery or injections, as well as to detect inconsistencies that might warrant more detailed investigation. Five of these categories of inconsistencies, called Waddell's signs, signify a non-organic or psychological component of LBP. These signs are superficial or non-anatomical tenderness, pain elicitation with sham maneuvers (e.g., downward pressure on shoulders), less pain with distraction (i.e., positive supine but negative sitting straight leg raising test), widespread and non-dermatomal weakness and sensory loss, and overreaction. The presence of three or more of these five signs has been shown to correlate with psychological distress, disability, and treatment failure.[9]

Inspection might reveal alignment problems or findings indicative of other pathology (e.g., lipomas might denote spina bifida). Absent or reduced lordosis can signify muscle spasm, whereas exaggerated lordosis might be associated with weakened abdominal musculature. Sensory deficits are generally, but not always, present with radicular symptoms. True neurological weakness should be distinguished from "pain-induced" weakness, which can be present with both mechanical and neurological etiologies. Deep tendon reflexes are the only true "objective" measure of neurological function, but they are often only prominent for L4 (patellar) and S1 (Achille's). However, studies have shown that over 10 percent of individuals might have undetectable or asymmetric deep tendon reflexes. Systematic reviews have found the straight leg raising test to be the most sensitive sign for lower lumbar radiculopathy, but it is limited by low specificity (pooled sensitivity of 0.85, specificity of 0.52).[10] For upper lumbar radiculopathy, the femoral stretch test might be useful, but it is also limited by low specificity.

Spinal palpation is often used to evaluate LBP. Relative to motion assessments, palpation has better reliability, but neither test correlates well with function. Patients with pain from degenerative discs are more likely to report more midline than paraspinal tenderness (though the latter is still usually present), whereas individuals with facet joint or SI joint pain are more likely to have paraspinal tenderness. For discogenic and facetogenic pain, no physical exam test correlates well with diagnosis.

RED FLAGS

The term "red flag" is used to designate serious causes of LBP that warrant immediate attention. These include cancer, spondylodiscitis, acute vertebral fractures, and cauda equina syndrome. Careful attention must be paid to risk factors for each of these conditions, which include family history (cancer), older age (cancer, fractures), substance abuse (infection), and the severity of symptoms (cauda equina syndrome). Nearly half of all cases of cauda equina syndrome arise as a result of a disc herniation, with tumors and infections accounting for another 40 percent. Over three-fourths of patients with cauda equina syndrome present with bladder or bowel incontinence, and one-third have diminished sphincter tone. In persons with serious or progressive neurological findings, a rectal exam is essential to rule out cauda equina syndrome (see Figs. 8.3, 8.4 and Table 8.3).

Table 8.3 RED FLAGS SUGGESTING SERIOUS UNDERLYING PATHOLOGY OR NERVE ROOT PATHOLOGY

Red Flag	*Possible Underlying Condition(s)*	*Individuals at Increased Risk*	*Associated Signs and Symptoms*
Age > 50 years	Metastases, vertebral fractures, herpes zoster, and life-threatening conditions such as aortic rupture or perforated bowel	*Malignancy:* (+) family or previous cancer history, (+) smoking history, unremitting pain not relieved by recumbency *Zoster:* risk of acute infection and postherpetic neuralgia increase with age *Vertebral fracture:* h/o fall or other trauma *Abdominal pathology (aortic aneurysm):* h/o smoking, hypertension, vasculitis, abdominal trauma, (+) family history; prior surgery (ruptured bowel)	*Malignancy:* unexplained weight loss, unremitting pain not relieved by recumbency *Zoster:* history of rash *Abdominal pathology:* concomitant abdominal discomfort, peritoneal signs, nausea and vomiting

Age < 20 years	Might suggest congenital anomalies (e.g., spina bifida), early-onset disorders (e.g., Scheuermann's disease), or conditions associated with substance abuse (i.e., osteomyelitis)	*Congenital disorders:* neurological symptoms, (+) family history, other congenital abnormalities, systemic disease (e.g., diabetes, epilepsy, spina bifida) *Substance abuse:* males, depression or other psychiatric condition, poor school or work performance	*Congenital anomalies:* overlying birth marks, skin tags, patches of hair
Trauma	Vertebral fractures, SI joint pain	*Risk factors for vertebral factors:* old age, gait abnormalities, osteoporosis, female gender, previous fractures, corticosteroid use, Asian and Caucasian race	Fractures, ecchymoses, peritoneal signs
Systemic illness	Vertebral fractures, spinal infections, and metastases	*Risk factors for spinal infections:* recent infections, intravenous drug abuse, immunosuppresion, recent spinal procedures, diabetes, older age	*Spinal infections:* malaise, fever, chills, tenderness, leukocytosis, local signs of infection, elevated erythrocyte sedimentation rate.

(continued)

Table 8.3 (CONTINUED)

Red Flag	*Possible Underlying Condition(s)*	*Individuals at Increased Risk*	*Associated Signs and Symptoms*
Constitutional symptoms	Metastases and spinal infections	*Spinal metastases:* patients with breast, lung, prostate, and thyroid cancer	See above. Signs of discitis might be subtle; signs of meningitis can be fulminant and include meningeal signs.
Immunosuppresion or steroid use	Might predispose patients to infectious process, malignancy, or vertebral fractures	Patients with prolonged corticosteroid or immunosuppressive drug use (e.g., transplant recipients, autoimmune disease). Most common locations for vertebral fractures are mid-thoracic, thoracolumbar junction, and lower lumbar regions.	*Vertebral fracture:* focal tenderness, sudden onset, pain worsened by any movement and relieved by lying on back, height loss, and deformity

Widespread neurological symptoms	Cauda equina syndrome, myelopathy, multiple sclerosis	Patients with large disc hernation(s), recent (<48 hours) spinal procedures, traumatic injury, malignant and benign spinal tumors, spinal stenosis, and inflammatory conditions (e.g., ankylosing spondylitis and Paget's disease)	Marked motor and sensory deficits involving multiple nerve roots, gait disturbances, overflow incontinence, saddle anesthesia, and diminished reflexes and sphincter tone
Unrelenting pain	Psychogenic pain/somatoform disorder, malingering, malignancy, life-threatening abdominal pathology	*Psychogenic pain*: h/o depression, anxiety, psychosocial stressors, multiple somatic complaints, drug and/or alcohol problems	*Psychogenic pain:* Signs of non-organic pathology (i.e., Waddell's signs), changes in appetite or sleep habits, difficulty concentrating, irritability, irrational fears, panic attacks

Modified from Cohen SP, Argoff CE, Carragee EJ. Management of low back pain. *BMJ*. 2008;337:a2718.

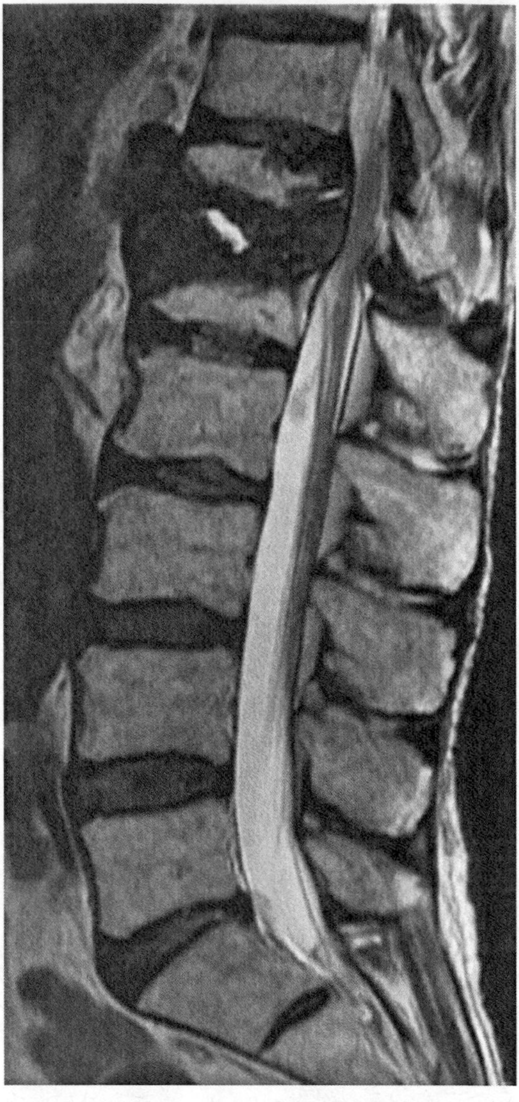

Figure 8.3. Sagittal MRI demonstrating T12–L1 spinal tuberculosis with bony destruction and abscess. From Cohen SP, Argoff CE,Carragee EJ. Management of low back pain. *BMJ*. 2008;337:a2718.

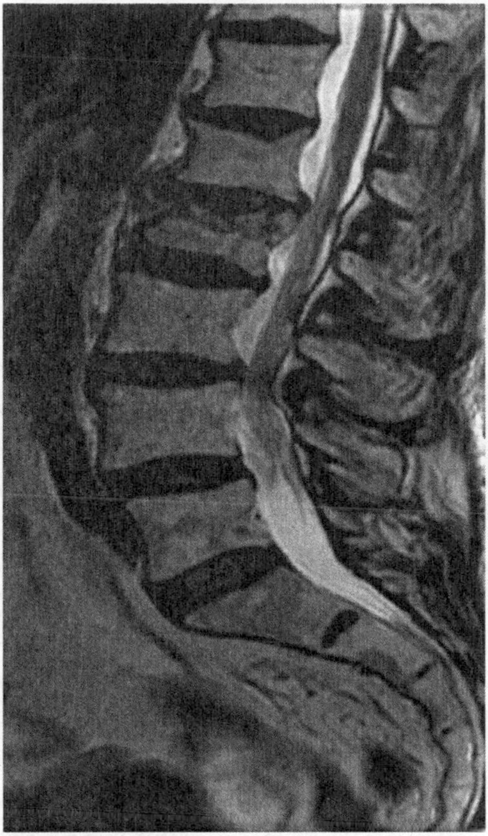

Figure 8.4. Sagittal MRI demonstrating an L2 vertebral fracture. From Cohen SP, Argoff CE, Carragee EJ. Management of low back pain. *BMJ*. 2008;337:a2718.

DIAGNOSTIC TOOLS

Imaging

Conventional imaging is useful in detecting fractures, scoliosis, spondyloarthropathies, and osteoporosis, but it is incapable of evaluating disc or soft-tissue pathology, which is best evaluated with magnetic resonance imaging (MRI). Yet MRI is characterized by a high rate of abnormalities in asymptomatic individuals and poor correlation with pain and function. Over half of individuals without LBP have bulging discs, and over 30 percent have herniations and/or annular tears. For all abnormalities, the prevalence rate increases with age. Clinical studies have shown that MRI does not generally affect decision making or improve outcomes in persons with LBP with or without radiculopathy,[11] and current recommendations are that it is indicated only in the presence of serious or progressive neurological deficits not trending toward improvement or when considering referral for injections or surgery.[12] A recent randomized study found that examining an MRI in patients referred for epidural steroid injections did not improve outcomes.[13]

Electrodiagnostic Studies

Electrodiagnostic studies such as electromyography (EMG) and nerve conduction studies are used to evaluate diseases involving muscles, nerve roots, and peripheral nerves. EMG directly assesses the physiologic integrity of a nerve root and can diagnose compressive and non-compressive radiculopathies. It can also measure the severity of disease. Nerve conduction studies cannot diagnose radiculopathy, but they can exclude polyneuropathy. Disadvantages of electrodiagnostic testing include the expense, a 2- to 4-week delay in their ability to identify pathology, and their unpleasantness.

Diagnostic Injections

Diagnostic injections are sometimes considered the reference standard for diagnosing many LBP disorders. Facet joint (nerve) blocks and SI joint blocks are frequently cited as the only way to identify the facet or SI joints as "pain generators," but they are subject to high false-positive rates.[14] Performing two or more blocks can reduce the false-positive rate but will inevitably also result in false-negative blocks, which translates to a lower "overall success rate" and a higher cost per effective treatment.[15] Discography operates under the premise that it is the only test that can correlate disc pathology with symptoms. However, it too is subject to a high false-positive rate and has not been proven to improve surgical outcomes.[14] Selective nerve root blocks are designed to identify the spinal nerve roots involved in radicular pain. They are most useful in patients with non-or multidermatomal symptoms and when imaging does not correlate with symptoms. Although there are no controlled trials evaluating the effect of selective nerve root blocks on surgical results, cohort studies suggest that they might improve decompression outcomes.[14]

CAUSES OF BACK PAIN

Although a broad spectrum of etiologies might result in LBP, in over 80 percent of cases no specific diagnosis can be rendered. Most of these cases are attributed to muscle and soft-tissue injuries. The most common etiologies of chronic LBP involve benign degenerative processes that have mechanical and/or neurogenic components secondary to abnormal stresses on vertebral (e.g., intervetebral discs, facet joints) or adjacent paraspinal structures (e.g., muscles, ligaments).

Myofascial Pain

Muscles constitute the largest structure in the spine, and myofascial pain can be a significant cause of LBP. Systematic reviews have found evidence of elevated electromyographic activity in LBP patients irrespective of the primary cause,[16] and controlled studies have demonstrated the efficacy of muscle relaxants.[17] But although a pain-spasm cycle may exist in LBP, whether this is the primary source or a protective mechanism cannot always be determined. Perhaps the strongest evidence for any treatment for LBP is for a multimodal exercise regimen that includes core stabilization, muscle strengthening, stretching, and aerobics.

Facet Arthropathy

Facetogenic pain accounts for between 10 percent and 15 percent of cases of mechanical LBP, increasing with age. The typical presentation is axial symptoms radiating into the upper leg accompanied by paraspinal tenderness. The only reliable way to make a diagnosis of facet joint pain is with local anesthetic blocks of the joints or medial branch nerves innervating them.

SI JOINT PAIN

SI joint pain accounts for between 15 percent and 25 percent of cases of axial LBP, with bimodal prevalence peaks in young adults and the elderly. SI joint pain is a heterogeneous condition that can include both intra-articular and extra-articular pathology, with the latter more common in younger people. Although some studies have found that a battery of provocative physical exam tests can identify a painful SI joint with reasonable accuracy,[18] the reference standard for diagnosing SI joint pain is a low volume anesthetic injection.

Internal Disc Disruption

Internal disc disruption (a.k.a. discogenic pain) accounts for between 20 percent and 45 percent of patients with mechanical LBP, and it is more common in younger adults. The classic presentation of discogenic pain is axial pain worsened by sitting, which might radiate into the leg(s) in a non-dermatomal pattern. Unlike facetogenic and SI joint pain, discogenic pain is more likely to be associated with midline, rather than paraspinal, tenderness. Risk factors for disc degeneration include occupation stress, obesity, and genetics. Non-surgical interventions are likely to benefit only a small subset of patients. Surgical treatments (e.g., spinal fusion and disc replacement) generally result in long-standing pain relief and functional improvement in only a minority of patients.

Herniated Disc

Herniated disc is the most common cause of radiculopathy in younger people, with a peak prevalence occurring in patients between 35 and 50 years of age. It is important to recognize that over two-thirds of herniated discs will resorb spontaneously within a year. The treatment of herniated disc is similar to that of spinal stenosis, though treatments tend to be more effective. The main advantage of decompression surgery over conservative therapy is that the resolution of symptoms might be faster.

Spinal Stenosis

Spinal stenosis can be classified into central, lateral recess, and foraminal, with the latter two more likely to cause unilateral pain. Among the three, foraminal stenosis is the most common. Specific etiologies for stenosis can include disc bulges, ligamentous and/or facet hypertrophy, osteophyte formation, and spondylolisthesis (which frequently results in axial pain). The diagnosis is generally made based on history and radiological studies. The classical presentation is an elderly person with pain extending into the calves or feet that is relieved by bending forward or rest. In individuals older than 60 years of age, nearly 20 percent have spinal stenosis, compared to <2 percent in those younger than 60 years. The straight leg raising test is less sensitive for neuropathic back pain caused by narrowing of the spinal canal than a herniated disc.

Visceral/Other

Visceral pain arising from internal organs can be referred to the low back secondary to the convergence of pain signals in the spinal cord. Visceral LBP accounts for at most 2 percent of LBP cases and can result from gastrointestinal disease (e.g., inflammatory bowel disease or diverticulitis), renal disease (e.g., nephrolithiasis), vascular disease (e.g., abdominal aortic aneurysm), and pelvic visceral disease (e.g., pelvic inflammatory disease, endometriosis, or prostatitis).

Psychogenic Pain

Chronic pain is often associated with psychological distress secondary to sleep abnormalities, impaired function, and financial insecurity. In addition, psychiatric and functional disorders, such as depression, can sometimes present as chronic LBP. Psychological assessment should be performed to identify conversion disorder, somatization disorder, factitious disorder, malingering, and adjustment disorder, if symptoms dictate. Regardless of whether psychopathology plays a primary or contributing role, psychological interventions designed to alleviate anxiety (e.g., biofeedback) and correct unhealthy thought and behavioral patterns (e.g., cognitive-behavioral therapy) can provide significant benefit in patients. A multi-disciplinary approach to care can be critical to improve patient outcomes in these difficult-to-treat cases.

TREATMENT

Most patients with LBP self-treat with over-the-counter medications and lifestyle modifications and do not seek medical care. Once a determination has been made that a patient's pain is not due to a serious source, modalities such as physical therapy and exercise should be initiated. Stretching, ice, and heat might prove effective in a subset of patients. After the first 24 hours of presentation, bed rest should be avoided. The advice to stay active is supported by a Cochrane review that demonstrated a beneficial effect for pain reduction and functional improvement in patients with acute non-specific back pain.[19]

Pharmacotherapy

The safest effective medication for acute LBP is acetaminophen. Acetaminophen has less efficacy than non-steroidal anti-inflammatory drugs (NSAIDs); however, when used in proper dosages it has a better side-effect profile. There is strong evidence supporting NSAIDs for mechanical LBP, but their use is limited by their ceiling effect, propensity for side effects with long-term use, and lack of efficacy for neuropathic pain.

Both benzodiazepine and non-benzodiazepine muscle relaxants can provide significant relief and functional improvement for acute and occasionally chronic LBP, but neither is beneficial for neuropathic symptoms. Especially for benzodiazpeines, the high incidence of side effects (e.g., cognitive effects, dependence) warrants caution. A substantial body of literature supports the short-term effectiveness of opioids for moderate to severe pain, but the evidence for long-term benefits is weak. In view of the high risks associated with long-term opioid use, they should be used cautiously only when other medications and interventions have failed, and with proper monitoring for analgesia, functional improvement, and aberrant behaviors.

Several reviews suggest that tricyclic antidepressants are more effective than placebo for chronic non-specific LBP, but the effect size is small, and few studies have assessed long-term benefits.[12,20] Antidepressants and anticonvulsants, particularly gabapentin, have also been shown in controlled studies to be effective for radicular pain.[2,20] Tricyclic antidepressants tend to be more effective than serotonin-norepinephrine reuptake inhibitors, but they are associated with less favorable side-effect profiles. In view of their comparable efficacy but lower incidence of adverse effects relative to amitriptyline, nortriptyline and imipramine are often prescribed as first-line agents. Caution should be utilized when prescribing antidepressants and/or anticonvulsants to the elderly because of their cognitive and psychomotor effects.

Complementary and Alternative Medicine Treatments

The World Health Organization (2012) defines complementary and alternative medicine (CAM) as "a broad set of healthcare practices that are not part of a country's own tradition and are not integrated into the dominant healthcare system."[21] The use of CAM to treat pain has grown significantly over the past few decades, with some studies showing utilization rates approaching 50 percent. Although CAM can include such arcane therapies as reflexology, mainstream treatments account for a substantial majority. There is substantial evidence to support massage therapy for acute and chronic back pain, but no evidence that it provides long-term benefit.[22] For spinal manipulation, there is moderate evidence supporting short- but not long-term benefit for axial and radicular pain.[22] For acupuncture, there is moderate evidence supporting a modest intermediate-term treatment effect for both axial and radicular pain, with studies comparing acupuncture to no treatment showing a greater effect than those comparing it to sham acupuncture.[22,23] With respect to herbal medications, there is some evidence to support a small, short-term effect in nonspecific LBP.[23] There is weak evidence for short-term benefit with transcutaneous electrical nerve stimulation, and negative evidence for the use of traction.[22]

Procedural Interventions

Nerve blocks might provide diagnostic and theurapeutic value in patients whose symptoms persist after 6 weeks. Epidural steroid injections are considered by some to be a first-line treatment for radiculopathy[24] and were shown in one well-designed controlled study to reduce the need for surgery.[25] Epidural steroid injections tend to work best in those with a short duration (less than 6 months) of pain, leg pain that is greater than back pain, and intermittent symptoms. In individuals who fail to respond to epidural steroids, pulsed radiofrequency of the dorsal root ganglia might provide benefit. Corticosteroid injections can also provide short-term relief for SI joint pain, but there is no evidence to support their use for facet joint pain, degenerated discs, or myofascial pain. Radiofrequency denervation, which entails lesioning the small nerves that innervate painful joints, is the reference standard for treating facet joint and SI joint pain in those who respond to diagnostic blocks. In patients with acute or subacute vertebral fractures, vertebroplasty or kyphoplasty may be considered. There are few effective treatments for failed back surgery, but randomized studies have demonstrated the effectiveness of spinal cord stimulation in those with predominantly radicular symptoms.

Psychotherapy and Exercise

Support groups, counseling, and relaxation therapy can be beneficial to some patients in the appropriate clinical setting. For behavioral therapy, there is evidence that both operant and cognitive therapy can alleviate pain, but there is little evidence to support one type of treatment over another.[22] Intensive multimodal exercise programs have proven to be beneficial for subacute and chronic spinal pain for up to 6 months after treatment cessation, but there is conflicting evidence supporting back schools.[22]

Surgery

For acute LBP, surgery is considered only for serious spinal pathology or progressive nerve root dysfunction due to a herniated disc. In patients with persistent radiculopathy secondary to a herniated disc, decompressive surgery can improve symptoms relative to conservative treatment for up to 6 months, but most studies show no significant differences after 2 years.[26] In well-selected individuals with spinal stenosis or spondylolisthesis, the benefits of surgery can last for at least 2 years. For mechanical LBP pain secondary to non-specific degenerative pathology, only 15 percent to 40 percent of individuals can expect significant functional improvement.[2] Absolute indications for open surgery for LBP include (1) bowel or bladder incontinence or sexual dysfunction, (2) loss of reflexes or motor weakness resulting in falls, and (3) incapacitating pain unresponsive to more conservative measures.

CONCLUSIONS

LBP is a common complaint that poses an enormous social and economic burden. Most symptoms will resolve spontaneously with little intervention, but recurrence is common. Understanding when referrals for imaging and interventions are indicated can be enhanced by obtaining a thorough history and physical exam, though neither is associated with high specificity. Imaging studies should be minimized because of their low specificity, which can lead to "over-diagnosis"; however, they should be obtained in patients with progressive neurologic deficits, patients with failure to improve, and those at risk for serious pathology. In individuals who fail to respond to conservative treatment, procedural interventions can provide benefit to a subset of patients, but they tend to be more effective in those with radicular pain of short duration.

REFERENCES

1. Deyo RA, Mirza SK, Martin BI. Back pain prevalence and visit rates: estimates from U.S. national surveys, 2002. *Spine (Phila Pa 1976)*. 2006;31(23):2724–2727.
2. Cohen SP, Argoff CE, Carragee EJ. Management of low back pain. *BMJ*. 2008;337:a2718.
3. Postacchini F, Lami R, Pugliese O. Familial predisposition to discogenic low-back pain. An epidemiologic and immunogenetic study. *Spine (Phila Pa 1976)*. 1988;13(12):1403–1406.
4. Von Korff M, Saunders K. The course of back pain in primary care. *Spine (Phila Pa 1976)*. 1996;21(24):2833–2837; discussion 2838–2839.
5. Livshits G, Popham M, Malkin I, et al. Lumbar disc degeneration and genetic factors are the main risk factors for low back pain in women: the UK twin spine study. *Ann Rheum Dis*. 2011;70(10):1740–1745.
6. Cohen SP, Hurley RW, Christo PJ, Winkley J, et al. Clinical predictors of success and failure for lumbar facet radiofrequency denervation. *Clin J Pain*. 2007;23(1):45–52.
7. Merskey H, Bogduk N. *Classification of Chronic Pain: Descriptions of Chronic Pain Syndromes and Definition of Pain Terms*. 2nd ed. International Association for the Study of Pain (IASP); 1994.
8. Freynhagen R, Baron R, Tolle T, et al. Screening of neuropathic pain components in patients with chronic back pain associated with nerve root compression: a prospective observational pilot study (MIPORT). *Curr Med Res Opin*. 2006;22(3):529–537.

9. Waddell G, McCulloch JA, Kummel E, Venner RM. Nonorganic physical signs in low-back pain. *Spine (Phila Pa 1976)*. 1980;5(2):117–125.
10. Rubinstein SM, van Tulder M. A best-evidence review of diagnostic procedures for neck and low-back pain. *Best Pract Res Clin Rheumatol*. 2008;22(3):471–482.
11. Chou R, Fu R, Carrino JA, Deyo RA. Imaging strategies for low-back pain: systematic review and meta-analysis. *Lancet*. 2009;373(9662):463–472.
12. Chou R, Qaseem A, Snow V, et al. Diagnosis and treatment of low back pain: a joint clinical practice guideline from the American College of Physicians and the American Pain Society. *Ann Intern Med*. 2007;147(7):478–491.
13. CohenS, Gupta A, Strassels S, et al. Does MRI affect outcomes in patients with lumbrosacral radiculopathy referred for epidural steroid injections? A randomized, double-blind, controlled study. *Arch Intern Med* 2012;172:134–142.
14. Cohen SP, Hurley RW. The ability of diagnostic spinal injections to predict surgical outcomes. *Anesth Analg*. 2007;105(6):1756–1775.
15. Cohen SP, Williams KA, Kurihara C, et al. Multicenter, randomized, comparative cost-effectiveness study comparing 0, 1, and 2 diagnostic medial branch (facet joint nerve) block treatment paradigms before lumbar facet radiofrequency denervation. *Anesthesiology*. 2010;113(2):395–405.
16. Geisser ME, Ranavaya M, Haig AJ, et al. A meta-analytic review of surface electromyography among persons with low back pain and normal, healthy controls. *J Pain*. 2005;6(11):711–726.
17. Browning R, Jackson JL, O'Malley PG. Cyclobenzaprine and back pain: a meta-analysis. *Arch Intern Med*. 2001;161(13):1613–1620.
18. Szadek KM, van der Wurff P, van Tulder MW, et al. Diagnostic validity of criteria for sacroiliac joint pain: a systematic review. *J Pain*. 2009;10(4):354–368.
19. Hagen KB, Hilde G, Jamtvedt G, Winnem MF. The Cochrane review of bed rest for acute low back pain and sciatica. *Spine (Phila Pa 1976)*. 2000;25(22):2932–2939.
20. Staiger TO, Gaster B, Sullivan MD, Deyo RA. Systematic review of antidepressants in the treatment of chronic low back pain. *Spine (Phila Pa 1976)*. 2003;28(22):2540–2545.
21. World Health Organization. Traditional medicine: Definitions. Available at: http://www.who.int/medicines/areas/traditional/definitions/en/index.html. Last accessed October 21, 2012.
22. Chou R, Huffman LH, American Pain Society, American College of Physicians. Nonpharmacologic therapies for acute and chronic low back pain: a review of the evidence for an American Pain Society/American College of Physicians clinical practice guideline. *Ann Intern Med*. 2007;147(7):492–504.
23. Rubinstein SM, van Middelkoop M, Kuijpers T, et al. A systematic review on the effectiveness of complementary and alternative medicine for chronic non-specific low-back pain. *Eur Spine J*. 2010;19(8):1213–1228.

24. Wilkinson IM, Cohen SP. Epidural steroid injections. *Curr Pain Headache Rep.* 2012;16:50–59.
25. Riew KD, Park JB, Cho YS, et al. Nerve root blocks in the treatment of lumbar radicular pain. A minimum five-year follow-up. *J Bone Joint Surg Am.* 2006;88:1722–1725.
26. Peul WC, van Houwelingen HC, van den Hout WB, et al. Surgery versus prolonged conservative treatment for sciatica. *N Engl J Med.* 2007;356(22):2245–2256.

9

Neck and Upper Extremity Pain

TOMAS KUCERA AND ROBERT W. HURLEY

> CERVICAL RADICULAR PAIN
>
> A 32-year-old woman presents to your office with persistent neck pain that radiates down her arms past the elbows to the hands. She describes the pain in the arms as sharp, electric-like, and relieved by placing her hands behind her head. Her neck pain, but not arm pain, is relieved by non-steroidal anti-inflammatory drug (NSAID) therapy. She has no significant medical history except for a motor vehicle collision (MVC) 4 years ago in which she was the restrained driver in a stationary vehicle that was rear-ended by a car travelling at 40 mph. Her pain has been present constantly since then and is occasionally worse with neck movement.

BACKGROUND

Cervical radiculopathy is a neurologic condition associated with neck and upper extremity pain caused by dysfunction of the nerves of the cervical spine. The lay population commonly refers to radiculopathic pain as "pinched" or "compressed" nerves. Symptoms are broad and include true neurological muscle weakness, numbness, paresthesias, and/or pain in the distribution of single or multiple nerve roots. Radiculopathic pain describes a neurologic condition wherein a patient has accompanying weakness or numbness due to impeded conduction along a nerve pathway. Radicular pain is caused by irritation of the nerve(s) that results in pain in a dermatomal distribution. It is distinguished from radiculopathic pain by the preservation of motor and sensory function.

PREVALENCE

Epidemiological data on cervical radiculopathy are not precisely defined. However, the limited data that do exist suggest an incidence of around 83.2/100,000 that is slightly higher in male than female (107.3 and 63.5, respectively) patients.[1] An Italian study found a point prevalence rate of 3.5 cases per 1000 people but did not note the annual incidence.[2] Both studies found the peak incidence to be in the 50-to-60-year-old age group.

HISTORY AND PHYSICAL EXAMINATION

The history and physical evaluation of the patient are key diagnostic indicators. Determining the presence or absence of emergent signs of spinal cord compression such as the sudden loss of bowel or bladder continence is essential. In our patient with stable symptoms for 4 years, this is unlikely. However, this information still must be obtained in order to rule out subsequent progression to a neurosurgical emergency. A complete description of the patient's pain pattern, timing of the symptoms, and inciting injury can help with the development of a preliminary diagnosis. In this case study, the young woman has "electrical" pain beginning in her neck and extending down her arms past her elbows. This pattern suggests radicular pain. Moreover, her MVC involved a high-speed rear-impact accident that occurred when her car was not in motion. This suggests a mechanism of cervical spine injury that could result in intervertebral disc herniation. The use of anatomic drawings of nerve distribution can be used to delineate the nerve injury pattern. On further questioning, our patient states that her pain covers the medial aspect of her forearm and ends in the fourth and fifth digits of her hand. This pain distribution suggests involvement of the C8 nerve root. The most commonly affected nerve roots are C7 and C6, and their injury usually results in symptoms extending into the lateral hand and forearm. Because our patient reports minimal axial neck pain and pain that radiates below her elbows, it is unlikely that her primary pain etiology is secondary to the cervical facet joints or disc pathology without nerve root involvement.

An important element of the history is functional pain assessment to include positions or activities that exacerbate or alleviate the neck pain. For example, disc herniations that result in narrowing of the foramina in which the spinal nerves exit might cause many patients to complain of pain that is exacerbated by neck extension or lateral bending, which cause the foramina to narrow. Patients with radiculopathy commonly state that their pain is improved when they place one or both hands behind their head, which causes abduction of their shoulders and decreased stretching of the impinged nerve, and therefore pain relief. Other important details of the history that are relevant include any associated injuries; pain acuity defined as acute, subacute (less than 6 months) or chronic; a previous history of similar pain; social history including occupation, pending litigation, workman's compensation, and pending disability claims; and substance dependence. Neurologic red flags include cervical myelopathy symptoms such as bowel, bladder, or gait dysfunction.

Physical Examination

The components of a thorough physical examination include observation, palpation, motor examination, sensory examination, deep tendon reflexes, and provocation tests. Observation of the patient in neutral posture during conversation is the first step of the physical examination. Palpation for tenderness, trigger points, and spasticity is important, with tenderness occasionally noted in the area of the affected nerve root(s). Understanding the significance of motor and sensory testing and deep tendon reflexes, along with their respective nerve root distributions, enables accurate diagnosis (Table 9.1).

Table 9.1 THE ACCURACY OF THE HISTORY AND PHYSICAL EXAM FOR CERVICAL RADICULOPATHY

Test or Symptom	*Sensitivity, %*	*Specificity*
Arm pain	99	–
Sensory deficits	85	–
Neck pain	79	–
Reflex deficits	71	–
Motor deficits	68	–
Scapular pain	52	–
Spurling's test	45	95 percent
Shoulder abduction (relief) sign	46	90 percent
Neck distraction test	42	100 percent
Lhermitte's sign	<28	"High"
Hoffman's sign	58	78 percent

Provocation tests are manual maneuvers used to reproduce the patient's pain. The Spurling test, or foraminal compression test, is a manual test useful in confirming cervical radiculopathy. The patient is positioned seated, and the head is extended and rotated while the clinician applies downward pressure on the top of the head. Pain radiating down the ipsilateral limb during rotation of the head is considered positive. Tong et al. found the test to be 93 percent specific, but only 30 percent sensitive, for diagnosing radiculopathy.[3] It is therefore *not* a useful screening test, but it can be helpful for the confirmation of cervical radiculopathy. Physical signs suggestive of myelopathy include Hoffman's sign and the Babinski test.

ADDITIONAL DIAGNOSTIC TESTING MODALITIES

Radiology

The American College of Radiology (ACR) Appropriateness Criteria recommend that patients of any age with chronic neck pain with or without a history of remote trauma should initially undergo a five-view radiographic examination (anteroposterior [AP], lateral, open mouth, both obliques).[4] Patients with normal radiographs and no neurologic signs or symptoms do not need further imaging. Patients with normal radiographs and neurologic signs or symptoms should undergo cervical magnetic resonance imaging (MRI) that includes the craniocervical junction and the upper thoracic region. If there is a contraindication to MRI examination, such as a cardiac pacemaker or severe claustrophobia, computed tomography (CT) myelography with multi-planar reconstruction is recommended (see Table 9.2).

Table 9.2 PREVALENCE OF CERVICAL SPINE PATHOLOGY IN ASYMPTOMATIC VOLUNTEERS

Decrease in signal intensity	81 percent
Disc degeneration	29 percent
Disc space narrowing	22 percent to 34 percent
Disc protrusion	69 percent to 79 percent
Spinal stenosis	5 percent
Any abnormality	>90 percent

Electromyography/Nerve Conduction Velocity

Electromyography (EMG) is an electrodiagnostic study that is composed of nerve conduction studies and a needle-electrode examination. According to the North American Spine Society clinical guidelines on cervical radiculopathy, the evidence is insufficient for making a recommendation for or against the use of EMG in patients who still have an unclear diagnosis after clinical examination, radiographs, and cervical MRI.[5] However, when clinical suspicion of nerve compression or injury is high, nerve conduction studies evaluating the conduction velocity, amplitude, and latency of motor and sensory nerves can help pinpoint which spinal nerves are affected.

Selective Nerve Root Blocks

Diagnostic selective nerve root blocks (SNRBs) entail injecting a small amount of local anesthetic directly onto a spinal nerve root (not into the epidural space) to identify symptomatic spinal nerves. North American Spine Society clinical guidelines on cervical radiculopathy recommend using SNRB in patients who have multiple lesions on MRI or CT myelography in order to clarify the symptomatic levels.[5] SNRB may also be considered for use in patients whose clinical symptoms are discordant with their radiologic findings. In one large retrospective study evaluating the ability of SNRB to improve surgical outcomes, Sasso et al. reported an 83 percent success rate for lumbar or cervical decompression surgery in patients with a positive SNRB, compared to 60 percent in those with a negative block.[6] Another study found that SNRB was more accurate in identifying a symptomatic nerve root based on surgical exploration than either EMG or myelography.[7]

TREATMENT

The flow chart in Fig. 9.1 summarizes the treatment of cervical radicular pain. The foundation and first step in most cases is physical therapy and treatment with NSAIDs which may help with mechanical neck pain. Spinal (chiropractic) manipulation of the neck is generally not recommended in most cases. Massage therapy and physical therapy have been shown to improve patient symptoms.[8] Medical management and interventions are often performed in conjunction with physical therapy. In those patients in whom radicular symptoms persist, epidural steroid injections or adjuvant medications should be considered.

Cervical Facet Pain

A 55-year-old man presents to your office with persistent neck pain that occasionally radiates down to his shoulder on the right side and above his elbow on the left side, in addition to a decreased range of motion. He is a smoker and denies any trauma to his neck. In his youth, while in the armed services, he boxed for exercise.

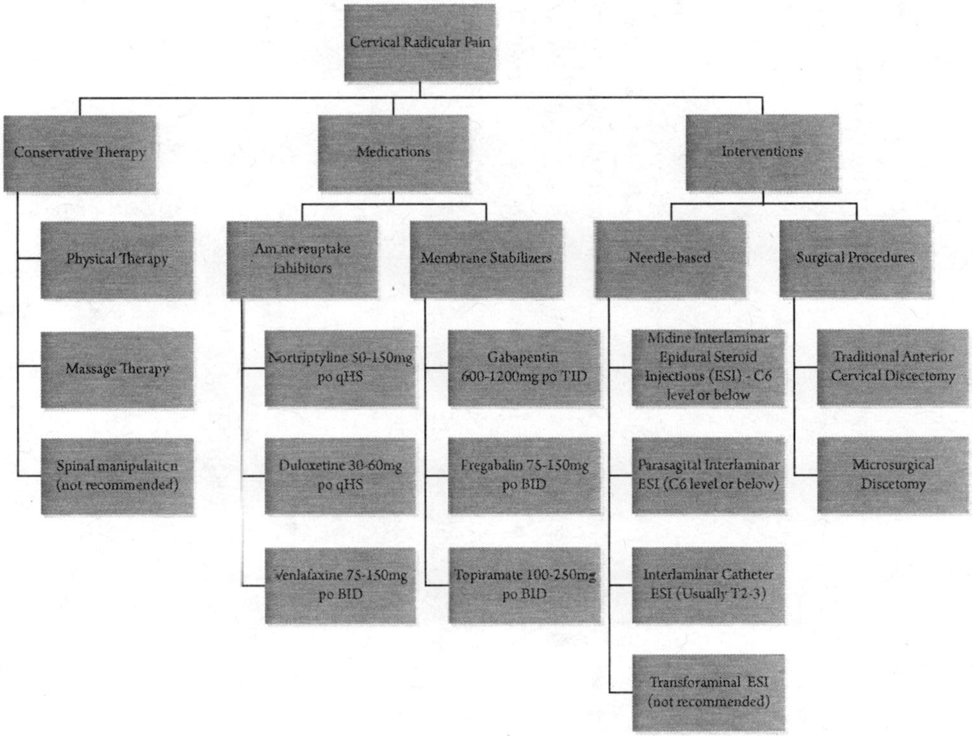

Figure 9.1. Flow chart demonstrating conservative, pharmacological and interventional treatment for cervical radicular pain.

BACKGROUND

Cervical facet pain or syndrome is a condition that results from inflammation or injury to the vertebral facet or zygapophyseal joints. These articular joints share the axial load of the head with the intervertebral discs and guide and limit motion in the neck. Cervical facet pain is typically experienced as a result of whiplash injuries, osteoarthritis, or occupational stressors associated with repetitive vibration.

PREVALENCE

The epidemiology of cervical facet pain, including incidence, has not been well studied, with much of the data coming from discrete groups of investigators that have published numerous studies. Aprill and Bogduk identified the zygapophyseal joint as the primary cause of pain in approximately 25 percent of patients with chronic non-radicular neck pain, whereas Manchikanti estimated the prevalence at about 36 percent in a similar population.[9,10] In patients with chronic pain following whiplash injury, epidemiological studies conducted using controlled blocks suggest a prevalence rate of between 50 percent and 60 percent.[12]

HISTORY AND PHYSICAL EXAMINATION

Patients with cervical facet joint pain, also called cervical facet syndrome, often present with complaints of neck pain, decreased range of motion, and headaches when the C2–3 facet joint (or the atlanto-axial and/or the atlanto-occipital joints) is involved. Patients commonly describe the pain as a dull, aching discomfort in the posterior neck that might radiate to the head, shoulder, or even arms, depending on the level(s) involved. As in the case above, cervical facet pain can mimic radicular pain in that it might travel into the arms; however, it rarely extends below the elbows, and it typically occurs in a variable, non-dermatomal distribution.

Common patterns of cervical facet pain that patients classically describe include morning stiffness and worse pain upon waking, similar to other osteoarthritic conditions. Patients frequently report that their pain is aggravated by turning their head to the side, especially when driving. They might describe pain that is increased by looking down or up. It is common for patients to have a history of previous whiplash injury or the repetitive strain associated with occupations such as a boxer (as in the case example), a service member (who must wear a Kevlar helmet), or a construction worker who uses pneumatic tools frequently. Younger patients commonly report a history of an athletic injury or MVC.

On physical examination, manual palpation, range of motion, and testing the joints through provocative stress maneuvers are important components that can suggest a clinical diagnosis of cervical facet syndrome. It is common for these patients to experience tenderness upon deep palpation of the facet joints along the paraspinous musculature (rather than midline tenderness, which is more common with disc pathology). Range of motion testing often demonstrates pain with movement to the side or looking down, as is the case for the patient described above.

ADDITIONAL DIAGNOSTIC MODALITIES

Diagnostic Imaging

As in the first case, patients who present with chronic neck pain or a history of remote trauma should initially undergo a five-view radiographic examination (AP, lateral, open mouth, both oblique) as recommended by the ACR.[4] Patients with normal radiographs and no neurologic signs or symptoms do not require further imaging. Patients with normal radiographs and neurologic signs or symptoms should undergo a cervical MRI if there are no contraindications, or CT myelography if they are unable to undergo an MRI. It should be noted that many experts and guidelines do not recommend routine x-rays for non-specific chronic neck pain in the absence of neurological signs or symptoms, a history of trauma, or red flags that might suggest serious pathology (e.g., metastases or infection). Advanced radiological imaging (e.g., MRI) has low sensitivity for detecting facetogenic pain, as identified by diagnostic injections.[11]

Diagnostic Testing

Diagnostic Injections

Diagnostic cervical facet joint nerve (medial branch) blocks are recommended in patients who meet certain criteria. According to some guidelines, diagnostic facet injections should be used in patients who have at least moderate non-radicular neck pain or headache for more than 3 months, failed conservative management, and have no contraindications to injections. The test is positive if the patient experiences greater than 50 percent relief and is able to perform previously painful movements without deterioration of the relief (see Fig. 9.2).[11]

TREATMENT

The reference standard for treating cervical facet joint pain is radiofrequency denervation, which is effective in approximately 60% of patients who respond positively to diagnostic blocks. Similar to other forms of mechanical neck pain, NSAIDs and other medications, and some alternative treatments such as acupuncture may provide significant benefit, though the evidence supporting these treatments is largely anecdotal.

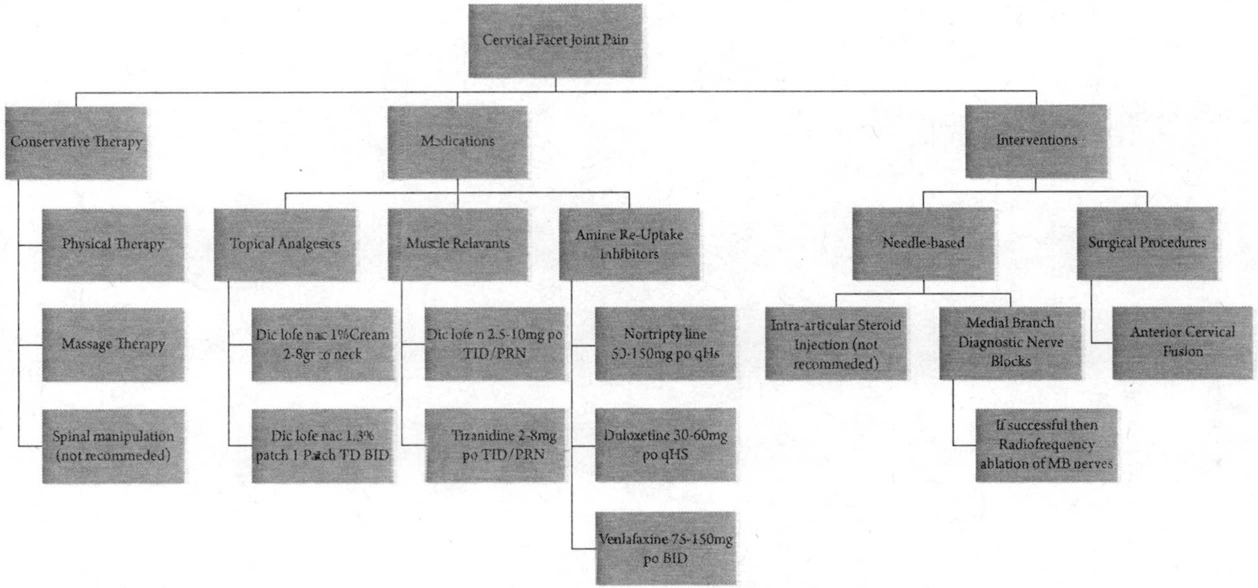

Figure 9.2. Flow chart demonstrating conservative, pharmacological and interventional treatment for cervical facet joint pain.

Cervical Discogenic Pain

A 48-year-old man who was a former college football player presents to your office with chronic neck pain that is diffuse and dull. He describes the pain as worse when he bends his neck forward or nods his head. The pain awakens him at night, and he must change position in order to obtain relief.

BACKGROUND

Cervical discogenic pain is a mechanical pain condition caused by degeneration of the intervertebral discs. Cervical disc disorders that can lead to pain include endplate fractures and annular tears and fissures. Discs that are degenerated require less stress in order for herniation to occur. A herniated nucleus pulposus occurs when the internal disc contents extend beyond the posterior margin of the vertebral body. This can result in axial "discogenic pain," but when it involves neuropathic pain secondary to nerve root inflammation, it is more appropriately referred to as radicular pain. On radiological imaging, degenerative disc disease may manifest as disruptions in the annulus fibrosis, degradation of the nucleus, and/or loss of disc height. Internal disc disruption is caused by annular tears with preservation of the external disc structures.

HISTORY AND PHYSICAL EXAMINATION

Discogenic pain that does not involve the nerve root is generally vague and diffuse. Patients often present with neck pain that is aggravated by movement, commonly flexion-extension and head rotation. They might complain that the pain awakens them from their sleep, as is the case with the above-mentioned football player. If a nerve root is involved, patients might have radicular pain, numbness, and/or weakness in the distribution of the affected nerve root.

On physical examination, the patient will usually have localized or diffuse tenderness over the neck, shoulders, and upper back, depending on the affected discs. One hallmark that is often used to distinguish discogenic from facetogenic pain is the location of the most prominent tenderness, which tends to be more midline with discogenic pain. When discogenic pain does not involve a nerve root, patients usually present with decreased range of motion with a normal neurologic examination.

RADIOLOGY

As in the preceding two cases, patients who present with chronic neck pain should initially undergo a five-view radiographic examination as recommended by the ACR.[4] Those with normal radiographs and no neurologic signs or symptoms do not require further imaging. Patients with normal radiographs and neurologic signs or symptoms should undergo a cervical MRI if there are no contraindications, or CT myelography if they are unable to undergo MRI. Multiple studies have demonstrated a high prevalence rate (>50 percent) of disc pathology in asymptomatic volunteers (i.e., lack of specificity), which has led many experts to conclude that advanced imaging should be reserved only for those individuals with serious or progressive neurological deficits or who are being referred for consideration of surgery or other procedural interventions.[13]

DISCOGRAPHY

Based on a systematic review by the National Guideline Clearinghouse, cervical discography is indicated only when certain criteria are met. Cervical discography is not used as often, and has not been studied as widely, as lumbar discography because of the potential complications. Discography is advocated by some experts as the only test that can connect symptoms to pathology. Candidates for cervical discography typically include patients who have persistent neck pain with inconclusive imaging and no neurological findings. Discography is considered positive if the injection of low volume contrast reproduces the patient's typical pain and at least one adjacent disc does not reproduce the pain.[14] Cervical discography is associated with a high false-positive rate in certain individuals (e.g., those with psychiatric problems and previous spine surgery) and carries the potential risk of injury to the trachea, esophagus, and spinal cord, as well as discitis. One recent study performed on the lumbar spine also raised the possibility of discography's predisposing patients to accelerated disc degeneration and/or herniation years after the procedure.[15] This is consistent with animal studies, which demonstrate that needle penetration of the annulus may induce subsequent pathology.

Treatment

The flow diagram in Fig. 9.3 outlines the treatment algorithm for discogenic pain. The surgical procedure of artificial disc replacement was recently approved by the United Stated Food and Drug Administration (FDA). There are currently several industry-sponsored, randomized, multicenter, U.S. Food and Drug Administration–approved trials comparing anterior cervical discectomy and fusion (ACDF) to artificial cervical disc arthroplasty (ACDA). The early results of 2-year follow-up suggest that ACDF and ACDA are comparable in their results, with some studies showing weak evidence that ACDA is superior to ACDF.[16]

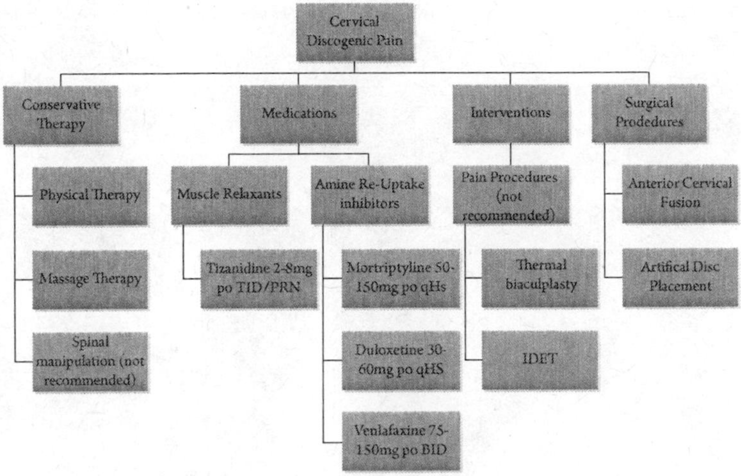

Figure 9.3. Flow chart demonstrating conservative, pharmacological and interventional treatment for cervical discogenic pain.

MYOFASCIAL PAIN

Myofascial pain is, as the name implies, pain related to the muscle and surrounding fascia. Cervical myofascial pain can be caused by any of the neck muscles (levator scapulae, rhomboids, supraspinatus, infraspinatus, and/or trapezius) and is often the result of trauma or overuse. The diagnosis is made based on clinical symptoms and examination. Cervical myofascial pain may be characterized by the presence of trigger points in any of the supporting muscles of the neck. Trigger points are palpable, taut muscle bundles that are painful and irritable on palpation during clinical examination.

Treatment

The hallmark of treatment for cervical myosfascial pain consists of physical therapy maneuvers that may include deep tissue massage,

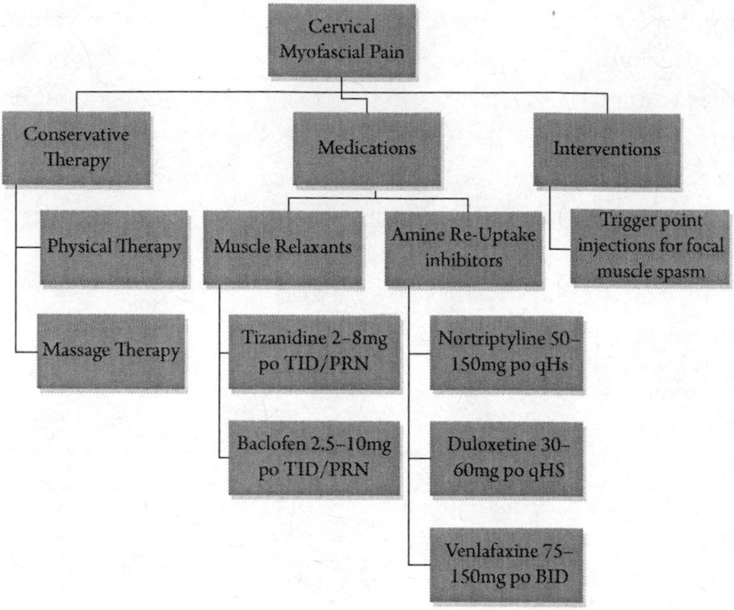

Figure 9.4. Flow chart demonstrating conservative, pharmacological and interventional treatment for cervical myofascial pain.

range of motion exercises, and stretching. If biomechanical causes such as abnormal posture are suspected, ergonomic modification and muscle re-training might be helpful. Muscle relaxants such as cyclobenzaprine, tizanidine, and baclofen might be useful, though they tend to work better for acute pain. Studies have also found tricyclic antidepressants and serotonin-norepinephrine reuptake inhibitors to be beneficial in some patients. When discrete trigger points are identified, trigger point injections can provide sustained relief.

SUMMARY

Cases 1 through 3 highlight the common presenting complaints that a healthcare practitioner might encounter in patients with overlapping neck and upper extremity pain complaints. In case 1, the patient presented with a history of trauma and radicular symptoms that included weakness and pain in a nerve root distribution extending down the arm. The facet joint pain noted in case 2 might sometimes mimic radicular pain, but it rarely radiates past the elbows and is usually non-dermatomal in pattern. Facetogenic pain is usually described as "dull and diffuse" and is frequently exacerbated by turning the head, as often occurs during driving. The discogenic pain observed in case 3 might also present as dull, aching neck pain. It is commonly encountered in athletes and other individuals whose occupations require repetitive motion. These patients usually complain of increased pain during flexion and extension of the neck. Myofascial pain is typically characterized by diffusely elevated muscle tone, localized or diffuse spasm, or discrete tender trigger points that elicit pain upon palpation. This pain is often related to either biomechanical stressors (e.g., a computer operator or truck driver) or a specific traumatic inciting event.

REFERENCES

1. Radhakrishnan K, Litchy WJ, O'Fallon WM, Kurland LT. Epidemiology of cervical radiculopathy. A population-based study from Rochester, Minnesota, 1976 through 1990. *Brain*. 1994;117(Pt 2):325–335.
2. Salemi G, Savettieri G, Meneghini F, et al. Prevalence of cervical spondylotic radiculopathy: a door-to-door survey in a Sicilian municipality. *Acta Neurol Scand*. 1996;93(2–3):184–188.
3. Tong HC, Haig AJ, Yamakawa K. The Spurling test and cervical radiculopathy. *Spine*. 2002;27(2):156–159.
4. American College of Radiology. ACR Appropriateness Criteria: chronic neck pain. National Guideline Clearinghouse. http://guideline.gov/summary/summary.aspx?doc_id=8297.
5. North American Spine Society. Diagnosis and treatment of cervical radiculopathy from degenerative disorders. Burr Ridge, IL: North American Spine Society; 2010.
6. Sasso RC, Macadaeg K, Nordmann D, Smith M. Selective nerve root injections can predict surgical outcome for lumbar and cervical radicu-

lopathy: comparison to magnetic resonance imaging. *J Spinal Disord Tech.* 2005;18:471–478.

7. Haueisen DC, Smith BS, Myers SR, Pryce ML. The diagnostic accuracy of spinal nerve injection studies. Their role in the evaluation of recurrent sciatica. *Clin Orthop Relat Res.* 1985;198:179–183.
8. Gross AR, Goldsmith C, Hoving JL, et al.; Cervical Overview Group. Conservative management of mechanical neck disorders: a systematic review. *J Rheumatol.* 2007;34(5):1083–1102.
9. Aprill C, Bogduk N. The prevalence of cervical zygapophyseal joint pain. A first approximation. *Spine.* 1992;17(7):744–747.
10. Manchikanti L, Boswell MV, Singh V, Pampati V, Damron KS, Beyer CD. Prevalence of facet joint pain in chronic spinal pain of cervical, thoracic, and lumbar regions. *BMC Musculoskelet Disord.* 2004;5:15.
11. Comprehensive evidence-based guidelines for interventional techniques in the management of chronic spinal pain. National Guideline Clearinghouse. http://guideline.gov/content.aspx?id=15136&search=facet+injection.
12. Cohen SP, Huang JH, Brummett C. Facet joint pain-advances in patient selection and management. *Nature Rev Rheumatol* 2012; Nov 20. doi: 10.1038/nrrheum.2012.198. [Epub ahead of print]
13. Barnsley L, Lord SM, Wallis BJ, Bogduk N. The prevalence of chronic cervical zygapophysial joint pain after whiplash. *Spine.* 1995;20(1):20–25; discussion: 26.
14. Matsumoto M, Fujimura Y, Suzuki N, et al. MRI of cervical intervertebral discs in asymptomatic subjects. *J Bone Joint Surg Br.* 1998;80:19–24.
15. Manchikanti L, Boswell MV, Singh V, et al. Comprehensive evidence-based guidelines for interventional techniques in the management of chronic spinal pain. *Pain Physician.* 2009;12(4):699–802.
16. Carragee EJ, Don AS, Hurwitz EL, Cuellar JM, Carrino JA, Herzog R. Does discography cause accelerated progression of degeneration changes in the lumbar disc: a ten-year matched cohort study. *Spine (Phila Pa 1976).* 2009;34:2338–2345.
17. Cepoiu-Martin M, Faris P, Lorenzetti D, Prefontaine E, Noseworthy T, Sutherland L. Artificial cervical disc arthroplasty: a systematic review. *Spine (Phila Pa 1976).* 2011;36(25):E1623–E1633.

10

Osteoarthritis

KRISTINE PHILLIPS

Case Presentation

A 53-year-old woman with right knee pain presents to her local primary care physician for evaluation and treatment. The knee pain has occurred almost daily for 6 months and is localized to the medial aspect of the knee. She rates her current pain as 4 on a scale of 0 to 10, with 10 being the worst level of pain. She has taken daily over-the-counter maximum strength acetaminophen for over 4 weeks and, subsequently, daily maximum strength naproxen for a 6-week period, but this has not relieved her symptoms. Her pain fluctuates daily, ranging from 3 to 6, and is worse when she is going down stairs. She has some associated symptoms, including worsening fatigue and occasional sleep disturbance. She reports no symptoms of chronic anxiety or depression but admits that stress is associated with worsening symptoms. Physical exam is notable for a body mass index of 32 and bony prominence of the right knee. Bilateral standing radiographs indicate mild to moderate degenerative joint disease of the right knee, with cartilage loss on the medial aspect of the knee, moderate sclerosis, and osteophyte formation.

Osteoarthritis (OA) is the most prevalent form of arthritis, affecting more than 21 million adults in the United States. During the development of OA, degradation of the cartilage matrix occurs initially. It is typically slowly progressive, with cartilage degeneration and the resulting loss of joint space proceeding at a pace that is not continuous. Once the collagen network has been degraded, it does not return to its original state. Periarticular bone changes can occur, with resulting osteophyte formation. There also appears to be an inflammatory component to some forms of OA, with resulting stiffness, swelling, and synovitis. The pain experienced by an individual does not necessarily correspond to the degree of cartilage loss or OA findings obtained via imaging modalities, although in a single individual worsening pain might correlate inversely with joint space width. Risk factors for OA include age, trauma (i.e., anterior cruciate ligment tear), biomechanical overloading (i.e., obesity), and genetic cartilage defects.

OA as a disease not only is associated with significant pain but also contributes to disability in adults. The disability associated with OA has a significant impact on the quality of life of patients with OA. Based on demographic trends, the impact on U.S. patients is expected to worsen in the near future. The combination of an aging population and increasing obesity has resulted in rapid growth in the number of patients undergoing knee replacement surgery for the treatment of pain associated with OA, a trend that will only increase in the upcoming decades.[1,2] Total knee replacement can improve function and yields significant pain relief for the many patients who undergo the procedure.[3,4] However, there are significant numbers of patients who have mild to moderate OA for whom non-surgical nociceptive treatments might be more appropriate. In addition, the modest association between radiographic joint damage and pain in OA suggests that there might be other components of pain such as inflammation or abnormal central pain processing. A proportion of patients have ongoing pain postoperatively, again suggesting that factors other than peripheral, nociceptive pain mechanisms are involved.[5–7] As is the case with many chronic pain diseases, OA patient populations likely have distinct subgroups based on neurobiologic, psychological, and cognitive features.[8,9]

There are no known treatments that have been shown to reverse the progression of OA, although some treatments might slow the rate of progression. In addition to pain relief, the preservation of function is an important consideration. Pain related to underlying OA can result in decreased quality of life and progressive disability.[10] Current studies are aimed at developing an approach to pain and disability management in OA that takes into account the total joint as an organ, with a focus on patient symptoms that will have a significant impact on the human and medical costs associated with chronic arthritis pain.

DIAGNOSIS

Musculoskeletal pain is the most common reason for medical appointments in the United States, amounting to millions of visits and billions of dollars each year in healthcare costs and lost productivity. All groups of persons, regardless of age, gender, ethnicity, or cultural background, experience unrelieved pain at some point, but women are significantly more likely to develop chronic pain disorders. Despite significant strides in understanding acute pain and developing effective treatments, the development and treatment of chronic musculoskeletal pain is not fully understood.

OA is one potential contributing factor to chronic musculoskeletal pain. Most patients presenting with chronic joint pain will have a radiograph of the affected joint to evaluate for OA, bony masses, or internal derangement. Standard views of the joint are usually the best starting point; in addition, radiographs of the opposite, unaffected joint might be helpful in evaluating anatomy and degree of cartilage loss. Bilateral standing views of the knees can be very helpful in assessing the extent of degenerative joint disease and the relative degree of cartilage loss. Although radiographs provide important information about alignment and cartilage, magnetic resonance imaging is suitable for better evaluation of not only cartilage but also soft tissue contrast and complex geometry. Several ongoing longitudinal studies will eventually provide important information regarding cartilage morphology and the timing of surgical treatment.[11]

Every experienced clinician realizes that pain is highly variable among individuals. In chronic OA pain, there is often dissociation between pain perception and underlying pathology. The degree of pain might not correspond to the radiographic findings at the time of evaluation, and this should be kept in mind when evaluating an individual patient. Significant pain that is disproportionate to objective findings is challenging to treat and frustrating for patients and clinicians alike.

TREATMENT

Treatments for OA are aimed primarily at alleviating patients' symptoms and improving physical function. The case outlined above is fairly typical for initial self-management of OA symptoms. This patient has several options and might have an approach individualized for her care that includes weight loss, increased physical activity, or medially directed non-pharmacologic therapies in addition to optimizing her pharmacologic treatment.

There have been many advances in understanding pain that localizes to a specific joint, but the disease is heterogeneous, and what works for one patient might not address the needs of a different patient. More work is needed to address some of the critical questions related to prevention, treatment, and monitoring of knee OA pain that is personalized for an individual with symptoms. Most treatments for OA have thus far been developed for peripheral nociceptive factors. Pain in OA has been historically attributed in part to joint damage, and nearly all therapies have been aimed at treating the pain derived from this peripheral structural problem, including exercise, topical analgesics, oral non-steroidal anti-inflammatory drugs (NSAIDS) and opioids, local injections, and eventually joint replacement. Although there are numerous interventions for OA nociceptive pain, there is no known cure for the cartilage and bone changes, and many patients experience progression of significant symptoms over the course of many years.

Recent data from an international study conducted by a task force of Osteoarthritis Research Society International and Outcome Measures in Rheumatology suggest that decisions regarding total joint arthroplasty cannot be predicted on the basis of the severity of the patients' pain or physical limitations.[12] Total knee replacement certainly can improve function and yields significant pain relief for many patients who undergo the procedure.[13,14] However, there is evidence that some patients might have a significant component of centrally mediated pain that might be improved following joint replacement.[15]

General Approach

The American College of Rheumatology (ACR) completed a recent update of the recommendations for therapies for OA.[16] The guidelines for management of hip and knee OA were originally published in 2000, and additional recommendations were provided in 2005. The updated recommendations published in 2012 were developed using the Grades of Recommendation Assessment, Development and Evaluation approach,[17] which represents an advance in methodology over previously employed measures.[18] These recommendations were made based on a systematic approach to the best available evidence of safety and benefit.

A summary of the recommendations of the ACR for hip and knee OA are outlined in Tables 10.1–10.3. Recommendations were classified as "conditional" or "strong." Using a 5-point Likert scale, expert panelists were asked to make a recommendation for each modality in the setting of a clinical scenario. The scale provided to panelists included the following choices: strong recommendation to use, weak (or conditional) recommendation to use, no recommendation, weak (or conditional) recommendation not to use, and strong recommendation not to use. The strength of a recommendation is meant to serve as a proxy for the quality of the evidence supporting the use of the intervention, as well as the extent to which one can be confident in desirable effects. Non-pharmacologic interventions included in the strong recommendations are listed in Table 10.1.

Patients with OA might benefit from weight loss, even in small amounts. Cardiovascular exercise should be encouraged if not otherwise contraindicated. There is no preference for aquatic versus land based exercises, and any exercise regimen may be optimized for patient

Table 10.1 AMERICAN COLLEGE OF RHEUMATOLOGY GUIDELINES 2012: STRONG RECOMMENDATIONS FOR NON-PHARMACOLOGIC MANAGEMENT OF KNEE OR HIP OA

Participation in cardiovascular (aerobic) and/or resistance land-based exercise
Participate in aquatic exercise
Weight loss for persons who are overweight

preference and compliance. Avoidance of excessive weight gain and caution with load-bearing exercise should also be counseled. Non-pharmacologic conditional recommendations are listed in Table 10.2.

Assistive devices such as canes, supports, and braces might take some of the stress off of the affected joint. The use of medially directed patellar taping may be considered, in addition to instruction and participation in Tai Chi programs. Patients with medial compartment OA may consider wearing laterally wedged subtalar strapped insoles, and patients with lateral compartment OA may consider wearing medially wedged insoles. In addition to these recommendations,

Table 10.2 AMERICAN COLLEGE OF RHEUMATOLOGY GUIDELINES 2012: CONDITIONAL RECOMMENDATIONS FOR NON-PHARMACOLOGIC MANAGEMENT OF KNEE OR HIP OA

Participate in self-management programs
Manual therapy and supervised exercise
Psychosocial interventions
Instruction on the use of thermal agents
Use of walking aids as needed
For knee OA:
Use patellar taping that is medially directed
Wear medially wedged insoles for lateral compartment OA
Wear laterally wedged subtalar strapped insoles for medial compartment OA
Tai Chi programs
For moderate to severe knee OA:
Consideration of Chinese acupuncture
Transcutaneous electrical stimulation

patients might be able to treat pain flares with the application of cold for no longer than 15 min of contact time; this may be repeated as needed. For other patients with significant stiffness, the application of moderate heat might be of benefit. Good nutrition and avoidance of trauma to the joint are also essential. The treatment of associated aggravating factors such as secondary bursitis also should be considered if warranted. Recent studies have shown alterations in pain processing that indicate a component of central nervous system mediation of pain (e.g., the presence of hyperalgesia) among people with knee and hip OA. It remains unclear how pain processing affects coping strategies to manage pain and perform activities. As with any chronic pain state, reducing stress or addressing relaxation strategies might prove beneficial.

Analgesics

Pharmacologic treatments are outlined in Table 10.3.

Acetaminophen (or paracetamol outside of the United States) is available without a prescription and is recommended for patients as a first-line pharmacologic therapy. Acetaminophen is relatively

Table 10.3 AMERICAN COLLEGE OF RHEUMATOLOGY GUIDELINES 2012: CONDITIONAL RECOMMENDATIONS FOR PHARMACOLOGIC MANAGEMENT OF KNEE OR HIP OA

Acetaminophen
Oral NSAIDs
Topical NSAIDs for knee OA
Tramadol
Intra-articular corticosteroid injections

well tolerated when taken on a regular basis. Doses of 500 mg to 750 mg taken two to three times daily might provide significant relief. Caution should be used in patients with known liver disease. Patients should be counseled not to exceed 3000 mg of acetaminophen per day per updated recommendations, and they should note the content of mixed cold and flu remedies, as they might contain acetaminophen. Topical analgesic treatments contain salicylate and are available over the counter, and they might provide temporary relief. Patients who are allergic to aspirin or patients who take blood thinners should not use salicylate-based topical treatments until they have discussed potential side effects with their doctor. Capsaicin, made from chili pepper seeds, is another topical agent. Anecdotal reports suggest that capsaicin works best on joints that are close to the skin (i.e., fingers).

Anti-inflammatory Medications

NSAIDs target cyclooxygenase-1 and cyclooxygenase-2 (COX-2) and can provide relief from acute pain in patients with OA. However, they can cause or worsen gastritis, gastrointestinal hemorrhage or ulcers, renal insufficiency, congestive heart failure, hypertension, and cardiovascular disease. Also, many patients with arthritis have comorbidities; the use of NSAIDs is limited by their potential for interaction with other medications, in addition to their impact on underlying disease. Per ACR guidelines, topical NSAIDs, rather than oral NSAIDs, are recommended for consideration in persons older than 75 years of age.

COX-2-specific agents are approved in the United States by the U.S. Food and Drug Administration (FDA) and in Europe for use in arthritis patients. The gastrointestinal safety profile is more favorable for these agents, and they do not interfere with platelet activity, so they may be used in patients on warfarin. They should be used with caution in patients with renal or cardiovascular disease. The favorable gastrointestinal safety profile of COX-2 inhibitors is attenuated with the co-administration of aspirin.

Nonacetylated Salicylates

Nonacetylated salicylate compounds include choline magnesium trisalicylate. Doses of 500 to 750 mg two or three times daily are effective therapy for many patients and have been used by rheumatologists for the treatment of arthritis symptoms for many years. These medications have fewer adverse gastrointestinal side effects than regular aspirin compounds or NSAIDs.

Corticosteroids

Chronic systemic steroids should not be used for the management of OA. Local intra-articular injection of corticosteroids might provide significant relief of pain and stiffness, and despite the evidence in randomized trials, anecdotal reports suggest that some patients have long-lasting pain relief from a single injection.

The injection of corticosteroids into any joint should be performed in a sterile manner by physicians experienced with this technique; potential risks include infection, bleeding, bruising, lipodystrophy, and osteonecrosis. These complications are rare with careful technique in experienced hands. Patients might experience improvement of symptoms immediately after injection, and improvements might be greatest in those with joint effusion from whom synovial fluid is withdrawn prior to injection. Any synovial fluid present should be aspirated, if possible, with an aseptic technique before injection. The fluid should be sent for Gram stain, culture, cell count, and differential, and experienced personnel should perform an examination for crystals. Limited studies of some forms of intra-articular injections have shown no effect on the progression of radiographic disease.

Viscosupplementation

Viscosupplements such as injectable hyaluronate are approved by the FDA and might provide modest relief. These were not included in the recommendations set out by the ACR.

Alternative Treatments

Many patients with OA use alternative therapies to try to relieve their symptoms. Many non-prescription supplements have not shown significant results in limited studies. Glucosamine and chondroitin sulfate are by far the most studied agents in this category, but their mechanism of action is unknown. Glucosamine and chondroitin sulfate at a dose of 1200 to 1500 mg daily appears to be safe in most patients with OA, and some studies suggest that their efficacy is similar to that of NSAIDs and acetaminophen. The ACR guidelines conditionally recommended *against* the use of glucosamine and chondroitin sulfate for patients with knee OA, citing significant heterogeneity in effect size in published trials.

Acupuncture, although used by many patients, has not been shown to be of consistent benefit in trials. Risks include reports of hepatitis transmission and pneumothorax.

Traditional Chinese acupuncture was recommended for consideration only in the setting of chronic pain and moderate to severe OA for which there is a relative or absolute contraindication to surgery.

Instruction in the use of transcutaneous electrical stimulation was similarly conditionally recommended only if the patient has moderate to severe pain and is a candidate for knee arthroplasty but is unwilling or unable to undergo the procedure.

Narcotic Analgesics

Narcotic analgesics should not be routinely used for patients with chronic OA, although they may serve a short-term role as a bridge to surgical intervention for patients with advanced joint disease. They may also be reserved for patients with severe joint disease and intolerable suffering who are not candidates for other therapeutic interventions. Lower potency medications, such as combination tramadol/acetaminophen or acetaminophen with codeine, should be tried first. Usual precautions should be taken when prescribing these, such as counseling patients about their correct use, sedative effects, and addictive potential. Additional caution should be used with older patients or patients with more co-morbidities. In the case of presumed tolerance or minimal efficacy with low-dose opioids, referral to a pain specialist or rheumatologist is warranted, as higher doses of opioids will seldom provide long-term benefit.

Centrally Acting Agents

"Central pain" is used to describe any central nervous system dysfunction or pathology that might be contributing to the development or maintenance of chronic pain. Central mechanisms that enhance the perception or modulation of pain differentially have also been referred to as central augmentation or amplification. This type of pain mechanism was originally thought to be confined to individuals with idiopathic or functional pain syndromes, such as fibromyalgia, headache, irritable bowel syndrome, temporomandibular joint disorder, and interstitial cystitis. These pain syndromes have been shown to be familial/genetic (e.g., the risk of developing fibromyalgia is eight times higher in first-degree relatives of patients with fibromyalgia). This type of pain often co-aggregates with other centrally mediated symptoms such as fatigue, memory difficulties, and mood disturbances.[19] Recent twin studies support a genetic basis of pain, as well as this cluster of co-aggregating symptoms.

Central factors might play a role in pain related to OA. Emerging research suggests that many patients with OA demonstrate signs of generalized hyperalgesia and faulty central pain modulatory processing similar to those seen with other idiopathic pain disorders.[20] Further work to establish the optimal means of quantifying and predicting pain is needed, particularly in patients with diffuse pain syndromes and OA. The recent FDA approval of a dual reuptake antidepressant (duloxetine) for musculoskeletal pain such as OA highlights the considerable amount of data that supports this approach.[21]

OA may also be viewed in some cases as a mixed pain state, with some individuals possessing more prominent features of central pain. In some patients, central factors might be superimposed upon the more traditional peripheral factors, leading to the need for a broader and more flexible approach to diagnosis and treatment. Patients with OA demonstrate signs of generalized hyperalgesia and faulty central pain modulatory processing similar to those seen with other idiopathic pain disorders.[20]

Because OA is a potentially mixed pain state, there are tremendous opportunities to move toward individualized analgesia by identifying individuals with OA who have a primary central component of pain that would likely preferentially respond to therapies known to be effective in central pain states such as centrally acting analgesics (e.g., dual reuptake inhibitors, gabapentinoids) and non-pharmacological therapies (exercise or cognitive behavioral therapy). Duloxetine is now approved for musculoskeletal pain, including OA.[21] Additional centrally acting agents that might be of benefit include gabapentin, pregabalin, or other dual reuptake inhibitors such as milnacipran. Low doses of amitriptyline or nortriptyline might prove beneficial, particularly for nighttime pain. Additional studies in this area are needed to guide treatment options in this area.

Surgical Intervention

Arthroscopy is under review by the ACR and is not recommended in European League Against Rheumatism guidelines.[22] It may still be used on a case-by-case basis for specific indications. Osteotomy is another surgical treatment for OA that is aimed at delaying disease progression, but additional studies with long-term follow-up are needed.

Arthroplasty is now used to treat many patients with severe OA, especially in those for whom more-conservative measures have failed. The life of a joint replacement is typically 10 to 20 years, although some patients do well for much longer. The reported failure rate following hip arthroplasty (due to pain) is quite high at approximately 10 percent, and it is even higher (approximately 15 percent to 20 percent) for knee replacement surgery.[23,24] This severe pain persists at least 3 to 4 years after surgery in some patients and is not thought to have a peripheral neuropathic component.[24] Replacement after the original joint arthroplasty surgery might be more complex and can have higher failure and infection rates than initial total joint replacement.

CONCLUSIONS

OA is the most common form of arthritis in the United States, and chronic pain related to underlying OA increases with advancing age. Many patients can achieve relief of their symptoms of chronic joint pain with appropriate care; however, further research is needed in order to improve the long-term outcomes of this disease. Advances in joint replacement surgery have made this an excellent treatment for many patients with more-severe disease. Additional studies are needed to further characterize disease-specific molecular pathways that may serve as potential targets for intervention.

REFERENCES

1. Lawrence RC, Felson DT, Helmick CG, et al. Estimates of the prevalence of arthritis and other rheumatic conditions in the United States. Part II. *Arthritis Rheum.* 2008;58:26–35.
2. Kurtz SM, Ong KL, Schmier J, et al. Future clinical and economic impact of revision total hip and knee arthroplasty. *J Bone Joint Surg Am.* 2007;89 Suppl 3:144–151.
3. Dunbar MJ. Subjective outcomes after knee arthroplasty. *Acta Orthop Scand Suppl.* 2001;72:1–63.
4. Jones CA, Voaklander DC, Johnston DW, Suarez-Almazor ME. Health related quality of life outcomes after total hip and knee arthroplasties in a community based population. *J Rheumatol.* 2000;27:1745–1752.
5. Baker PN, van der Meulen JH, Lewsey J, Gregg PJ. The role of pain and function in determining patient satisfaction after total knee replacement. Data from the National Joint Registry for England and Wales. *J Bone Joint Surg Br.* 2007;89:893–900.
6. Dickstein R, Heffes Y, Shabtai EI, Markowitz E. Total knee arthroplasty in the elderly: patients' self-appraisal 6 and 12 months postoperatively. *Gerontology.* 1998;44:204–210.
7. Robertsson O, Dunbar M, Pehrsson T, Knutson K, Lidgren L. Patient satisfaction after knee arthroplasty: a report on 27,372 knees operated on between 1981 and 1995 in Sweden. *Acta Orthop Scand.* 2000;71:262–267.
8. Edwards RR, Haythornthwaite JA, Smith MT, Klick B, Katz JN. Catastrophizing and depressive symptoms as prospective predictors of outcomes following total knee replacement. *Pain Res Manag.* 2009;14:307–311.
9. Sullivan M, Tanzer M, Stanish W, et al. Psychological determinants of problematic outcomes following total knee arthroplasty. *Pain.* 2009;143:123–129.
10. Losina E, Walensky RP, Reichmann WM, et al. Impact of obesity and knee osteoarthritis on morbidity and mortality in older Americans. *Ann Intern Med.* 2011;154:217–226.
11. Knoop J, van der Leeden M, Thorstensson CA, et al. Identification of phenotypes with different clinical outcomes in knee osteoarthritis: data from the Osteoarthritis Initiative. *Arthritis Care Res (Hoboken).* 2011;63:1535–1542.
12. Gossec L, Paternotte S, Maillefert JF, et al. The role of pain and functional impairment in the decision to recommend total joint replacement in hip and knee osteoarthritis: an international cross-sectional study of 1909 patients. Report of the OARSI-OMERACT Task Force on total joint replacement. *Osteoarthritis Cartilage.* 2011;19:147–154.
13. Callaghan JJ, Bracha P, Liu SS, Piyaworakhun S, Goetz DD, Johnston RC. Survivorship of a Charnley total hip arthroplasty. A concise follow-up, at

a minimum of thirty-five years, of previous reports. *J Bone Joint Surg Am.* 2009;91:2617–2621.

14. Callaghan JJ, Wells CW, Liu SS, Goetz DD, Johnston RC. Cemented rotating-platform total knee replacement: a concise follow-up, at a minimum of twenty years, of a previous report. *J Bone Joint Surg Am.* 2010;92:1635–1639.
15. Graven-Nielsen T, Wodehouse T, Langford RM, Arendt-Nielsen L, Kidd BL. Normalisation of widespread hyperesthesia and facilitated spatial summation of deep-tissue pain in knee osteoarthritis patients after knee replacement. *Arthritis Rheum.* 2012;64(9):2907–2916.
16. Hochberg MC, Altman RD, April KT, et al. American College of Rheumatology 2012 recommendations for the use of nonpharmacologic and pharmacologic therapies in osteoarthritis of the hand, hip, and knee. *Arthritis Care Res (Hoboken).* 2012;64:465–474.
17. Guyatt GH, Oxman AD, Schunemann HJ, Tugwell P, Knottnerus A. GRADE guidelines: a new series of articles in the *Journal of Clinical Epidemiology. J Clin Epidemiol.* 2011;64:380–382.
18. Recommendations for the medical management of osteoarthritis of the hip and knee: 2000 update. American College of Rheumatology Subcommittee on Osteoarthritis Guidelines. *Arthritis Rheum.* 2000;43:1905–1915.
19. Murphy SL, Lyden AK, Phillips K, Clauw DJ, Williams DA. Subgroups of older adults with osteoarthritis based upon differing comorbid symptom presentations and potential underlying pain mechanisms. *Arthritis Res Ther.* 2011;13:R135.
20. Phillips K, Clauw DJ. Central pain mechanisms in chronic pain states—maybe it is all in their head. *Best Pract Res Clin Rheumatol.* 2011;25:141–154.
21. Chappell AS, Ossanna MJ, Liu-Seifert H, et al. Duloxetine, a centrally acting analgesic, in the treatment of patients with osteoarthritis knee pain: a 13-week, randomized, placebo-controlled trial. *Pain.* 2009;146:253–260.
22. Harris WH, Sledge CB. Total hip and total knee replacement (2). *N Engl J Med* 1990;323:801–807, 725–731.
23. Wylde V, Blom AW, Whitehouse SL, Taylor AH, Pattison GT, Bannister GC. Patient-reported outcomes after total hip and knee arthroplasty: comparison of midterm results. *J Arthroplasty* 2009;24:210–216.
24. Wylde V, Hewlett S, Learmonth ID, Dieppe P. Persistent pain after joint replacement: prevalence, sensory qualities, and postoperative determinants. *Pain* 2011;152:566–572.

11

Neuropathies: DPN, HIV, Idiopathic

CHRISTINA M. ULANE AND THOMAS H. BRANNAGAN III

Case Presentation

A 59-year-old man with a history of right hip replacement and coronary artery disease is referred for evaluation of pain and paresthesias in his hands and feet. His symptoms began approximately 5 months ago, initially with numbness, tingling, and sharp radiating pain in his feet; his pain later involved his fingers. He notes that the left side is more symptomatic than the right, and that the numbness is constant but the pain and paresthesias are intermittent. His initial evaluation revealed vitamin B12 deficiency due to pernicious anemia from *H. pylori* gastritis. He was started on B12 injections, and his symptoms stabilized. However, his symptoms progressed from involving just the feet to including the ankles, and from just the fingers to his entire hands. His symptoms are worse at the end of the day. He denies weakness. He was given a trial of pregabalin for the pain and paresthesias, but he experienced no improvement, so this was discontinued.

His neurological exam is notable for normal muscle bulk and strength and reflexes. He has loss of sensation to pinprick and temperature in a stocking-and-glove distribution, to the mid-calves and in the fingertips. There is allodynia to light touch, and vibration sense is decreased in the toes and ankles. Laboratory evaluation revealed mildly impaired glucose tolerance (IGT) on the 2-hour glucose tolerance test (fasting glucose, 101 mg/dL [abnormal = 100–125 mg/dL]; 2 hours post 75 g oral dextrose, 151 mg/dL [abnormal = 140–199 mg/dL]) and slightly elevated hemoglobin A1C at 6.0 percent (normal < 5.7 percent) but was otherwise unremarkable. Electrophysiologic testing revealed a large-fiber, axonal, sensory polyneuropathy with a mild left median neuropathy at the wrist, consistent with carpal tunnel syndrome. Based on the clinical picture and supplementary data, he was diagnosed with peripheral neuropathy due to B12 deficiency and IGT. He was counseled regarding diet, exercise, and the importance of glycemic control to prevent further progression and possibly improve his symptoms.

He remained stable for 1 year, but at follow-up evaluation the numbness had progressed from the feet to the knees, and he had begun to experience a new burning pain. This traveled around, at times on his lips, and at other times on his thigh or scalp. He also complained of increased sensitivity to pressure and touch, which he noticed when he lightly stubbed his toe. In addition, he noticed muscle fatigue and aching in the forearms and ankles. Pregabalin was prescribed in the setting of the new symptoms of evoked pain and dysesthesias, this time with notable benefit.

DIAGNOSIS OF PAINFUL PERIPHERAL NEUROPATHY

The International Association for the Study of Pain (IASP) recently redefined neuropathic pain as "pain arising as a direct consequence of a lesion or disease affecting the somatosensory system."[1] The IASP proposes a grading system with the following key features: pain in a neuroanatomically plausible distribution, history suggesting a lesion or disease affecting the somatosensory system, demonstration of a neuroanatomically plausible distribution by at least one confirmatory test, and demonstration of the lesion or disease by at least one confirmatory test. Based on these criteria, patients can be classified as having definite, probable, or possible neuropathic pain. The prevalence of painful peripheral neuropathy is difficult to accurately assess, given the variability in presentation, definition, and patient reporting; however, studies suggest that up to 10 percent of the general population experiences neuropathic pain.

Neuropathic pain has certain qualities and anatomic distribution patterns that distinguish it from mechanical or nociceptive pain, and which might identify an etiology. Neuropathic pain is often described by patients as electric-shock-like, shooting, or burning. It can occur spontaneously in the absence of stimuli, in response to non-noxious or noxious stimuli (sincehyperalgesia is increased pain to noxious stimulation), or accompanied by paresthesias (non-painful abnormal sensations, such as "pins and needles"). Furthermore, neuropathic pain can also be vague, diffuse, and asymmetric. These qualities may be found with neuropathic pain of either central or peripheral origin, and the neuroanatomic distribution can help delineate the origin. For example, in painful peripheral neuropathies, pain will often follow the pattern of the neuropathy. In length-dependent peripheral neuropathies (such as diabetic neuropathy), pain often begins in the toes and feet and progresses more proximally. Because the longer nerves of the lower extremities are more vulnerable to metabolic and toxic injuries, early involvement of the hands should make one consider other diagnoses, such as coexistent carpal tunnel syndrome.

Additional information that supports the diagnosis of peripheral neuropathic pain is evidence of a lesion or damage to the somatosensory system. Neurological exam might reveal an area of sensory deficit to one or more modalities (even in the presence of allodynia). Electrodiagnostic studies can also provide useful information regarding the presence and nature of peripheral neuropathy. These objective findings indicating damage to the peripheral sensory system are often found in the same or overlapping regions as the neuropathic pain.

WORK-UP AND ETIOLOGY OF PERIPHERAL NEUROPATHY

There are over 200 known causes of peripheral neuropathy, yet in up to 40 percent of patients an identifiable cause is not found. The possible etiologies for peripheral neuropathy are diverse and include metabolic, nutritional, infectious, immune-mediated, and hereditary causes. Diabetes mellitus is the most common cause of neuropathy, but others to consider include vitamin deficiency (especially of B12), monoclonal gammopathy (due to myelodysplastic syndromes or amyloidosis), human immunodeficiency virus (HIV), alcohol toxicity, paraneoplastic, inflammation (acute or chronic inflammatory demyelinating neuropathies), autoimmune disease (e.g., Sjogren's syndrome), other connective tissue diseases, toxic neuropathies (e.g., chemotherapy, antifungal agents, lead poisoning), and vasculitis. It is beyond the scope of this chapter to review these causes and their detailed work-ups; however, general principles and a list of practical screening tests are recommended. As with any medical condition, a detailed history and examination are necessary, including a focused neurological exam testing all sensory modalities. Clinically, peripheral neuropathies can be categorized based on pattern (focal or diffuse), fiber-type involvement (large or small, motor, sensory, or mixed), and electrophysiologic findings (axonal or demyelinating). Focal neuropathies are typified by median neuropathy and the clinical syndrome of carpal tunnel syndrome, or by compression neuropathies (radial nerve palsy). Diffuse neuropathies are typically length dependent, starting in the feet and progressing proximally, with later involvement of the hands; they are most often symmetric. Neurological examination should include tests for muscle strength, reflexes (especially ankle jerks), pinprick and temperature sensation (small-fiber), vibratory and joint position sense (large-fiber), and Romberg sign. Sensory testing might elicit paresthesias or allodynia.

There are various laboratory tests that can be obtained when screening for neuropathy, but it is neither efficient nor cost-effective to screen for all possible causes. When a patient is identified as having a length-dependent symmetric neuropathy, current recommendations for screening laboratory tests suggest blood glucose and/or glucose tolerance tests, vitamin B12 (and metabolites), and serum protein immunofixation.[2] Further laboratory tests to consider include hemoglobin A1C, complete blood count, liver function tests, creatinine, erythrocyte sedimentation rate, and vitamin B6 (either in excess or deficiency). A rheumatologic work-up and cerebrospinal fluid analysis might help identify or rule out inflammatory causes.

Electrodiagnostic testing (nerve conduction studies and electromyography, performed together) can further delineate and specify the type of fiber involvement and pattern of neuropathy as an extension of the neurological exam, and it often can detect abnormalities before they are clinically apparent. Nerve conduction studies distinguish axonal and demyelinating injuries, and electromyography assesses whether there is ongoing denervation or chronic neurogenic changes. Importantly, electrodiagnosis provides an assessment of the large fibers only, and thus in a purely small-fiber neuropathy, testing can be completely normal. Small-fiber neuropathy can be assessed via skin biopsy, which might reveal decreased epidermal nerve fiber density. Evaluation for neuropathy is important even in patients with

STEP 1: History and Exam

- Co-morbidities
- Family history
- Acute, subacute or chronic onset
- Pattern of sensory abnormalities and pain
- Fiber-type involvement (pain and temperature or vibration and joint-position sense)
- Pattern of involvement – symmetrical, multifocal, or proximal weakness

⇓

STEP 2: Laboratory Testing

- Hemoglobin A1C, Fasting Glucose, 2h glucose tolerance test, B12, methylmalonic acid, B6, serum immunofixation,
- Consider: thyroid stimulating hormone, erythrocyte sedimentation rate, anti-nuclear antibody
- Consider lumbar puncture if one suspects neoplastic, infectious or inflammatory etiology (or if there are demyelinating findings on electrodiagnostics)

⇓

STEP 3: Further Studies

- Electrodiagnostic studies (axonal vs demyelinating, symmetrical vs multifocal)
- Consider skin biopsy (if suspect small-fiber neuropathy *and* all other testing is negative)

Figure 11.1. Evaluation of peripheral neuropathy.

known diabetes mellitus, as these patients might have additional causes of neuropathy. On average, 25 percent of all neuropathies and 50 percent of small-fiber neuropathies are idiopathic (see Fig. 11.1).

In the case presented above, the patient had symptoms consistent with both small- and large-fiber neuropathy. His vitamin B12 levels were initially low and appropriately corrected. Deficiency in vitamin B12 can cause myriad neurological symptoms, but it often affects the large fibers of peripheral nerves, which are responsible for vibration and joint-position sense, rather than pain and temperature.

In addition, he was also found to have IGT, which can cause a painful, small-fiber sensory neuropathy.

Although diabetes mellitus is by far the most common cause of peripheral neuropathy, there is growing evidence that the pre-diabetic state of IGT is also associated with small-fiber peripheral neuropathy.[3] A causal relationship and the identification of mechanisms have not been clearly delineated, yet there is a general consensus that an association between IGT and peripheral neuropathy exists. There are also some data that suggest that attaining near-normal glycemic control can delay the progression of neuropathy and relieve painful neuropathy symptoms.[4] Eighty percent of patients with diabetic neuropathy have no symptoms; however, for some patients who have pain, it might be severe.

HIV sensory neuropathy may be caused by the HIV virus itself, coexisting infection related to immunosuppression (e.g., cytomegalovirus), or treatment with nucleoside reverse transcriptase inhibitors (e.g., stavudine, didanosine). These etiologies might coexist in a single patient and are clinically indistinguishable. With the advent of antiretroviral treatment, morbidity and mortality for HIV have declined significantly. Neurological complications of HIV are also on the decline, yet peripheral neuropathy has become the most common neurological symptom seen.

When treating painful peripheral neuropathy, clear expectations should be discussed with the patient. In this case, despite B12 supplementation, the patient continued to have symptoms requiring treatment. It is crucial for patients and physicians to realize that the complete elimination of pain is often not possible (especially with severe and long-standing symptoms), but pain reduction and functional improvement are achievable. One study showed that in patients with all types of chronic pain (neuropathic and other), 50 percent experienced at least 30 percent reduction in pain severity.[5] As each patient is different, time and patience are required in order to obtain the most effective pain treatment regimen.

MECHANISMS OF PERIPHERAL NEUROPATHIC PAIN

Under physiologic circumstances, pain arises when peripheral nociceptive afferents are activated by either actual or potential tissue damage. Neuropathic pain occurs when this system is activated in the absence of adequate stimulation. There are multiple mechanisms that can cause neuropathic pain, and different disease processes can share similar mechanisms. Multiple mechanisms of neuropathic pain can be present in one individual, and different mechanisms can lead to similar clinical symptoms. Research has identified several potential mechanisms of neuropathic pain that include changes in sodium channel expression, the accumulation and redistribution of sodium channels, central sensitization, peripheral sensitization, changes in α-adrenergic receptor expression, sympathetic sprouting, enhanced transmission, and reduced inhibition. This complex array of mechanisms leads to both spontaneous pain and abnormal evoked pain responses.[6] Although clinically difficult, the identification of neuropathic pain mechanisms is a growing area of research, given the widespread consensus that the mechanistic-based treatment of pain might be associated with better outcomes than etiologic-based therapy.[7]

Pain in the absence of appropriate physiological stimuli is generated by ectopic or spontaneous activity in injured and nearby nociceptive afferent fibers. Studies in animals and humans have suggested a role for the increased expression of sodium channels, which is hypothesized to lower the threshold for action potential firing. Potassium and potentially calcium channel modulation might also play a role. In the case presentation, the patient's initial spontaneous pain did not respond to pregabalin. It is therefore possible that his spontaneous pain was a result of ion channel dysfunction that was not targeted by pregabalin (which acts via voltage-gated calcium channels), which would explain why he did not initially respond.

Apart from peripheral ectopic activity, central sensitization can also occur. Primary pain afferents reach the spinal cord via the dorsal root ganglia, where they activate second-order nociceptive neurons. Continuous ectopic activity, inflammatory responses in the spinal cord, and the loss of inhibitory pathways (involving GABAergic interneurons in the spinal cord and descending monoaminergic and opiodergic pathways) all contribute to the development of chronic neuropathic pain. These mechanisms form the rationale for the treatment options that are currently available, as well as those under investigation.[8,9] In addition, pathways involved in central sensitization might be responsible for hyperesthesia, and this would provide a possible explanation as to why the patient responded to pregabalin after he developed the new symptoms of evoked pain and allodynia.[6]

Biologically active molecules implicated in chronic neuropathic pain include excitatory amino acids, spinal nitric oxide, and the melanocortin system, all of which are under investigation as potential therapeutic targets. More directly linked to currently available treatments are pathways involving spinal inflammatory cytokines such as tumor necrosis factor-α and interleukin-1; prostaglandin-mediated stimulation of peripheral afferent fibers (and their role in central sensitization); endogenous opioids involved in central inhibition; the noradrenergic and serotonergic systems; and GABAergic spinal inhibitory pathways. In some of the aforementioned systems, mechanisms of action (e.g., norepinephrine) are complex and can be either activating or inhibitory, depending on the site of action.[9]

TREATMENT OF PAINFUL PERIPHERAL NEUROPATHY

In evaluating and treating patients with peripheral neuropathy, the first goal is to identify the cause of the peripheral neuropathy, in hopes of finding a reversible or treatable condition. For some patients, such as those with idiopathic neuropathy, there is no effective treatment for the nerve damage itself. For others, recovery might be slow and dependent on nerve regeneration, so their treatment is directed at the symptoms of pain. Peripheral neuropathic pain is resistant to traditional analgesics such as non-steroidal anti-inflammatories and acetaminophen, though these tend to be amongst the most commonly prescribed drugs for the conditions. There are several consensus criteria and treatment algorithms for neuropathic pain. Some criteria group all types of neuropathic pain together regardless of etiology or whether the pain is central or peripheral in origin, whereas others separate out the various types of neuropathic pain. In general, treatment principles are similar (see Fig. 11.2): first-line agents include tricyclic antidepressants (TCAs), calcium channel binding antiepileptics (e.g., gabapentin and pregabaline), and in some instances serotonin and norepinephrine reuptake inhibitors (SNRIs), and second-line agents include opioids and tramadol.

Certain differences do exist, particularly with respect to postherpetic neuralgia (see Chapter 12). With regard to painful peripheral neuropathy, treatment algorithms are similar, with exceptions for diabetic neuropathy and HIV neuropathy. For HIV neuropathy, only 8 percent topical capsaicin patch (Neurogesx or Qutenza) and lamotrigine have proven effective.[10] Many studies have shown negative results for treating HIV neuropathy with agents that work for other causes of neuropathy. Negative results have been reported for pregabalin, gabapentin, and amitriptyline in HIV neuropathy.[11]

Important components of treating painful peripheral neuropathy are the global assessment and co-morbidities of the patient. For instance, given the debilitating nature of chronic neuropathic pain, depression, anxiety, and insomnia often coexist in these patients,

Diagnosis of Peripheral Neuropathic Pain

Patient identified with signs and symptoms of painful peripheral neuropathy (neurological exam, diagnostics)

⇩

1st Line Agents:

- ***TCAs*** (tricyclic antidepressants: nortriptyline, amitriptyline,)
- ***SNRIs*** (serotonin and norepinephrine reuptake inhibitors: duloxetine, venlafaxine)
- ***Calcium channel a2-δligands*** (pregabalin, gabapentin)
- ***Topical lidocaine*** (5%)
- ****DPN*-pregabalin, SNRIs
- ****HIV*-lamotrigine, topical capsaicin (8%)

⇩

2nd Line Agents:

- ***Tramadol***
- ***Opioids***
- ***Antiepileptics*** (lamotrigine, oxcarbazepine)

Figure 11.2. Management of peripheral neuropathic pain.

and this might help the physician tailor treatment. In addition, medical co-morbidities such as obesity and heart disease will also contribute to treatment choice based on certain side-effect profiles (see Table 11.1).

Antidepressants

Within this group, the TCAs and SNRIs are most often utilized. This class of agents might be particularly helpful in patients suffering from co-morbid depression or anxiety. In general, the

Table 11.1 PERIPHERAL NEUROPATHIC PAIN MEDICATION PROFILES

Drug	*Mechanism*	*Side Effects*	*Dosing*	*Additional Benefits*
TCAs (nortriptyline, amitriptyline)	Serotonin and/or norepinephrine reuptake inhibition in descending pathways; sodium channel, adenosine, and *N*-methyl-D-aspartate receptor blockade; anticholinergic effects; activation of α-2 receptors (sympatholysis)	Sedation Anticholinergic effects (dry mouth, urinary retention) Weight gain *Caution:* Cardiac disease (check electrocardiogram) Glaucoma Epilepsy Concomitant use of tramadol (serotonin syndrome)	Amitriptyline: • Start 10 to 25 mg qhs • Maintenance on 50 to 150 mg/d Nortriptyline: • Start 10 to 25 mg qhs • Maintenance on 50 to 150 mg/d	Helpful for insomnia, depression

α2-δ ligands (pregabalin, gabapentin)	neurotransmitters by binding to voltage-gated calcium channels on primary afferent nociceptors	Dizziness Peripheral edema Weight gain *Caution:* Adjust dose for renal insufficiency	• Start 75 mg bid • Maintenance on 150 to 300 mg bid *Gabapentin:* • Start 100 mg tid • Maintenance on 300 mg tid to 1200 mg qid	significant drug interactions
SNRIs (duloxetine, venlafaxine, milnacipran)	Serotonin and norepinephrine reuptake inhibition	Nausea *Caution:* Hepatic dysfunction, renal insufficiency, alcohol abuse (duloxetine) Cardiac disease, withdrawal syndrome with abrupt discontinuation (venlafaxine) Concomitant use of tramadol (serotonin syndrome)	Duloxetine: • Start 20 to 30 mg daily • Maintenance on 60 to 120 mg/d Venlafaxine: • Start 37.5 mg daily • Maintenance on 150 to 375 mg/d Milnacipran: • Start 12.5 mg daily • Maintenance on 50 to 100 mg/d	Helpful for depression

(continued)

Table 11.1 (CONTINUED)

Drug	*Mechanism*	*Side Effects*	*Dosing*	*Additional Benefits*
Topical capsaicin (0.025 percent to 0.075 percent)	TRPV1 receptor agonism, blockade of voltage-activated calcium channels, depletion of substance P	Transient site erythema, pain with initial applications	Must apply three to four times per day. Beneficial effects might not be noted for >1 week	No systemic effects
Topical capsaicin (8 percent)	TRPV1 receptor agonism, causing influx of calcium and impaired local nociceptor function	Can cause transient site erythema, pain	Pretreat with topical anesthetic; apply up to four patches to affected area for 60 min Repeat application q3 months	No systemic effects
Topical lidocaine (5 percent)	Sodium channel blockade	Can cause transient site erythema, rash	Start one patch for 12 hours Maintenance: one to three patches for 12 hours	No systemic effects

Opioids (controlled-release [CR] oxycodone, methadone)	μ-receptor agonism (also κ-receptor agonism for oxycodone)	Nausea/vomiting Constipation Dizziness *Caution:* History of substance abuse Suicide risk Driving impairment	Oxycodone CR: • Start 10 mg daily • Maintenance on 40 mg daily Methadone: • Start 5 mg daily • Maintenance on 10 to 20 mg daily	Rapid onset
Tramadol	μ-receptor agonism, serotonin and norepinephrine reuptake inhibition	Nausea/vomiting Constipation Dizziness *Caution:* History of substance abuse Suicide risk Driving impairment Concomitant use of SNRI, TCA (serotonin syndrome)	Start 25 mg daily Maintenance on 200 to 400 mg daily	Rapid onset

(continued)

Table 11.1 (CONTINUED)

Drug	*Mechanism*	*Side Effects*	*Dosing*	*Additional Benefits*
Antiepileptics (lamotrigine, oxcarbazepine)	Lamotrigine: voltage-dependent sodium channel blocker Oxcarbazapine: sodium-channel blocker	Lamotrigine: Risk of rash and Stevens-Johnson Syndrome Oxcarbazapine: Somnolence Dizziness Gait disturbance Rarely, leukopenia, rash, hepatotoxicity, hyponatremia	Lamotrigine: • Start 25 mg daily • Maintenance on 100 to 250 mg bid Oxcarbazepine: • Start 75 mg qhs • Maintenance on 300 to 1200 mg bid	Lamotrigine might be beneficial in patients with bipolar disease

dosages employed, blood levels required for a therapeutic effect, and onset of effect are all lower and shorter for the treatment of pain than of depression. Thus, the side-effect profiles of these drugs might be more favorable for treating pain than for treating depression. TCAs have several modes of action, including inhibition of the reuptake of serotonin and/or norepinephrine, which might increase the activity of inhibitory pathways. Clinical trials for selective serotonin reuptake inhibitors such as fluoxetine have mostly been negative, suggesting that both norepinephrine and serotonin reuptake inhibition are required for analgesia. Although their analgesic properties are thought to be independent of their antidepressant effects, as alluded to earlier, the latter is likely to contribute to their success in some circumstances. Side effects are mainly due to anticholinergic and antihistaminergic properties, which cause symptoms such as dry mouth and somnolence. Before initiating therapy with TCAs, an electrocardiogram to screen for a prolonged QT interval and a thorough cardiac history should be obtained.

Similarly, the SNRIs inhibit the reuptake of serotonin and norepinephrine. Duloxetine was the first medication to be approved by the U.S. Food and Drug Administration to treat diabetic neuropathic pain; however, it is used for other types of neuropathic pain as well, and it can be very effective. The main benefit of SNRIs over TCAs, which are more efficacious, is their better side-effect profile.

Anti-epileptics

Within this group, gabapentin and pregabalin are the most effective, best-studied, and most widely used agents for treating neuropathic pain. Both molecules act on calcium channels. Because of their favorable side-effect profile and minimal interactions with other medications, gabapentin and pregabalin are safe and effective. The main side effect is sedation, but gradual titration to therapeutic dose, with caution in the elderly, generally makes these drugs well tolerated. Other side effects include weight gain, which is more pronounced in the first 6 months. Pregabalin can be very effective in patients with painful diabetic neuropathy, as it is supported by "level A" evidence.[12]

When gabapentinoid drugs are poorly tolerated or ineffective, other anticonvulsants that act via different mechanisms can be considered. These include valproic acid, which modulates γ-aminobutyric acid pathways and multiple ion channels; lamotrigine, which blocks sodium channels and decreases the release of glutamate; oxcarbazepine, which acts as an antagonist at sodium and possibly calcium and potassium channels, and which might also reduce glutamate release; and, more recently, lacosamide, which also exerts its analgesic effects through sodium channels.

Opioids

The opioid system is another important component of pain pathways. There are three opioid receptors: μ (involved in supraspinal analgesia), κ, and δ (both involved in spinal analgesia). Opiate receptors are found both on peripheral nociceptive afferents and in the central nervous system, where they reside in the spinal cord, brainstem (periaqueductal gray), and higher limbic system. Opioids have been shown to reduce neuropathic pain of various etiologies (albeit in higher doses than typically employed for mechanical or visceral pain), with efficacy similar to the TCAs and gabapentin. However, because of their side-effect profile and concerns about misuse and abuse, opioids are not considered as first-line agents.[13]

Treatment Guidelines

Multiple consensus guidelines exist for the treatment of neuropathic pain. In general, first-line agents to be considered include TCAs (nortriptyline, amitriptyline, desiprimine), calcium channel ligands (gabapentin, pregabalin), SNRIs in the elderly (duloxetine, venlafaxine), and topical lidocaine patches for evoked pain (i.e., allodynia). Second-line agents include opioids (methadone, morphine sulfate, and oxycodone) and tramadol.

Recent studies have demonstrated that combination treatment with membrane stabilizers (e.g., gabapentin) and either TCAs or opioids can provide superior pain relief at lower doses, and with fewer side effects, than either agent given individually.[14,15] However, many individuals prefer to maximize one agent prior to starting another so as to better discern which drug is responsible for the beneficial and/or adverse effects.

SUMMARY

In conclusion, neuropathic pain is a common symptom for which patients will seek medical attention, often initially in the primary care setting. If a patient is suspected of having a peripheral neuropathy, a screening evaluation should be employed in order to appropriately treat underlying correctable conditions. Elimination of pain due to peripheral neuropathy is not always possible, but there are various treatment options that can be highly beneficial.

REFERENCES

1. Treede RD, Jensen TS, Campbell JN, et al. Neuropathic pain: redefinition and a grading system for clinical and research purposes. *Neurology*. 2008;70(18):1630–1635.

2. England JD, Gronseth GS, Franklin G, et al. Practice parameter: evaluation of distal symmetric polyneuropathy: role of autonomic testing, nerve biopsy, and skin biopsy (an evidence-based review). Report of the American Academy of Neurology, American Association of Neuromuscular and Electrodiagnostic Medicine, and American Academy of Physical Medicine and Rehabilitation. *Neurology*. 2009;72(2):177–184.
3. Rajabally YA. Neuropathy and impaired glucose tolerance: an updated review of the evidence. *Acta Neurol Scand*. 2011;124(1):1–8.
4. Smith AG, Singleton JR. Impaired glucose tolerance and neuropathy. *Neurologist*. 2008;14(1):23–29.
5. Turk DC. Clinical effectiveness and cost-effectiveness of treatments for patients with chronic pain. *Clin J Pain*. 2002;18(6):355–365.
6. Woolf CJ. Central sensitization: implications for the diagnosis and treatment of pain. *Pain*. 2011;152(3 Suppl):S2–S15.
7. Woolf CJ. Pain: moving from symptom control toward mechanism-specific pharmacologic management. *Ann Intern Med*. 2004;140(6):441–451.
8. Baron R, Binder A, Wasner G. Neuropathic pain: diagnosis, pathophysiological mechanisms, and treatment. *Lancet Neurol*. 2010;9(8):807–819.
9. Kumar S, Ruchi R, James SR, Chidiac EJ. Gene therapy for chronic neuropathic pain: how does it work and where do we stand today? *Pain Med*. 2011;12(5):808–822.
10. de Leon-Casasola O. New developments in the treatment algorithm for peripheral neuropathic pain. *Pain Med*. 2011;12(Suppl 3):S100–S108.
11. Phillips TJ, Cherry CL, Cox S, Marshall SJ, Rice AS. Pharmacological treatment of painful HIV-associated sensory neuropathy: a systematic review and meta-analysis of randomised controlled trials. *PLoS One*. 2010;5(12):e14433.
12. Bril V, England JD, Franklin GM, et al. Evidence-based guideline: treatment of painful diabetic neuropathy—report of the American Association of Neuromuscular and Electrodiagnostic Medicine, the American Academy of Neurology, and the American Academy of Physical Medicine & Rehabilitation. *Muscle Nerve*. 2011;43(6):910–917.
13. Dworkin RH, O'Connor AB, Audette J, et al. Recommendations for the pharmacological management of neuropathic pain: an overview and literature update. *Mayo Clin Proc*. 2010;85(3 Suppl):S3–S14.
14. Gilron I, Bailey JM, Tu D, Holden RR, Jackson AC, Houlden RL. Nortriptyline and gabapentin, alone and in combination for neuropathic pain: a double-blind, randomised controlled crossover trial. *Lancet*. 2009;374(9697):1252–1261.
15. Gilron I, Bailey JM, Tu D, Holden RR, Weaver DF, Houlden RL. Morphine, gabapentin, or their combination for neuropathic pain. *N Engl J Med*. 2005;352(13):1324–1334.

SUGGESTED READING

Brannagan TH III. Peripheral neuropathy pain: mechanisms and treatment. *J Clin Neuromuscul Dis.* 2003;5(2):61–71.

Dyck PJ, Thomas PK. *Peripheral Neuropathy*. 4th ed. Philadelphia: Saunders; 2005.

Brannagan T III. *Neuropathic pain.* In: Rowland LP, Pedley TA, Merritt HH, eds. *Merritt's Eurology.* 12th ed. Philadelphia: Lippincott Williams & Wilkins; 2010.

12

Chronic Post-surgical Pain

CHAD M. BRUMMETT AND SRINIVAS CHIRAVURI

Case Presentation

A 65-year-old male presents 8 months following a video-assisted thoracoscopic surgery (VATS) wedge resection for a lung mass. He describes burning and numbness in the areas around the puncture sites for his surgery. He prefers to not wear a shirt because of the irritation and holds his arm fixed away from his body. He has tried a variety of non-steroidal anti-inflammatory drugs (NSAIDs) and opioids, with only minimal improvement in his pain.

BACKGROUND

Chronic pain following surgery has likely occurred since the times of the first surgeries. Some surgeries are associated with higher rates of pain, but chronic pain has been reported in virtually every surgical condition in which it has been investigated. Despite the knowledge that chronic pain following surgery is common, physicians' ability to predict when patients are at risk in order to implement means of prevention is poor. There are many ongoing studies of the predictors of post-surgical pain, but we are likely many years away from meaningful improvement of the understanding of its development. Until that time, patients will continue to develop chronic pain and seek care for long-term management.

EPIDEMIOLOGY

As with most types of chronic pain, estimating the true incidence is exceedingly challenging. The most common conditions described include pain following inguinal hernia repair, breast surgery, thoracic surgery, amputation of a lower extremity, and coronary artery bypass surgery (CABG). The estimated prevalence of pain does vary some with the surgery performed; however, there are high rates noted in all of the commonly studied conditions (Table 12.1).[1]

Table 12.1 ESTIMATED INCIDENCE OF CHRONIC POSTOPERATIVE PAIN AND DISABILITY AFTER SELECTED SURGICAL PROCEDURES

	Estimated Incidence of Chronic Pain, %	*Estimated Chronic Severe (Disabling) Pain (>5 out of score of 10), %*	*U.S. Surgical Volumes (1000s)*[a]
Amputation[b]	30 to 50	5 to 10	159 (lower limb only)
Breast surgery (lumpectomy and mastectomy)[c]	20 to 30	5 to 10	479
Thoracotomy[d]	30 to 40	10	Unknown
Inguinal hernia repair[e]	10	2 to 4	609

(continued)

Table 12.1 (*CONTINUED*)

	Estimated Incidence of Chronic Pain, %	*Estimated Chronic Severe (Disabling) Pain (>5 out of score of 10), %*	*U.S. Surgical Volumes (1000s)*[a]
Coronary artery bypass surgery[f]	30 to 50	5 to 10	598
Caesarean section[g]	10	4	220

Note: Gall bladder surgery not included, because the preoperative diagnosis of pain specifically from gall bladder is difficult and persistent postoperative pain could therefore be related to other intra-abdominal disorders.

[a]National Center For Health Statistics, Ambulatory and Inpatients Procedures, USA, 1996.

[b]Data from Sandroni P, Benrud-Larson LM, McClelland RL, Low PA. Complex regional pain syndrome type I: incidence and prevalence in Olmsted County, a population-based study. *Pain.* 2003;103(1–2):199–207.

[c]Data from Bourne RB, Chesworth BM, Davis AM, Mahomed NN, Charron KD. Patient satisfaction after total knee arthroplasty: who is satisfied and who is not? *Clin Orthop Relat Res.* 2010;468(1):57–63.

[d]Data from Nikolajsen L, Brandsborg B, Lucht U, Jensen TS, Kehlet H. Chronic pain following total hip arthroplasty: a nationwide questionnaire study. *Acta Anaesthesiol Scand.* 2006;50(4):495–500; Gotoda Y, Kambara N, Sakai T, Kishi Y, Kodama K, Koyama T. The morbidity, time course and predictive factors for persistent post-thoracotomy pain. *Eur J Pain.* 2001;5(1):89–96; Wildgaard K, Ravn J, Nikolajsen L, Jakobsen E, Jensen TS, Kehlet H. Consequences of persistent pain after lung cancer surgery: a nationwide questionnaire study. *Acta Anaesthesiol Scand.* 2011;55(1):60–68; and Steegers MA, Snik DM, Verhagen AF, van der Drift MA, Wilder-Smith OH. Only half of the chronic pain after thoracic surgery shows a neuropathic component. *J Pain.* 2008;9(10):955–961.

[e]Data from Brummett CM. Chronic pain following breast surgery. *Techniques in Regional Anesthesia and Pain Medicine.* 2011;15(3):124–132; Gartner R, Jensen MB, Nielsen J, Ewertz M, Kroman N, Kehlet H. Prevalence of and factors associated with persistent pain following breast cancer surgery. *JAMA.* 2009;302(18):1985–1992; and Mikkelsen T, Werner MU, Lassen B, Kehlet H. Pain and sensory dysfunction 6 to 12 months after inguinal herniotomy. *Anesth Analg.* 2004;99(1):146–151.

[f]Data from Grant AM, Scott NW, O'Dwyer PJ. Five-year follow-up of a randomized trial to assess pain and numbness after laparoscopic or open repair of groin hernia. *Br J Surg.* 2004;91(12):1570–1574; Flor H. Phantom-limb pain: characteristics, causes, and treatment. *Lancet Neurol.* 2002;1(3):182–189; and Nikolajsen L, Jensen TS. Phantom limb pain. *Br J Anaesth.* 2001;87(1):107–116.

[g]Data from Eisenach JC, Pan PH, Smiley R, Lavand'homme P, Landau R, Houle TT. Severity of acute pain after childbirth, but not type of delivery, predicts persistent pain and postpartum depression. *Pain.* 2008;140(1):87–94.

Between 10 percent and 50 percent of patients will report chronic pain, and approximately 2 percent to 10 percent of the patients will describe the pain as severe or disabling. Complex regional pain syndrome (CRPS) can occur following distal extremity surgery.[2] CRPS is covered in Chapter 14.

When describing chronic pain after surgery, the above conditions are most commonly considered; however, there are also many patients having surgery to treat a painful condition who either fail to derive analgesic benefit or worsen after surgery. Total knee and hip arthroplasty are two such procedures with rates of failure to derive benefit estimated to be between 20 percent and 30 percent and between 10 percent and 20 percent, respectively.[3,4] The present chapter focuses on new chronic post-surgical pain; arthroplasties are described further in the osteoarthritis chapter (Chapter 10).

Although pain can present after any surgery, there are some particular surgical conditions that merit further discussion.

Thoracic Surgery

Chronic pain following thoracotomy has long been known to be a significant problem and has been the source of many studies of regional anesthesia and surgical techniques to prevent chronic pain.[5] Researchers and surgeons had hoped that the transition from thoracotomy to VATS would decrease the incidence of chronic pain; however, studies to date have demonstrated similar rates of chronic pain (25 percent to 47 percent).[6,7] Although there are no data for the prevalence of pain following robotic surgery (smaller trocars) and rates seem similar for VATS and thoracotomy, there are some data to suggest that pain after VATS might be less severe.[6] The rationale for the transition to VATS and robotic surgeries is based in large part on other measures of surgical recovery and will likely drive the use of these less invasive surgical techniques.

The type of pain reported after thoracic surgery is often neuropathic in nature. This is thought to be due to damage of the intercostal nerves during surgery. Thoracic surgery is sometimes performed for cancer, and patients often have chemotherapy and/or radiation following surgery. Either of these treatments has the potential to cause chronic pain independent of surgery.

Breast Surgery

Early recognition and improvements in treatment for breast cancer have led to an increased number of survivors. As a result, some of the focus in breast cancer therapy has transitioned from the treatment of the cancer to the long-term sequelae of cancer and its treatment. Chronic pain after breast surgery is now recognized as a common problem, with an estimated prevalence of between 29 percent and 47 percent.[1,8,9] The prevalence of severe or disabling pain is more challenging to estimate but might be as high as 10 percent to 13 percent. Despite the transition from radical mastectomies to less invasive surgeries (lumpectomy, partial mastectomy), the report of chronic pain remains high. Even more so than with other surgical conditions, the multiple treatment modalities that follow breast surgery, including radiation, chemotherapy, and hormonal therapies, likely impact the report of pain. There are no good data available that estimate the causal factors or contributions from each of the therapies, as most of the data come from survey studies done at delayed time points after surgery. Such studies have inherent limitations of recall bias and are unable to assess the temporal associations between treatment and the development of pain. Some researchers have speculated that the fear of cancer recurrence might drive some of the pain complaints.[8]

As with thoracic surgery, pain following breast surgery is commonly neuropathic in nature. Patients can have local tissue damage causing localized breast pain. Others can have pain in the axilla, upper arm, distal arm, and/or hand due to damage of the brachial plexus or intercostobrachial nerve during lymph node dissection or radiation.[8,9] Other potential causes of pain in breast cancer survivors include widespread arthralgias from aromatase-inhibitor therapy and chemotherapy-induced peripheral neuropathy.[8] Although it is important to understand the potential causes of the pain complaint, the therapeutic approaches are often quite similar once the patient has developed chronic pain.

Inguinal Hernia Repair

Although less common than some of the other described surgical conditions, pain following inguinal hernia surgery can be debilitating. The prevalence is estimated to be between 10 percent and 28 percent.[1,10] There are some prospectively collected data guiding these estimates. Pain following laproscopic surgery might be less common; however, surgical technique does not fully explain the varied patient outcomes.[11] The described pain is frequently neuropathic in nature and involves one or more of the sensory distributions of the groin, including the ilioinguinal, iliohypogastric, and genitofemoral nerves. Some experts believe that the chronic pain reported after inguinal hernia repair was present prior to surgery and possibly represents an inappropriate reason for surgery.

Post-amputation Pain

Chronic pain after amputation can present in a number of ways.[12,13] The most common presentation is neuropathic pain at the distal site of the amputation. Although not always present, neuromas at the amputation site can be a source of great discomfort and make it almost impossible for patients to tolerate prostheses (stump pain). Phantom limb pain after traumatic or surgical amputation can be extremely troubling and frustrating. The estimated incidence of post-amputation pain is between 30 percent and 50 percent, with approximately 5 percent to 10 percent of patients describing severe pain. The population of patients varies greatly, with some patients requiring amputation for vascular disease and/or infection (diabetes) and an increasing number of war veterans with pain from traumatic amputation.[13]

Caesarian Section

Approximately one-third of deliveries are performed by caesarian section (C-section); therefore, it is concerning that an estimated 10 percent of women complain of chronic pain after C-section. Relative to the average surgical population, obstetric patients are younger and healthier, yet chronic pain remains a problem for them. Whether this has a surgical cause or is due to the many structural and hormonal changes of pregnancy is unclear. One study found that the severity of acute pain, but not the method of delivery, was predictive of pain 2 months postpartum.[14] More data are certainly needed in order for us to better understand the incidence and predictors of pain in this population.[15]

CABG

The high reported rates of chronic pain after CABG are surprising to some clinicians, as patients tend to recovery incredibly well realtive to those who have undergone other surgeries of the thorax. Some of the injuries described include neurological changes from stretching of the brachial plexus during surgery; however, this is still relatively rare and does not explain much of the chronic pain reported. Studies estimate that the incidence of pain after CABG is between 30 percent and 50 percent, with a rate of severe pain of between 5 percent and 10 percent.[1,16,17]

PAIN-PRONE PHENOTYPE

Although the surgery performed certainly plays a role in the potential for the development of chronic pain, there are patient factors that are possibly more important to consider. Given that only some patients undergoing the same surgery and perioperative pain regimen will develop pain, patient factors clearly play an important role in the outcomes. Studies of chronic post-surgical pain have found pain in other locations of the body to be a predictor of the report of chronic post-surgical pain.[3,4,6,9] There have also been multiple descriptions of psychological predictors, as well as higher risk in females.[1,18] Although acute post-surgical pain is frequently described as an independent predictor, there might be close links between acute and chronic pain sensitivity.[1,4] Therefore, severe acute pain might not be "causal" in the development of chronic pain.

There are some phenotypic (i.e., observable physical or biochemical characteristics of a person or the expression of a trait) and likely genotypic characteristics that are predictive for the development of chronic post-surgical pain, and possibly all chronic pain states. Female sex, psychological co-morbidities, and pain in other locations are phenotypic characteristics associated with chronic pain disorders of the central nervous system. The best studied of the disorders of central nervous system pain processing, or centralized pain, is fibromyalgia.[19–21] Patients with centralized pain are known to have increased central nervous system levels of neurotransmitters associated with the facilitation of pain (e.g., glutamate, Substance P), along with lower levels of those that down-regulate pain (e.g., norepinephrine, serotonin, γ-aminobutyric acid). As is described in the chapter on fibromyalgia (Chapter 20), these central nervous system changes mirror those seen in many chronic pain conditions, including chronic post-surgical pain. Certainly, the preoperative phenotypic predictors previously described paint a picture of a patient with a fibromyalgia-like phenotype. Whether pre-surgical phenotypes and/or genotypes of altered central pain processing can predict a high-risk population is not known, but this question is the subject of ongoing research.

TRANSITION FROM ACUTE TO CHRONIC PAIN

Acute nociception is expected by patients, doctors, and nurses; however, the associations between the transition from acute pain to chronic disease are clear. Many studies have described severe acute post-operative pain as a predictor of chronic pain. The link between acute and chronic pain is widely accepted, and some believe that patients prone to severe acute pain are the same as those likely to develop chronic pain. Regardless of whether acute pain itself is predictive of poor long-term outcomes, there are neuroplastic changes that occur and help to describe the neuropathic symptoms often reported.

Preclinical and clinical studies have helped elucidate the changes and some of the mechanisms behind "central sensitization." Normally, there is a separation between low-threshold mechanoceptors (nerve fibers mediating light touch and proprioception) and nociceptors (pain fibers). In pain conditions, like chronic post-surgical pain, neuroplastic changes occur that cause the nociceptors to respond in an exaggerated fashion to painful stimuli (hyperalgesia) and mechanoceptors to express pain in response to non-painful stimuli (allodynia). Figure 12.1 shows some of the changes that occur with central sensitization, including the loss of inhibitory control. Although the full pathophysiology is not fully understood, there are known changes in the peripheral nervous system, spinal cord, and brain driving these abnormalities. The pathophysiology of central sensitization is covered in an outstanding review by Dr. Clifford Woolf.[21] Whether some of the features and

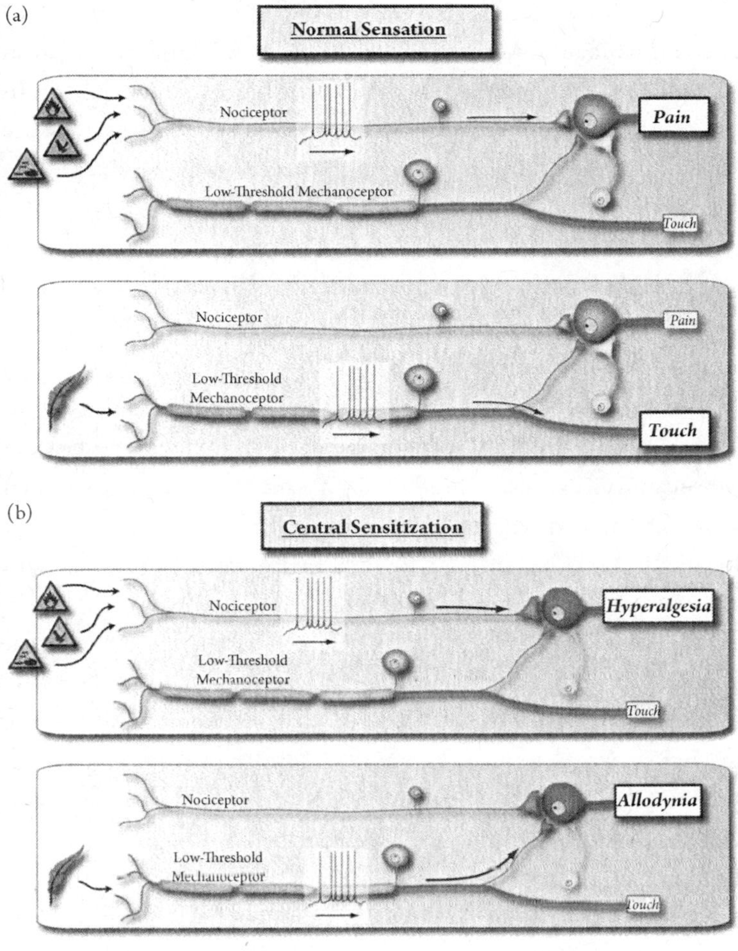

Figure 12.1. *A*, neuroplastic changes in the transition from acute to chronic pain. In normal sensation, the parallel pathways of nociceptors and mechanoceptors do not intersect because of strong synaptic inputs and inhibitory neurons. In this way, the central nervous system can distinguish noxious from non-noxious stimuli. *B*, in central sensitization there is an enhanced responsiveness to noxious stimuli in the nociceptive pathways (hyperalgesia). In addition, somatosensory pathways intersect with nociceptive pathways, and there is a loss of inhibition (allodynia, or pain in response to a non-noxious stimulus). Reproduced with permission from Woolf CJ. Central sensitization: implications for the diagnosis and treatment of pain. *Pain.* 2011;152(3 Suppl):S2–S15.

neurophysiologic abnormalities associated with chronic post-surgical pain are sometimes present prior to surgery in a different fashion, as described above in the "Pain-prone Phenotype" section, is not well understood, but data suggest that this might be true.

ASSESSMENT AND TREATMENT OF CHRONIC POST-SURGICAL PAIN

The treatment of pain following surgery requires a careful history and physical examination in order for the clinician to better understand the location, severity, descriptors, and other sequelae associated with the pain. Because complete resolution of the pain is frequently unlikely, it is very important to determine the patient's goals and create fair expectations and goals.

Pain Assessment and Differential Diagnosis

Although it is important to conduct a thorough history and physical examination to rule out other diagnoses, the temporal association and location of pain following surgery normally narrow the differential diagnosis. It is important, however, to ensure that there is not ongoing damage or a new disorder in the surgical area. For the purposes of this chapter, it is not possible to create a complete differential diagnosis list for all surgical conditions. In patients with a history of cancer, concerns about recurrence can be a issue when pain continues after surgery. In the breast cancer population, some have suggested that the fear of recurrence constitutes some of the reason for the described high incidence and can also affect the reported pain intensity.[8] In the case described at the beginning of the chapter, a work-up for cancer recurrence likely is not necessary, as it would be unlikely to present in a dermatomal fashion around the areas of incision.

There are multiple ways to assess the degree of neuropathic pain symptoms. Many clinicians do this through eliciting pain descriptors from the patient, including words such as "burning," "tingling," "pins and needles," etc. There are, however, easy-to-administer patient report measures, such as the PainDETECT[22] or McGill Pain Questionnaire,[23] which can help elucidate whether the pain is likely to be neuropathic in nature. Our clinic uses the PainDETECT, as there are available normative data, as well as a great deal of ongoing research in determining patient response to therapy based on responses to the questionnaire.[22]

TREATMENT

As with the treatment of most chronic pain states, a multi-disciplinary and multimodal treatment approach is often superior. Treatments can include medications, psychotherapy, complementary and alternative medicine, minimally invasive interventional modalities, and surgery.

Medications

The choice of medications for pain should be tailored to the individual patient. Acute and sub-acute pain (within 3 months of surgery) should be differentiated from chronic pain (≥3 months), as pain following surgery is normally expected to improve. The patient in the case description had previously tried opioids and NSAIDs without much benefit. There can be a role for opioids in chronic post-surgical pain, but doses should be limited, and chronic therapy is often associated with tolerance and treatment failure. Higher doses of opioids might worsen pain, potentially by causing opioid-induced hyperalgesia, as described in Chapter 1.

As noted in the "Pain Assessment" section, many of the surgical conditions are associated with descriptions of neuropathic pain. Neuropathic pain conditions tend to respond best to medications in the anticonvulsant and antidepressant classes. As in the case described, patients normally have tried only opioids and NSAIDs prior to presenting to a pain medicine clinic. Trials of medications for neuropathic pain, such as gabapentin or nortriptyline, can produce meaningful improvements in pain. Tailoring these medications so as to find maximal benefit with an acceptable side-effect profile is often the greatest challenge. Although simultaneous initiation might worsen side effects, there are data to support the concept that membrane stabilizers and antidepressant pain medications (not selective serotonin reuptake inhibitors) have additive, if not synergistic, effects in neuropathic pain.[24]

The use of compounded medication creams has become more popular in recent years, likely because they are thought to be relatively safe. There is essentially no regulatory oversight for the production and compounding of most topical therapies beyond branded patches such as the lidocaine patches. Despite a relative lack of efficacy and safety data in post-surgical pain driving the use of topical creams, the concept is reasonably well founded, and they are likely safe with reasonable dosing. It is recommended that physicians discuss evidence and safety with the compounding pharmacies prior to considering widespread usage without experience.

There are certainly many other classes of medications that can be considered should simple measures fail because of a lack of efficacy or intolerable side effects. General guidelines for the treatment of chronic post-surgical pain are shown in Fig. 12.2. We recommend that a pain specialist be contacted for assistance if conservative measures fail.

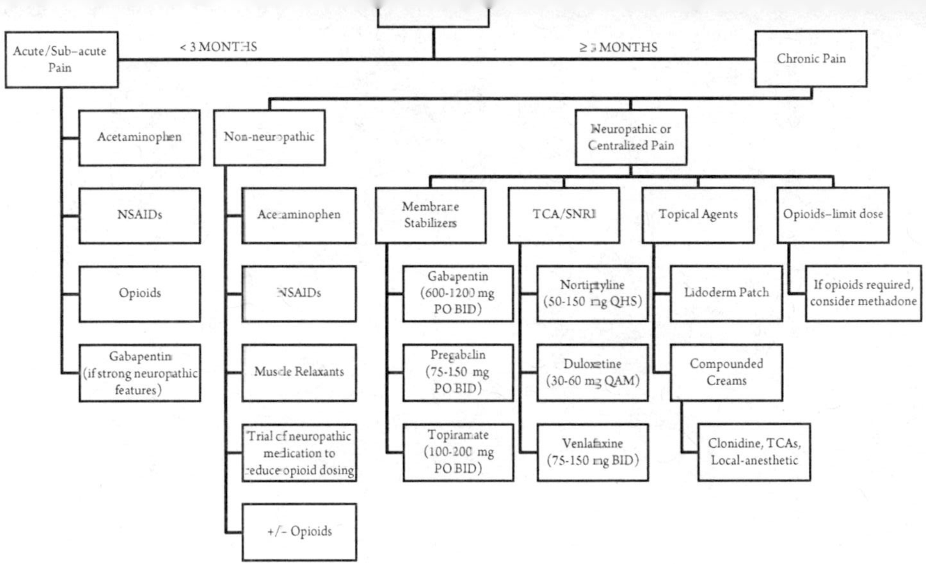

Figure 12.2. Algorithm for the medical management of chronic post-surgical pain. Acute and subacute pain (<3 months duration) should be distinguished from a chronic post-surgical pain state. In acute/sub-acute pain, the focus should be on symptomatic management with the anticipation of resolution of the symptom. In chronic post-surgical pain, most patients complain of neuropathic features and have signs and symptoms of central sensitization. Patients with neuropathic/centralized pain features tend to respond better to medications that alter central pain processing, including tricyclic antidepressants (TCAs), serotonin-norepinephrine reuptake inhibitors (SNRIs), and gabapentinoids. General recommendations and dosing guidelines are provided, but analgesic and side effects will vary greatly among patients and will need to be individualized. Most centrally acting medications require slow dose escalation so as to avoid side effects.

Psychotherapy

As with virtually all chronic pain states, psychological factors are often present in chronic post-surgical pain. These factors might be thought of as important in predictive modeling for disease prevention studies, but once the patient develops chronic pain, psychological factors should be addressed regardless of when they presented. Depression and anxiety are associated with higher pain intensity and lesser physical function and should be appropriately treated. In the case described, the patient could be expected to have some situational depression associated with the loss of function. When the pain limits normal social interaction (for example, this patient does not want to wear a shirt because of allodynia), depression and/or anxiety are common.

As is noted in Chapter 4, there are techniques such as cognitive-behavioral therapy and biofeedback that can be considered as alternatives or adjuncts to medications and interventions regardless of a patient's psychological status. Despite demonstrated effect sizes greater than those seen with many medications for chronic pain, many insurers will not authorize such therapies. The average patient often cannot afford the out-of-pocket expenses. Some groups are developing Web-based behavioral interventions to allow for widespread free access.

Complementary and Alternative Medicine

Complementary and alternative medicine therapies are described in Chapters 3 and 5. These therapies should be tailored to the patient and condition, but they can certainly be a portion of the treatment plan.

Interventions

There are some minimally invasive techniques that are performed for chronic post-surgical pain. These interventions range from perineural injections of local anesthetic and steroid to neuroablative (e.g., radiofrequency ablation or cryoablation) and neuromodulatory (e.g., spinal cord or peripheral nerve stimulation) procedures. There are limited data to support the efficacy of many of these interventions in chronic post-surgical pain, with most data existing in the form of case series. The lack of Level 1 evidence, however, does not itself imply a lack of efficacy. More data are certainly needed in order to better elucidate the efficacy of the interventions used. For some patients, conservative measures such as medications and cognitive-behavioral therapy will not suffice, and more advanced therapies should be considered. As interventions are not a focus of this textbook, we recommend consulting with a board-certified pain physician if conservative measures fail to provide benefit.

Surgery

Patients will frequently request that the pain simply be "cut out"; however, surgical options in chronic post-surgical pain are often incredibly limited. In this case, there are no recommended surgeries for pain following thoracic surgery or many of the other commonly described surgical conditions commonly associated with pain. Some experts believe that additional surgery can sometimes benefit patients with pain following inguinal hernia repair, although it is a controversial concept. The mesh can cause entrapment or local irritation of the nerves of the inguinal region. Whether surgery to remove the mesh or ligate the nerves will improve pain is unclear. It is recommended that conservative measures be considered prior to considering surgery.

FUTURE DIRECTIONS

Although the true incidence is debated and large prospective studies are still lacking, there is no doubt that chronic post-surgical pain affects many patients each year and is a source of significant morbidity. Future studies are needed to better identify high-risk populations, and there is a need for efficient clinical trials of preventative therapies in the perioperative period. Although multimodal analgesia in the perioperative period is championed by many in the pain community, the exact medications to use and the duration of treatment are still in question.

CONCLUSIONS

Chronic post-surgical pain is a frustrating disease for patients and treating physicians. When well managed, pain and function can normally be improved, but complete resolution of the pain is frequently not possible. Until we have the potential to prevent its development, physicians will be left to manage the multifaceted issues that occur in chronic post-surgical pain.

REFERENCES

1. Kehlet H, Jensen TS, Woolf CJ. Persistent postsurgical pain: risk factors and prevention. *Lancet.* 2006;367(9522):1618–1625.
2. Sandroni P, Benrud-Larson LM, McClelland RL, Low PA. Complex regional pain syndrome type I: incidence and prevalence in Olmsted County, a population-based study. *Pain.* 2003;103(1–2):199–207.
3. Bourne RB, Chesworth BM, Davis AM, Mahomed NN, Charron KD. Patient satisfaction after total knee arthroplasty: who is satisfied and who is not? *Clin Orthop Relat Res.* 2010;468(1):57–63.
4. Nikolajsen L, Brandsborg B, Lucht U, Jensen TS, Kehlet H. Chronic pain following total hip arthroplasty: a nationwide questionnaire study. *Acta Anaesthesiol Scand.* 2006;50(4):495–500.
5. Gotoda Y, Kambara N, Sakai T, Kishi Y, Kodama K, Koyama T. The morbidity, time course and predictive factors for persistent post-thoracotomy pain. *Eur J Pain.* 2001;5(1):89–96.

6. Wildgaard K, Ravn J, Nikolajsen L, Jakobsen E, Jensen TS, Kehlet H. Consequences of persistent pain after lung cancer surgery: a nationwide questionnaire study. *Acta Anaesthesiol Scand.* 2011;55(1):60–68.
7. Steegers MA, Snik DM, Verhagen AF, van der Drift MA, Wilder-Smith OH. Only half of the chronic pain after thoracic surgery shows a neuropathic component. *J Pain.* 2008;9(10):955–961.
8. Brummett CM. Chronic pain following breast surgery. *Techniques in Regional Anesthesia and Pain Medicine.* 2011;15(3):124–132.
9. Gartner R, Jensen MB, Nielsen J, Ewertz M, Kroman N, Kehlet H. Prevalence of and factors associated with persistent pain following breast cancer surgery. *JAMA.* 2009;302(18):1985–1992.
10. Mikkelsen T, Werner MU, Lassen B, Kehlet H. Pain and sensory dysfunction 6 to 12 months after inguinal herniotomy. *Anesth Analg.* 2004;99(1):146–151.
11. Grant AM, Scott NW, O'Dwyer PJ. Five-year follow-up of a randomized trial to assess pain and numbness after laparoscopic or open repair of groin hernia. *Br J Surg.* 2004;91(12):1570–1574.
12. Flor H. Phantom-limb pain: characteristics, causes, and treatment. *Lancet Neurol.* 2002;1(3):182–189.
13. Nikolajsen L, Jensen TS. Phantom limb pain. *Br J Anaesth.* 2001;87(1):107–116.
14. Eisenach JC, Pan PH, Smiley R, Lavand'homme P, Landau R, Houle TT. Severity of acute pain after childbirth, but not type of delivery, predicts persistent pain and postpartum depression. *Pain.* 2008;140(1):87–94.
15. Nikolajsen L, Sorensen HC, Jensen TS, Kehlet H. Chronic pain following Caesarean section. *Acta Anaesthesiol Scand.* 2004;48(1):111–116.
16. Kalso E, Mennander S, Tasmuth T, Nilsson E. Chronic post-sternotomy pain. *Acta Anaesthesiol Scand.* 2001;45(8):935–939.
17. Bruce J, Drury N, Poobalan AS, Jeffrey RR, Smith WC, Chambers WA. The prevalence of chronic chest and leg pain following cardiac surgery: a historical cohort study. *Pain.* 2003;104(1–2):265–273.
18. Hinrichs-Rocker A, Schulz K, Jarvinen I, Lefering R, Simanski C, Neugebauer EA. Psychosocial predictors and correlates for chronic post-surgical pain (CPSP)—a systematic review. *Eur J Pain.* 2009;13(7):719–730.
19. Brummett CM, Clauw DJ. Fibromyalgia: a primer for the anesthesia community. *Curr Opin Anaesthesiol.* 2011;24(5):532–539.
20. Williams DA, Clauw DJ. Understanding fibromyalgia: lessons from the broader pain research community. *J Pain.* 2009;10(8):777–791.
21. Woolf CJ. Central sensitization: implications for the diagnosis and treatment of pain. *Pain.* 2011;152(3 Suppl):S2–S15.
22. Freynhagen R, Baron R, Gockel U, Tolle TR. painDETECT: a new screening questionnaire to identify neuropathic components in patients with back pain. *Curr Med Res Opin.* 2006;22(10):1911–1920.

23. Boureau F, Doubrere JF, Luu M. Study of verbal description in neuropathic pain. *Pain.* 1990;42(2):145–152.
24. Gilron I, Bailey JM, Tu D, Holden RR, Weaver DF, Houlden RL. Morphine, gabapentin, or their combination for neuropathic pain. *N Engl J Med.* 2005;352(13):1324–1334.

13

Herpes Zoster and Postherpetic Neuralgia

JULIE H. Y. HUANG, ANDREI D. SDRULLA, AND MARK WALLACE

Case Presentation

An 82-year-old retired salesman with a history of hypertension, hyperlipidemia, and coronary artery disease presents to the clinic with acute onset of a painful vesicular rash on his right flank. The patient recalls having chicken pox when he was 3 years old. On exam there is an erythematous vesicular eruption in a dermatomal pattern most consistent with herpes zoster. What are the issues to consider in the acute and long-term care of this patient?

Herpes zoster, or shingles, is a viral infection resulting from the reactivation of the varicella-zoster virus (VZV) that lies dormant in the dorsal root sensory, cranial nerve, or autonomic ganglia following resolution of an initial primary varicella infection. The most common complication following herpes zoster infection is postherpetic neuralgia (PHN), a neuropathic pain condition that develops in approximately 15 percent of afflicted individuals. The disease most commonly occurs as a result of an age-related decline in cell-mediated immunity. PHN is associated with acute and sometimes persistent pain, which substantially reduces the day-to-day functioning and quality of life of affected individuals, particularly older adults. The lifetime risk of herpes zoster is approximately 20 percent to 30 percent, and up to 50 percent in those ≥80 years of age.[1] Individuals over 50 years of age are at nearly 15-fold increased risk of developing PHN relative to their younger counterparts. Understanding the pathophysiology, clinical presentation, prevention, and advances in treatment for PHN is therefore important for the primary care physician, given that PHN will annually afflict millions of older adults worldwide and can cause significant, often disabling, pain.

CLINICAL PRESENTATION

Herpes zoster typically begins with a prodrome of fatigue, flu-like symptoms, headache, fever, and malaise about 3 to 7 days prior to the appearance of a rash. The replication of the reactivated VZV occurs in the sensory ganglion and travels to the nerve endings at the dermoepidermal junction, which leads to the classic appearance of vesicular eruptions in a unilateral dermatomal distribution. Up to 50 percent of all cases occur in the thoracic dermatomes, although cases are also frequently noted in the ophthalmic division of the trigeminal nerve; other cranial nerves; and cervical, lumbar, and sacral dermatomes.

Acute pain can often coincide with progression of the rash, from the initial formation of vesicles that progress to pustular lesions that crust over, with eventual healing over several weeks. This type of pain that occurs within 30 days of rash onset has been defined as acute herpetic neuralgia and resolves before the diagnosis of PHN can be made. PHN is pain that persists after the initial rash formation for

120 days or more. PHN characteristically varies from an aching or itching sensation to the more classic burning, stabbing, shooting, or lancinating pain typically associated with nerve damage. The pain may be constant or intermittent, associated with altered sensitivity to touch (paresthesia) that might become unpleasant (dysesthesia), associated with exaggerated responses to non-painful (hyperesthesia) or painful stimuli (hyperalgesia), evoked by normal stimuli (allodynia), or persist beyond the duration of the stimulus (hyperpathia). These characteristic abnormalities are important findings that can be used to correctly distinguish neuropathic pain syndromes from other chronic pain processes associated with an intact nociceptive system.[2] A clinical variant, zoster sine herpete, occurs in <5 percent of cases and presents with dermatomal pain in the absence of any skin lesions; serological testing can often be performed in the early course of the disease, though this condition is rarely diagnosed in a definitive manner.

PATHOPHYSIOLOGY

PHN is a neuropathic pain process that results from both peripheral and central pathophysiological mechanisms. Several pathophysiological mechanisms of PHN have been proposed based on findings of demonstrated damage of primary afferents with significant inflammation of the dorsal root ganglia (DRG) and nerve fibers supplying the affected dermatomes. Reactivated viral replication of herpes zoster leads to severe peripheral axonal loss that ultimately results in maladaptive central and peripheral sensitization to pain signaling. Abnormal sensitization of small unmyelinated C fiber cutaneous nociceptors might lead to spontaneous burning pain and heat hyperalgesia in patients with minimal sensory loss. PHN pain in some patients has been associated with small fiber deafferentation that results in profoundly impaired pain and temperature sensation. This mechanism might result in severe pain in response to light touch and other normally non-painful mechanical stimuli (allodynia), possibly due to the formation of new connections between large diameter primary afferents and central pain transmission neurons. Others with deafferentation present with severe spontaneous pain without hyperalgesia or allodynia, presumably due to the loss of both large- and small-diameter fibers. These individuals typically experience increased spontaneous activity in deafferented central neurons and/or reorganization of central connections.[2] A skin biopsy is not typically needed in clinical practice and should be reserved for difficult diagnoses. A better understanding of these underlying pathophysiological mechanisms has led to the development of pharmacologic agents with demonstrated efficacy for the treatment of PHN.

PREVENTION OF ACUTE HERPES ZOSTER

Several studies have shown the efficacy of antiviral therapy in decreasing the severity and duration of acute herpes zoster (AHZ) pain and the duration and incidence of PHN. This class of drugs impairs viral replication by inhibiting DNA polymerase, reduces the duration of viral shedding, and decreases the degree of resulting neural damage. Antiviral treatment, which includes acyclovir, famciclovir, and valacyclovir (all approved by the U.S. Food and Drug Administration [FDA]), should be started within 72 hours after the onset of rash. This recommendation does not apply to patients who are immunocompromised, have neurological complications, or present with disseminated zoster. Foscarnet, which is a noncompetitive inhibitor of viral DNA polymerase, is used in patients with known resistance to acyclovir secondary to lack of viral thymidine kinase, which has been found in patients with AIDS or prolonged exposure to acyclovir. Uncontrolled studies have also demonstrated a possible benefit when antiviral therapy is started beyond 72 hours after the onset of a rash.[3]

Because the pharmacologic treatment of PHN can be limited in efficacy, advances in the development of a herpes zoster vaccine have been pursued for preventing primary varicella (VZV) infection in childhood using a live attenuated Oka vaccine virus, as well as for increasing VZV-specific cellular immunity in adults. The adult vaccine is also a live attenuated Oka vaccine virus that establishes latency in sensory ganglia. In determining the efficacy and safety of the herpes zoster vaccine, the Shingles Prevention Study, a multicenter, randomized, double-blind, placebo-controlled trial of 40,000 adults aged 60 years or more, was conducted. In the initial study, the AHZ-vaccinated group had a 51 percent lower incidence of AHZ, a 67 percent reduction in PHN, and a 61 percent lower burden of illness. The results indicated that the vaccine decreased both the incidence and the severity of AHZ. Moreover, there was a 73 percent reduction in the number of cases of AHZ with severe and long-lasting pain. Over a 7-year follow-up, the live attenuated zoster vaccine showed sustained efficacy for a significantly reduced incidence of AHZ and reduced incidence of PHN, and it was associated with a lower burden of illness (a composite measure of the incidence, severity, and duration of pain and discomfort caused by AHZ).[4,5]

TREATMENT OF PHN

Pharmacotherapies that have been found to be effective in the management of PHN include antidepressants, particularly tricyclic antidepressants (TCAs); certain anticonvulsants (the calcium channel ligands); opioid analgesics; and topical lidocaine (Tables 13.1–13.6). Studies have evaluated the relative efficacy of these treatments, and consensus guidelines and recommendations for the treatment of

Table 13.1 ANTIVIRAL MEDICATIONS FOR HERPES ZOSTER

Drug	*Trade Name*	*Mechanism of Action*	*Typical Dose Range*	*Pharmacology*	*Indications*	*Common Adverse Side Effects*
Acyclovir	Zovirax	Incorporates into viral DNA and inhibits DNA polymerase	800 mg four to five times daily for 7 to 10 days; start within 72 hours of symptom onset (oral)	Liver metabolism and urine excretion, primarily; half-life = 2.5 to 3 hours	Shingles/acute herpes zoster (AHZ), genital or mucocutaneous herpes simplex virus (HSV), HSV encephalitis, HSV keratitis, varicella	Nausea, vomiting, diarrhea, headache, malaise, rash, dizziness, arthralgia, lethargy, confusion, injection site reaction, and photosensitivity
Famciclovir	Famvir	Selectively inhibits herpes viral DNA synthesis and replication; inhibits DNA	500 mg TID for 7 days (oral)	Liver metabolism, urine (primarily) and fecal excretion; half-life = 2 to 3 hours	AHZ, genital or orolabial HSV	Headache, nausea, diarrhea, vomiting, fatigue, pruritus, neutropenia, abnormal liver function tests (LFTs), paresthesias, and flatulence

Valacyclovir	Valtrex	Incorporates into viral DNA and inhibits DNA polymerase	1000 mg Q8h for 7 days (oral)	Gastrointestinal tract and liver metabolism, urine and fecal excretion; half-life < 30 minutes	AHZ, genital HSV, herpes labialis	Nausea, headache, vomiting, dizziness, abdominal pain, fatigue, depression, arthralgia, diarrhea, dysmenorrhea, decreased platelets, rash, elevated LFTs, photosensitivity, and decreased neutrophils
Foscarnet	Foscavir	Selectively inhibits viral DNA polymerase	40 mg/kg Q8–12 fcr 2 to 3 weeks (intravenous)	Liver metabolism, urine excretion primarily; half-life = 3 to 4 hours (plasma), 45 to 130 hours (terminal)	AHZ, cytomegalovirus retinitis, mucocutaneous HSV infection	Fever, nausea, anemia, vomiting, headache, seizures, diarrhea, renal impairment, hypokalemia, hypocalcemia, local burning or discomfort, nephrotoxicity, hypomagnesemia, hypo- or hyper-phosphatemia, and bone marrow depression

PHN currently indicate first-line pharmacotherapy as including tramadol, gabapentin, pregabalin, and topical liocaine. Second-line medications include the TCAs and opioids, largely because they are not tolerated as well in elderly patients.[6] Other modalities studied include capsaicin, which has been approved by the FDA for the management of PHN.[7] Invasive injections and surgical interventions are limited to patients refractory to conservative treatments.

Antidepressants: TCAs and Selective Serotonin and Norepinephrine Reuptake Inhibitors

TCAs—amitriptyline, nortriptyline, desipramine, and imipramine—provide analgesia independent of their antidepressive effects via multiple mechanisms, which include norepinephrine and serotonin reuptake inhibition in descending pathways. Of the two, serotonin reuptake inhibition is thought to be less important in analgesia; hence the comparatively decreased efficacy of selective serotonin reuptake inhibitors. Other active mechanisms include blockade of peripheral neural sodium channels, muscarinic and nicotinic acetylcholine receptors, α-adrenergic receptors, *N*-methyl-D-aspartate receptors, substance P release, and, to a lesser extent, even dopamine receptors.

Several studies investigating the use of antidepressants—specifically TCAs—for the treatment of AHZ and for the prevention and treatment of pain associated with PHN have shown benefit, with pooled analyses indicating a number-needed-to-treat (NNT) for TCAs ranging between 2.1 and 2.6.[8,9] Secondary amine tricyclics (e.g., nortriptyline and desipramine) are generally preferred, especially in elderly and frail patients, because they are better tolerated and have fewer side effects than amitriptyline. Desipramine has fewer sedative effects than amitriptyline and nortriptyline, but there is less evidence supporting its use. The other class of antidepressants used for neuropathic pain includes the selective serotonin and norepinephrine reuptake inhibitors (duloxetine, milnacipran and venlafaxine). Randomized controlled trials have demonstrated their efficacy in patients with diabetic and other peripheral neuropathies; however, they have not yet been studied for PHN.[10]

Dosing of TCAs is typically initiated at 25 mg at night and titrated slowly to a target dose of 50 to 100 mg in a single evening dose. A lower dose of 10 mg at night should be started in elderly patients. Minor side effects of TCAs include sedation, weight gain, dizziness, constipation, dry mouth, orthostatic hypotension, and urinary retention. Significant toxicities to monitor for include tachyarrhythmia, QT interval prolongation, and worsening of acute angle glaucoma. A baseline electrocardiogram should be reviewed prior to starting these medications, especially in elderly patients or those with cardiac risk factors. Patients should be monitored closely for concomitant use of selective serotonin reuptake inhibitor antidepressants, given their mechanism of action, because of an increased risk of developing serotonin syndrome and toxic tricyclic serum levels.

Anticonvulsants and Calcium Channel (α2-δ) Ligands (Gabapentin, Pregabalin)

Although several anticonvulsants have been used to treat PHN and other neuropathic pain syndromes, the calcium channel ligands, gabapentin and pregabalin, have been shown to have the greatest efficacy and fewer adverse effects. Pregabalin and gabapentin, analogues of γ-aminobutyric acid, exert their analgesic effects by acting on the α2-δ1 subunit of cellular calcium channels and blocking excitatory neurotransmitter release, including that of glutamate and norepinephrine. Their binding to calcium channels results in the suppression of abnormal neuronal discharges and an increased threshold for nerve activation. Although gabapentin and pregabalin are generally

Table 13.2 TRICYCLIC ANTIDEPRESSANTS

Drug	*Trade Name*	*Mechanism of Action*	*Typical Dose Range, mg/d*	*Pharmacology*	*Evidence of Efficacy*	*Common Adverse Side Effects*
Amitriptyline	Elavil, Endep	Inhibits norepinephrine (NE) and 5HT reuptake; muscarinic acetylcholine receptor antagonist, H1 receptor antagonist, α1 adrenergic receptor antagonist; blocks Na+ channels	10–150 in qhs dosing; starting dose of 25 to 75 mg po qhs; starting dose in elderly of 10 to 25 mg po qhs (oral)	Liver metabolism and urine (primarily) and fecal excretion; half-life = 10 to 26 hours	***Strong***—Diabetic neuropathy, postherpetic neuralgia (PHN), headache prophylaxis ***Moderate***—Central pain after spinal cord injury (SCI), central post-stroke pain (CPSP), chronic radiculopathy	Dry mouth, constipation, fluid retention, weight gain, difficulty concentrating, and cardiotoxicity

Nortriptyline	Pamelor	Inhibits NE and 5HT reuptake; muscarinic acetylcholine receptor antagonist; blocks Na+ channels	25–150 in qhs dosing; starting dose of 25 to 50 mg po qhs (oral)	Liver metabolism, urine (primarily) and fecal excretion; half-life = 18 to 44 hours	***Strong***—Diabetic neuropathy, PHN ***Moderate***—SCI, CPSP, chronic radiculopathy; headache prophylaxis	Drowsiness, dizziness, nausea, vomiting, insomnia, sweating, dry mouth, tachycardia, pruritus, weight gain, and constipation
Imipramine	Tofranil	Inhibits NE and 5HT reuptake; M2 muscarinic acetylcholine receptor antagonist, histamine H1 receptor antagonist; blocks Na+ channels, enhances dopaminergic activity	25–150, 0.2 to 3 mg/kg; starting dose of 0.2 to 0.4 mg/kg (oral)	Liver metabolism, urine excretion (primarily), and bile/feces; half-life = 11 to 25 hours	***Strong***—Diabetic neuropathy, PHN ***Moderate***—SCI, CPSP, chronic radiculopathy	Drowsiness, dizziness, nausea, vomiting, headache, insomnia, sweating, confusion, dry mouth, tachycardia, and constipation

(continued)

Table 13.2 (CONTINUED)

Drug	*Trade Name*	*Mechanism of Action*	*Typical Dose Range, mg/d*	*Pharmacology*	*Evidence of Efficacy*	*Common Adverse Side Effects*
Desipramine	Norpramin	Inhibits NE reuptake; muscarinic acetylcholine receptor antagonist; blocks Na+ channels	25–150; starting dose of 25 to 75 mg daily (oral)	Liver metabolism, urine excretion primarily; half-life = 12 to 27 hours	***Strong***—Diabetic neuropathy, PHN ***Moderate***—SCI, CPSP, chronic radiculopathy	Drowsiness, dizziness, nausea, vomiting, blurry vision, diaphoresis, confusion, dry mouth, tachycardia, and constipation

Table 13.3 SELECTIVE SEROTONIN AND NOREPINEPHRINE REUPTAKE INHIBITORS

Drug	*Trade Name*	*Mechanism of Action*	*Typical Dose Range, mg/d*	*Pharmacology*	*Evidence for Efficacy*	*Common Adverse Side Effects*
Duloxetine	Cymbalta	Inhibition of both norepinephrine (NE) and serotonin (5HT) reuptake	30–120; starting dose of 30 mg po daily; max 120 mg/d (oral)	Liver metabolism and urine excretion; half-life = 12 hours	***Strong***—Diabetic neuropathy	Nausea, dry mouth, constipation, fatigue, somnolence, insomnia, dizziness, diarhea, constipation, fatigue, sweating, vomiting, blurred vision, tremor, anxiety, elevated blood pressure, elevated liver enzymes, weight changes, hot flashes, syncope, and headache
Venlafaxine	Effexor, Effexor XR	Inhibition of NE, 5HT, and dopamine reuptake	37.5–225; starting dose of 37.5 mg po twice daily; max 375 mg/d (oral)	Liver metabolism, urine excretion; half-life = 5 hours	***Strong***—Diabetic neuropathy, headache prophylaxis	Nausea, headache, somnolence, insomnia, dry mouth, dizziness, sweating, constipation, anorexia, diarrhea, anxiety, blurred vision, vomiting, weight loss, tremor, paresthesias, rash, elevated blood pressure, chills, weight loss, vasodilation, tachycardia, and mydriasis

well tolerated, their most common side effects include dizziness, sedation, lightheadedness, somnolence, peripheral edema, gait or balance problems, and weight gain.

Randomized, placebo-controlled trials support the use of gabapentin in the treatment of PHN, with significant reductions in pain and improvements in quality of life seen with daily dosages ranging between 1800 and 3600 mg[11,12]; the pooled NNT for gabapentin in PHN is approximately 4.4.[8] Pregabalin has also been demonstrated in randomized, placebo-controlled trials to provide pain relief and improved sleep at doses ranging between 150 to 600 mg daily.[13,14]

The optimal dosing for gabapentin is not well-defined, and one common recommendation includes initiating treatment at 300 mg daily and titrating up at a rate of 300 mg every 3 to 4 days to a target of 1800 to 2400 mg daily (divided into 3 to 4 doses because of the short half-life) over a few weeks. With increased dosing, the bioavailability decreases. The maximum FDA-approved dose is 1800 mg/d; however, studies have shown that up to 3600 mg/d might be required. In the elderly, initial dosing can be started at 100 mg daily and titrated upwards at a slower rate every 3 to 4 days as tolerated. Dosages need to be adjusted in patients with renal insufficiency, such as starting a single dose of 100 mg one hour after dialysis on alternate days. Pregabalin has a comparable analgesic efficacy and side-effect profile, and it might be associated with better compliance than gabapentin secondary to its twice-daily dosing and faster titration, though at a higher cost at this time.

Opioids and Tramadol

Opioids have been used extensively for the treatment of chronic neuropathic pain. The analgesic effects of opioids are mediated via agonism at μ-type opioid receptors localized throughout the central and peripheral nervous systems. Opioids have been specifically

Drug	*Trade Name*	*Mechanism of Action*	*Typical Dose Range, mg/d*	*Pharmacology*	*Evidence of Efficacy*	*Common Adverse Side Effects*
Gabapentin	Neurontin	Binds α_2-δ_1 subunit of calcium channels, decreasing release of glutamate, norepinephrine (NE), and substance P	300–3600 in TID dosing; starting dose of 100 mg daily or TID	Urine excretion; half-life = 5 to 7 hours	***Strong***—Diabetic neuropathy, PHN, cancer-associated neuropathic pain ***Moderate***—Spasticity in patients with multiple sclerosis and spinal cord injury (SCI), fibromyalgia; headache prophylaxis ***Weak***—Chronic daily headache, myofascial pain, low back pain, muscle cramps	Dizziness, sedation, lightheadedness, somnolence, nausea, vomiting, and weight gain
Pregabalin	Lyrica	Binds α_2-δ_1 subunit of calcium channels, decreasing release of glutamate, NE, and substance P	50–450 in BID or TID dosing; starting dose of 50 mg BID (oral)	Negligible metabolism; urine excretion (90 percent); half-life = 6.3 hours	***Strong***—Diabetic neuropathy, PHN, SCI, fibromyalgia	Dizziness, somnolence, ataxia, weight gain, peripheral edema, headache, dry mouth, and blurred vision

investigated in PHN in randomized, placebo-controlled trials and have been found to be effective.[6] In one three-arm randomized controlled trial, a trend was found for morphine (or methadone) to provide better pain relief than nortripytline (or desipramine), with most patients preferring opioids.[15] Both treatments were more effective than placebo. Controlled-release oxycodone was shown to be better than placebo over 4 weeks in another randomized controlled trial.[16] In a non-randomized study, the addition of transdermal fentanyl to amitriptyline and gabapentin was associated with improved pain ratings and improved quality of life in patients with PHN.[17] The NNT to provide a significant analgesic benefit has been calculated as 2.7 for opioid therapy.[8] Despite the strong evidence supporting opioids for PHN, there are concerns regarding their long-term use. Opioids are associated with numerous undesirable side effects such as sedation, nausea, constipation, sleep disturbances, hypogonadism, addiction, and tolerance. Although the efficacy and tolerability of long-term chronic opioids have not been rigorously evaluated, there is some evidence that long-term opioids are effective in PHN and other chronic pain conditions.

Tramadol is a weak, centrally acting μ-opioid agonist and a reuptake inhibitor of norepinephrine and serotonin that has been shown to provide significant neuropathic pain relief. Given its shared chemical profiles as both an opioid and a serotonin reuptake inhibitor, its use carries an increased risk of serotonin syndrome with concomitant use of CYP2D6 inhibitors, such as antidepressant medications. Tramadol can cause seizures in patients who have a history of seizures or are taking seizure-threshold-lowering medications. Relative to placebo, tramadol provided better pain control and quality of life in an intermediate-duration randomized controlled trial, with the NNT being 4.8.[18] The maximum daily dose should not exceed 400 mg, and lower doses should be used in the elderly and patients with impaired renal function. Tramadol has a side-effect profile similar to those of opioids and antidepressants and can cause nausea, vomiting, constipation, urinary retention, headache, and sedation. Tapentadol, like tramadol, is also a reuptake blocker of norepinephrine and serotonin, but it is a stronger μ-opioid agonist.

General clinical guidelines for prescribing opioid analgesics for the treatment of PHN should include the following considerations. Treatment should start with the lowest effective dose, generally using short-acting opioid formulations (e.g., oxycodone). Once an effective regimen has been achieved, a transition to long-acting opioid formulations can be made (e.g., controlled-release oxycodone or morphine, fentanyl transdermal patch, or methadone). Common side effects should be proactively anticipated and aggressively managed, such as by using anti-emetics and laxatives for nausea and constipation, respectively. Frequent assessments of treatment efficacy and side effects should be followed; if not tolerated or ineffective, opioid doses should be tapered gradually to prevent withdrawal symptoms. Great care should be taken when prescribing opioids to the elderly, as they might not tolerate opioids as well as other age groups; thus, careful titration with frequent evaluation for side effects is recommended.

Topical Lidocaine or Patch

Topical 5 percent lidocaine provides analgesia by penetrating the skin to block voltage-gated sodium channels, resulting in membrane stabilization and decreased activity of injured nerves in the affected region. This modality is FDA approved for the treatment of PHN, and it is a commonly used therapy because of its excellent safety and tolerability profile. Adverse effects are mild and can include skin reaction at the site of placement. Lidocaine gel and patches were compared to placebo in multiple trials and were found to be efficacious, although many of those trials had methodological limitations.[6] In an open-label, randomized trial, 5 percent lidocaine patch was found to

Table 13.5 OPIOIDS

Drug	*Trade Name*	*Mechanism of Action*	*Typical Dose Range*	*Pharmacology*	*Evidence of Efficacy*	*Common Adverse Side Effects*
Tramadol	Ultram, Ryzolt	Binds to μ-opioid receptors and weakly inhibits norepinephrine and serotonin reuptake, producing analgesia (central opioid agonist)	50–100 mg po Q4–6 hours prn, max 400 mg/day (oral)	Liver metabolism and urine excretion primarily; half-life = 6.3 to 7.9 hours	***Strong***—Diabetic neuropathy, PHN, phantom limb pain ***Moderate***—Spinal cord injury (SCI), cancer-associated neuropathic pain	Nausea, vomiting, headache, flushing, dizziness, pruritus, somnolence, diarrhea, dyspepsia, and constipation
Oxycodone	Oxycontin, OxyFast	Binds to various opioid receptors, producing analgesia and sedation (opioid agonist)	5–30 mg po q4h prn (immediate release); 10–30 mg po q8–12h (extended	Liver metabolism and urine excretion; half-life = 3.2 hours (4.5 hours for extended-release	***Strong***—Diabetic neuropathy, PHN, phantom limb pain ***Moderate***—Chronic radiculopathy	Nausea, vomiting, constipation, headache, sedation, miosis, pruritus, rash, dysphoria, and

Fentanyl Transmucosal	Abstral, Actiq, Fentora, Onsolis	Binds to various opioid receptors, producing analgesia and sedation (opioid agonist)	100–400 mcg SL Q4h prn; max of four doses per day	Liver metabolism and urine excretion; half-life = 3.7 hours	***Strong***—Diabetic neuropathy, PHN, phantom limb pain ***Moderate***—Chronic radiculopathy	Nausa, vomiting, confusion, dry mouth, dizziness, pruritus, dyspnea, and constipation
Fentanyl Transdermal	Duragesic	Binds to various opioid receptors, producing analgesia and sedation (opioid agonist)	12.5–100 mcg/h patch q72h (transdermal)	Liver metabolism and urine excretion; half-life = 1 to 2 hours	***Strong***—Diabetic neuropathy, PHN, phantom limb pain ***Moderate***—Chronic radiculopathy	Nausa, vomiting, confusion, dry mouth, dizziness, pruritus, dyspnea, and constipation

(continued)

Table 13.5 (CONTINUED)

Drug	*Trade Name*	*Mechanism of Action*	*Typical Dose Range*	*Pharmacology*	*Evidence of Efficacy*	*Common Adverse Side Effects*
Morphine sulfate	Avinza, Kadian, MS Contin, Oramorph SR	Binds to various opioid receptors, producing analgesia and sedation (opioid agonist)	10–30 mg po Q3–4h prn (immediate release); 15–45 mg po Q8–12h prn (extended release); 2.5–10 mg Q2–6h prn (IV, IM, SC)	Liver metabolism and urine excretion; half-life = 2 to 4 hours	***Strong***—Diabetic neuropathy, PHN, phantom limb pain ***Moderate***—Chronic radiculopathy	Nausa, vomiting, miosis, confusion, dry mouth, pruritus, somnolence, dizziness, dyspnea, flushing, histamine release, and constipation
Hydromorphone	Dilaudid, Exalgo, Dilaudid-HP	Binds to various opioid receptors, producing analgesia and sedation (opioid agonist)	2–8 mg po Q3–4h prn (immediate release); 8–64 mg po Q24h (extended release); 0.2–4 mg Q3–6h (IV,	Liver metabolism and urine excretion; half-life = 2.5 hours (oral), 11 hours (oral ER), or 2.3 hours (IV)	***Strong***—Diabetic neuropathy, PHN, phantom limb pain ***Moderate***—Chronic radiculopathy	Nausea, vomiting, somnolence, pruritus, flushing, hyperhidrosis, xerostomia, muscle spasms, headache, rash, constipation,

Methadone	Dolophine, Methadose	Binds to various opioid receptors, producing analgesia and sedation (opioid agonist)	2.5–10 mg Q8–12h (oral) or 2.5–5 mg Q8–12h (SC, IM, IV); max 40 mg on day 1 and 100 mg/d thereafter	Liver metabolism and urine and fecal excretion; half-life = 8 to 59 hours (slow release from liver and other tissues)	***Strong***—Diabetic neuropathy, PHN, phantom limb pain ***Moderate***—Chronic radiculopathy	Nausea, vomiting, sedation, dizziness, lightheadedness, sweating, and constipation

Notes: extended release; IV, intravenous; IM, intramuscular; SC, subcutaneous.

provide slightly better pain relief to patients with PHN than pregabalin (62 percent vs. 47 percent) and was associated with fewer side effects.[19] Topical lidocaine may be considered as first-line therapy in the elderly, given its limited systemic side effects.[6] Recommended use includes up to three patches applied on and off for 12-hour intervals. The patches should be applied over the area of maximal pain and can be cut to fit the affected areas. Of note, topical lidocaine should not be applied to patients with active zoster lesions, and it is FDA approved only for the treatment of PHN.

Other Drugs (Capsaicin Cream or Patch, Botox)

Capsaicin is the active component of hot chili peppers and is a highly selective agonist of the TRPV1 receptor found on afferent nociceptor terminals. The activation of TRPV1 initially stimulates and then desensitizes and degenerates cutaneous nociceptive neurons, a process that has been referred to as "defunctionalization." This affects only peripheral endings and is transient, with most nerve fibers regenerating within a few months. Topical applications are available in two concentrations, 0.025 percent and 0.075 percent, with the 0.075 percent formulation being shown in randomized studies to provide significant pain relief relative to placebo.[6]

Recently, a high-concentration (8 percent) capsaicin patch (Qutenza) was approved by the FDA for PHN. This formulation was compared with a low-dose 0.04 percent capsaicin "control" patch in a series of randomized, double-blind trials for PHN, and the 8 percent patch was found to be superior.[7] The advantage of Qutenza is that it involves only a 60-minute application that can be repeated as needed after 3 months. Side effects are site related, and the most common are erythema and application site pain. One current recommendation is to apply topical lidocaine for one hour before the capsaicin patch in order to enhance tolerability, though some practitioners prefer to use sedation or nerve blocks for "anesthesia," because the pre-application of topical lidocaine is not always effective.[7] Patients should be advised to avoid contact with their eyes, which limits its use for facial PHN.

Botulinum toxin type A (BTX-A) has been evaluated recently for the treatment of PHN. BTX-A acts by inhibiting the release of neurotransmitters from presynaptic vesicles via the cleavage of key vesicle docking proteins, thereby preventing the release of neurotransmitters until new docking proteins are synthesized. The analgesic effects of BTX-A are thought to be mediated via the inhibition of neurogenic inflammation in the periphery. Randomized, placebo-controlled studies compared the efficacy of BTX-A with that of placebo and yielded significant reductions in pain scores and improved quality of life that were sustained for at least 3 months.[20] BTX-A should be considered for patients with focal, localized PHN refractory to other therapies.

Combination Therapy

Combination drug therapy (CDT) is often recommended when monotherapy provides insufficient relief. CDT selection should be based on complementary mechanisms of drug action and potential synergy. The goal of multimodal approaches is to minimize the adverse effects of individual medications due to lower drug doses when used in combination, but there is an increased risk of adverse effects with increasing polypharmacy. CDT makes sense given the complex peripheral and central mechanisms thought to be involved in the development of PHN, and a number of CDTs have been studied in clinical trials. Gabapentin and morphine combined achieved better analgesia in patients with painful diabetic neuropathy (PDN) or PHN than either agent alone, and at lower doses of each drug, albeit with a higher frequency of constipation and dry mouth.[21] In a similarly designed study,

Table 13.6 OTHER PHARMACOTHERAPIES

Drug	*Trade Name*	*Mechanism of Action*	*Typical Dose Range*	*Pharmacology*	*Evidence of Efficacy*	*Common Adverse Side Effects*
Lidocaine (3 percent cream or 5 percent ointment)	LidaMantle	Inhibits Na ion channels, stabilizing cell membranes and inhibiting nerve impulse initiation and conduction (amide local anesthetic)	Apply BID-TID, max 5 g of ointment/dose (topical)	Liver metabolism and urine excretion; half-life = 1.5 to 2 hours	***Strong***—PHN, mixed neuropathic pain	Local erythema, edema, abnormal sensations, and allergic reactions
Lidocaine (5 percent patch)	Lidoderm	Inhibits Na ion channels, stabilizing cell membranes and inhibiting nerve impulse initiation and conduction (amide local anesthetic)	Apply up to 12 h/d, max three patches at a time (transdermal)	Liver metabolism and urine excretion; half-life = 1.5 to 2 hours	***Strong***—PHN, mixed neuropathic pain	Application site reaction, local erythema, local edema, burning or discomfort, abnormal sensations, and urticaria

Botulinum Toxin A (BTX-A)	Botox	Inhibits ACh release from nerve endings, reducing neuromuscular transmission and local muscle activity (neurotoxin)	10 to 100 units per region divided among 5 to 40 sites with a 1 to 2 cm radius of skin (subcutaneous); max 200 units/total dose	Unknown metabolism and excretion; minimal to no systemic absorption; half-life unknown	***Strong***—Cervical dystonia, hyperhidrosis, migraine headache ***Moderate***—PHN	Injection site reaction, injection pain or discomfort, fatigue, muscle weakness, fever, infection, pruritus, and headache
Caspaicin (0.025 percent or 0.075 percent cream)	Zostrix, Capzasin, Salonpas Hot	Selectively binds nerve membrane TRPV1 receptors, initially stimulates and then desensitizes and degenerates cutaneous nociceptive neurons; substance P depletion might also reduce pain impulse transmission to the central nervous system (CNS)	Apply TID/QID (topical)	Unknown metabolism and excretion; minimal systemic absorption; half-life unknown	***Strong***—Post-traumatic neuralgia, PHN, diabetic polyneuropathy, mixed neuropathic pain	Burning, erythema, and thermal hyperalgesia

(continued)

Table 13.6 (CONTINUED)

Drug	*Trade Name*	*Mechanism of Action*	*Typical Dose Range*	*Pharmacology*	*Evidence of Efficacy*	*Common Adverse Side Effects*
Caspaicin (8% patch)	Qutenza	Selectively binds nerve membrane TRPV1 receptors, initially stimulates and then desensitizes and degenerates cutaneous nociceptive neurons; substance P depletion might also reduce pain impulse transmission to the CNS	1 to 4 patches at one time (topical); remove patches after 60 minutes; may repeat no more than q3 months; pre-treat with topical anesthetic	Unknown metabolism and excretion; minimal systemic absorption; half-life unknown	***Strong***—HIV neuropathy, PHN	Application site erythema, pain, pruritus, papules, edema, drying, nausea, HTN, nasopharyngitis, sinusitis, pruritis, vomiting, and bronchitis

nortriptyline and gabapentin decreased pain significantly more than either drug alone in patients with neuropathic pain (PDN or PHN), with dry mouth being the most common adverse effect.[22] A number of studies have examined the effect of adding a selected medication to an existing pain regimen (i.e., opioid therapy), and the outcomes have generally been positive, with better pain relief relative to control shown for gabapentin, pregabalin, and topical capsaicin 8 percent.[6]

Interventional Therapy

Interventional therapies play a limited role in the management of PHN and are utilized primarily for PHN refractory to conservative modalities. Although some randomized studies suggest that interventional procedures such as epidural and paravertebral steroid injections have the potential to prevent the development of PHN, one controlled study evaluating a single epidural steroid injection in subjects with AHZ found that although the injection provided superior pain reduction for one month, it did not prevent PHN.[23] Intrathecal injection of steroid and lidocaine successfully treated PHN in a randomized controlled trial, yet this modality has not been widely accepted because of potential adverse effects such as the development of adhesive arachnoiditis.[24] Spinal cord stimulation, a neuromodulatory technique commonly used for chronic, refractory neuropathic pain conditions, was found to provide long-lasting relief in 23 of 28 patients (4 patients with AHZ and 24 with PHN) refractory to pharmacological therapy,[25] but randomized studies are lacking. Neurosurgical approaches such as rhizhotomies have historically offered minimal relief without long-term benefit while imposing serious surgical risks. Given that there are more effective modalities for the treatment of PHN, neurosurgical approaches are generally contraindicated.

CONCLUSIONS

The treatment of AHZ and its most common complication PHN remains challenging, and these disorders affect millions of people annually. Pharmacologic therapies that have good evidence-based efficacy include TCAs, gabapentin and pregabalin, opioid analgesics, and topical lidocaine patches. Invasive modalities play a potential role for patients with pain refractory to more conventional modalities. Because chronic pain is associated with significant emotional co-morbidities, psychological interventions, including cognitive-behavioral therapy, may be incorporated in the treatment course on an individual basis. Presently, efforts should be aimed at preventing herpes zoster and PHN through vaccination and/or the use of antiviral agents. Ongoing research into the underlying mechanisms of these conditions will facilitate the development of improved treatments for both AHZ and PHN.

REFERENCES

1. Bennett GJ, Watson CP. Herpes zoster and postherpetic neuralgia: past, present and future. *Pain Res Manag*. 2009;14(4):275–282.
2. Baron R, Binder A, Wasner G. Neuropathic pain: diagnosis, pathophysiological mechanisms, and treatment. *Lancet Neurol*. 2010;9(8):807–819.
3. Quan D, Hammack BN, Kittelson J, Gilden DH. Improvement of postherpetic neuralgia after treatment with intravenous acyclovir followed by oral valacyclovir. *Arch Neurol*. 2006;63(7):940–942.
4. Oxman MN, Levin MJ, Johnson GR, et al. A vaccine to prevent herpes zoster and postherpetic neuralgia in older adults *N Engl J Med*. 2005;352(22):2271–2284.
5. Oxman MN, Levin MJ, Shingles Prevention Study Group. Vaccination against herpes zoster and postherpetic neuralgia *J Infect Dis*. 2008;197(Suppl 2):S228–S236.
6. Attal N, Cruccu G, Baron R, et al. EFNS guidelines on the pharmacological treatment of neuropathic pain: 2010 revision. *Eur J Neurol*. 2010;17(9):1113–e88.

7. Wallace M, Pappagallo M. Qutenza(R): a capsaicin 8% patch for the management of postherpetic neuralgia *Expert Rev Neurother*. 2011;11(1):15–27.
8. Hempenstall K, Nurmikko TJ, Johnson RW, A'Hern RP, Rice AS. Analgesic therapy in postherpetic neuralgia: a quantitative systematic review. *PLoS Med*. 2005;2(7):e164.
9. Rowbotham MC, Reisner LA, Davies PS, Fields HL. Treatment response in antidepressant-naive postherpetic neuralgia patients: double-blind, randomized trial. *J Pain*. 2005;6(11):741–746.
10. Collins SL, Moore RA, McQuay HJ, Wiffen P. Antidepressants and anticonvulsants for diabetic neuropathy and postherpetic neuralgia: a quantitative systematic review *J Pain Symptom Manage*. 2000;20(6):449–458.
11. Rice AS, Maton S, Postherpetic Neuralgia Study Group. Gabapentin in postherpetic neuralgia: a randomised, double blind, placebo controlled study. *Pain*. 2001;94(2):215–224.
12. Rowbotham M, Harden N, Stacey B, Bernstein P, Magnus-Miller L. Gabapentin for the treatment of postherpetic neuralgia: a randomized controlled trial. *JAMA*. 1998;280(21):1837–1842.
13. Freynhagen R, Strojek K, Griesing T, Whalen E, Balkenohl M. Efficacy of pregab alin in neuropathic pain evaluated in a 12-week, randomised, double-blind, multicentre, placebo-controlled trial of flexible- and fixed-dose regimens. *Pain*. 2005;115(3):254–263.
14. Gilron I, Wajsbrot D, Therrien F, Lemay J. Pregabalin for peripheral neuropathic pain: a multicenter, enriched enrollment randomized withdrawal placebo-controlled trial. *Clin J Pain*. 2011;27(3):185–193.
15. Raja SN, Haythornthwaite JA, Pappagallo M, et al. Opioids versus antidepressants in postherpetic neuralgia: a randomized, placebo-controlled trial. *Neurology*. 2002;59(7):1015–1021.
16. Watson CP, Babul N. Efficacy of oxycodone in neuropathic pain: a randomized trial in postherpetic neuralgia. *Neurology*. 1998;50(6):1837–1841.
17. Mordarski S, Lysenko L, Gerber H, Zietek M, Gredes T, Dominiak M. The effect of treatment with fentanyl patches on pain relief and improvement in overall daily functioning in patients with postherpetic neuralgia. *J Physiol Pharmacol*. 2009;60(Suppl 8):31–35.
18. Boureau F, Legallicier P, Kabir-Ahmadi M. Tramadol in post-herpetic neuralgia: a randomized, double-blind, placebo-controlled trial. *Pain*. 2003;104(1–2):323–331.
19. Baron R, Mayoral V, Leijon G, Binder A, Steigerwald I, Serpell M. 5% lidocaine medicated plaster versus pregabalin in post-herpetic neuralgia and diabetic polyneuropathy: an open-label, non-inferiority two-stage RCT study *Curr Med Res Opin*. 2009;25(7):1663–1676.
20. Ranoux D, Attal N, Morain F, Bouhassira D. Botulinum toxin type A induces direct analgesic effects in chronic neuropathic pain. *Ann Neurol*. 2008;64(3):274–283.

21. Gilron I, Bailey JM, Tu D, Holden RR, Weaver DF, Houlden RL. Morphine, gabapentin, or their combination for neuropathic pain. *N Engl J Med.* 2005;352(13):1324–1334.
22. Gilron I, Bailey JM, Tu D, Holden RR, Jackson AC, Houlden RL. Nortriptyline and gabapentin, alone and in combination for neuropathic pain: a double-blind, randomised controlled crossover trial. *Lancet.* 2009;374(9697):1252–1261.
23. van Wijck AJ, Opstelten W, Moons KG, et al. The PINE study of epidural steroids and local anaesthetics to prevent postherpetic neuralgia: a randomised controlled trial. *Lancet.* 2006;367(9506):219–224.
24. van Wijck AJ, Wallace M, Mekhail N, van Kleef M. Evidence-based interventional pain medicine according to clinical diagnoses. 17. Herpes zoster and post-herpetic neuralgia. *Pain Pract.* 2011;11(1):88–97.
25. Harke H, Gretenkort P, Ladleif HU, Koester P, Rahman S. Spinal cord stimulation in postherpetic neuralgia and in acute herpes zoster pain. *Anesth Analg.* 2002;94(3):694–700.

14

Complex Regional Pain Syndrome

SALIM M. HAYEK AND HENRY E. VUCETIC

Case Presentation

A 35-year-old female presents to clinic with complaints of severe burning electrical-like pain in her left ankle. The patient informs you that she fractured her ankle 6 months ago while trick-or-treating with her children. She underwent open reduction and internal fixation under general anesthesia. According to the surgeon, the fixation is stable and there is nothing more to be done surgically. The patient states that she has swelling episodes, especially with physical loading, and periods when her left ankle and foot become sweaty, hot, and discolored. The opioids prescribed by her surgeon do not provide her with adequate pain relief, she is unable to participate in physical therapy and has difficulty with simple daily chores (Fig. 14.1).

Complex regional pain syndrome (CRPS) is a chronic pain condition that can result in significant disabilities for the affected patient. CRPS patients often pose challenging presentations for the general

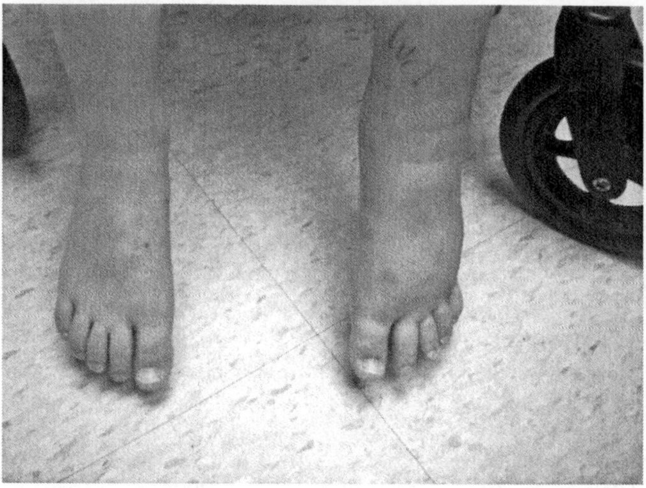

Figure 14.1. CRPS of the left lower extremity in a young patient following a minor foot injury. Note the swelling and skin mottling in the left foot region in contrast to the asymptomatic right foot.

practitioner and specialist.[1] Being able to identify a case of CRPS in a timely manner facilitates the implementation of appropriate treatment measures and might significantly improve outcomes, as well as the patient's overall future well-being.

HISTORY AND DIAGNOSIS

CRPS was first recognized in the United States. In 1864, army neurologist Silas Weir Mitchell described a painful condition afflicting injured Civil War soldiers. Soldiers with major peripheral nerve injuries experienced burning pain, swelling, and color changes in the affected limb. He coined the term "causalgia" in 1867 (derived from the Greek words *kausus* for heat and *algos* for pain) to describe the burning nature of the pain often experienced in this condition.[2]

Many decades later, J. A. Evans introduced the term "reflex sympathetic dystrophy" (RSD) to describe how the sympathetic nervous system (SNS) influenced extremity pain in a matching clinical entity that lacked clear nerve injury.[3] French surgeon Rene Leriche went on to highlight the involvement of the SNS in this entity by performing sympathetic blocks on affected limbs to provide pain relief. However, a variety of different names were used to describe the condition, and there was no consensus over diagnostic criteria. In 1994, a clearer definition and nomenclature for these two chronic pain conditions, RSD and causalgia, were developed by the International Association for the Study of Pain (IASP). The new term, "complex regional pain syndrome," was adopted to replace these older terms, and defined diagnostic criteria were established.[4] A distinction was made between the two original conditions. CRPS I, formerly known as RSD, is defined by the IASP as "a syndrome that usually develops after an initiating noxious event, is not limited to the distribution of a single peripheral nerve, and is apparently disproportionate to the inciting event. It is associated at some point with evidence of edema, changes in skin blood flow, abnormal sudomotor (i.e. sweating and swelling) activity in the region of the pain, or allodynia or hyperalgesia." CRPS II, formerly known as causalgia, added an identified major peripheral nerve injury to the above definition.[4] Clinically, the two conditions are indistinguishable.

PATHOPHYSIOLOGY AND MECHANISMS

The exact pathophysiology of CRPS remains unclear to expert practitioners and scientists studying the condition. Two theories have been proposed based on scientific evidence: one focuses on inflammatory processes, and the other emphasizes neuropathic mechanisms. A combination of both processes might be at play, with neurogenic inflammation leading to the complex sudomotor, sympathetic, deep tissue, and dermatologic manifestations. Neurogenic inflammation from a peripheral injury results in a spike in inflammatory factors including but not limited to substance P, calcitonin gene-related peptide, histamine, and cytokines. In patients with CRPS, these factors remain elevated for an prolonged period of time.[5,6] In response to injury, damaged afferent nociceptive neural fibers become coupled with adrenergic receptors. These receptors become up-regulated and produce the observed sympathetic signs.[7] Dysfunction in the somatic and autonomic nervous system strongly supports the theory that CRPS is a neuropathic condition. This explains why neuropathic pain symptoms are observed in a majority of patients with CRPS. However, many other factors, including genetic, psychological, and environmental factors, play an important modulatory role. Further, the intriguing recent notion that CRPS might be an autoimmune disorder gained some support when autoantibodies against a cholinergic receptor were identified in between 30 percent and 40 percent of CRPS patients.[8] In a follow-up study, the investigators identified immunoglobulin G autoantibodies in a subset of CRPS patients, but not in controls, directed against peptide sequences from the second extracellular loop of the β_2 adrenergic receptor and/or the muscarinic-2 receptor.[9]

EPIDEMIOLOGY

The largest epidemiologic study to date suggests that CRPS is not as infrequent as once thought. A study from the Netherlands reported that the incidence of CRPS was 26.2 cases per 100,000 people.[9] This was based on the diagnostic criteria set forth by the IASP in 1994, and the study reported a 4-fold higher rate than a study conducted by the Mayo Clinic in Olmsted County, MN.[10] Thus, with an estimated population of 300 million people in the United States, there might be more than 50,000 new cases annually. CRPS is found more commonly in females than males and has its highest incidence in individuals between 50 and 70 years of age. Upper extremity presentation is more common in adults, with fractures and sprains being the two most common inciting events.[7] CRPS manifests in 18 percent of patients with wrist fractures and >30 percent of individuals with ankle fractures.[11,12] However, in about 10 percent of cases, no inciting event or injury can explain the onset of symptoms.[9,13]

PRESENTATION

Patients presenting with CRPS affecting an extremity will often display a triad of sensory, autonomic, and motor signs and symptoms.[1] Sensory manifestations include mechanical and thermal allodynia, hyperalgesia in response to mechanical stimulation, and intense pain and hyperesthesia. The pain is often described as a burning, shooting, aching sensation that is localized in deep somatic tissues, is disproportionate to the injury, and lasts beyond the expected recovery time. The presenting symptoms are often unilateral and do not typically follow the distribution of any peripheral nerve.[14]

The autonomic manifestations include swelling, temperature and color changes, and sudomotor (sweating) abnormalities. These autonomic signs and symptoms are often brought on by weight–bearing, mechanical loading/stimuli to the affected extremity, or by environmental temperature changes.[15] More than 90 percent of patients will present with swelling in the affected area, color changes are observed in more than 70 percent of patients, and sudomotor changes affect 59 percent of patients with CRPS.[10]

Motor manifestations include weakness, tremor, muscle spasms, involuntary movements, dystonia, and paresis.[1] Patients will often acutely suffer from decreased range of motion in the affected limb, which might be secondary to joint effusion and/or pain. In those individuals with long-standing CRPS, contractures, fibrosis, hair and nail changes characterized by alterations in growth patterns, and glossy skin might ensue.[14] In most cases of CRPS types I and II, the signs and symptoms remain in the originally affected limb. However, in between 4 percent and 10 percent of cases, migration to other extremities occurs.[16] Contralateral spread (i.e., mirror image spread) is twice as likely to occur as ipsilateral spread to an arm or leg, with diagonal spread being the least common pattern of spread. When this ensues, it is usually attributed to new trauma.

DIAGNOSIS

CRPS is a clinical diagnosis made by the healthcare provider. The examiner should test for altered central pain processing when CRPS is suspected. Allodynia should be tested for by using a light brush or touching the affected area. Thermal allodynia is identified by using hot or cool objects in the affected area. Close attention needs to be paid to the skin, hair growth, and nails to identify any trophic changes present. Temperature asymmetry, observed in 56 percent of patients between the affected and unaffected limbs, needs to be documented as well. Finally, autonomic function can be identified via close examination of the skin. Sympathetic hypofunction often presents as hot, red, dry skin (warm CRPS), and sympathetic hyperfunction manifests as cold, blue, pale, and sweaty skin (cold CRPS).[13] Many radiologic and electrophysiologic tests have been proposed to help diagnose CRPS, including triple-phase bone scanning, electromyography, microneurography, somatosensory evoked potentials, qualitative sudomotor axon reflex testing, quantitative sensory testing, thermography, and laser Doppler flowmetry. However, none are clinically relevant, and all lack sufficient sensitivity and/or specificity.[15] Thus, CRPS remains a clinical diagnosis based on established diagnostic criteria.

In 1994, the IASP not only created new nomenclature but also established a set of diagnostic criteria for CRPS I and II (Table 14.1).[4] These original IASP criteria, however, have come under much criticism since their creation. Although highly sensitive (98 percent), they have been shown to lack sufficient specificity (36 percent).[17] In 2007, an attempt to improve the diagnostic criteria was made (the Budapest criteria [Table 14.1], named after the city in which they were proposed). The newer criteria included physical signs at the time of evaluation (rather than just patient report), new motor signs and symptoms added to the old criteria, and the separation of sudomotor and vasomotor signs (i.e., skin color and temperature) and symptoms from sensory manifestations.[18] These new criteria were clinically tested for validation and were found to retain a high level of sensitivity (99 percent) with increased specificity (68 percent). In 2012, the IASP website displayed the Budapest criteria as the official current diagnostic criteria for CRPS (http://www.iasp-pain.org/AM/Template.cfm?Section=Classification_of_Chronic_Pain&Template=/CM/ContentDisplay.cfm&ContentID=16275). These new criteria are divided into clinical and research criteria with the research criteria being more specific, but less sensitive than the clinical criteria.The research criteria require that four of the symptom categories and at least two sign categories be present (Table 14.1).

CLASSIFICATION

Traditionally, CRPS was hypothesized to have three distinct stages: an early inflammatory stage, a dystrophic stage, and a late atrophic stage. However, there is no evidence to support this staging pattern.[19] A large prospective study evaluating multiple signs and symptoms

Table 14.1 IASP DIAGNOSTIC CRITERIA FOR CRPS, OLD AND CURRENT

1994 IASP CRPS Diagnostic Criteria

CRPS I (Reflex Sympathetic Dystrophy)

1. The presence of an initiating noxious event or cause of immobilization.
2. Continuing pain, allodynia, or hyperalgesia which is disproportionate to any inciting event.
3. Evidence at some time of edema, changes in skin blood flow, or abnormal sudomotor activity in the region of pain.
4. This diagnosis is excluded by the existence of conditions that would otherwise account for the degree of pain and dysfunction.
   - Criteria 2–4 must be satisfied.

CRPS II (Causalgia)

1. The presence of continuing pain, allodynia, or hyperalgesia after a nerve injury, not necessarily limited to the distribution of the injured nerve.
2. Evidence at some time of edema, changes in skin blood flow, or abnormal sudomotor activity in the region of the pain.
3. This diagnosis is excluded by the existence of conditions that would otherwise account for the degree of pain and dysfunction.
   - All three criteria must be satisfied.

Current IASP Clinical Diagnostic Criteria for CRPS (Budapest Criteria)[a]

i. Continuing pain that is disproportionate to any inciting event.

ii. Must report at least one symptom in three of the four following categories:

1. Sensory: reports of hyperesthesia and/or allodynia.
2. Vasomotor: reports of temperature asymmetry and/or skin color changes and/or skin color asymmetry.
3. Sudomotor/edema: reports of edema and/or sweating changes and/or sweating asymmetry.

(continued)

Table 14.1 (*CONTINUED*)

4. Motor/trophic: reports of decreased range of motion and/or motor dysfunction (weakness, tremor, dystonia) and/or trophic changes (hair, nails, skin).

iii. Must display at least one sign at time of evaluation in two or more of the following categories:

1. Sensory: evidence of hyperalgesia (to pinprick) and/or allodynia (to light touch and/or deep somatic pressure and/or joint movement).
2. Vasomotor: evidence of temperature asymmetry and/or skin color changes and/or asymmetry.
3. Sudomotor/edema: evidence of edema and/or sweating changes and/or sweating asymmetry.
4. Motor/trophic: evidence of decreased range of motion and/or motor dysfunction (weakness, tremor, dystonia) and/or trophic changes (hair, nails, skin).

iv. There is no other diagnosis that better explains the signs and symptoms.

Source: Merskey H, Bogduk N. *Classification of Chronic Pain: Description of Chronic Pain Syndromes and Definition of Pain Terms*. IASP Press: Seattle, WA; 1994; and Harden RN, Bruehl S, Perez RS, et al. Validation of proposed diagnostic criteria (the "Budapest Criteria") for Complex Regional Pain Syndrome. *Pain*. 2010;150:268–274.

[a]Kohr D, Singh P, Tschematsch M, et al. Autoimmunity against the B2 adrenergic receptor and muscarinic-2 receptor in complex regional pain syndrome. *Pain*. 2011;152:2690–2700.

in 829 CRPS patients suggested that patients should be stratified based on clinical presentation into warm and cold CRPS subtypes.[13] Warm CRPS manifests as warm reddish skin, whereas cold CRPS presents with cool, shiny, and thin skin. In one study, only 13 percent of patients had cold CRPS upon presentation, further emphasizing the inflammatory role in CRPS, especially early in development.[13]

Another study found that that cold CRPS patients exhibited worse clinical outcomes and were more likely to experience progression of their disease 8 years after initial diagnosis.[20]

TREATMENT

Conservative

Treatments of CRPS patients can be very challenging, with the primary goal of management centering on restoration of function, pain control, and return to gainful employment.[21] Rehabilitation, desensitization, and normalization can be achieved in motivated patients through an interdisciplinary approach.[15,21,22] This often includes occupational therapy, physical therapy, interventional pain management, psychotherapy, and pharmacotherapy (Fig. 14.2). The purpose of some modalities is to treat the symptoms in order to facilitate rehabilitation (e.g., sympathetic nerve blocks to maximize physical therapy).[15]

Occupational and physical therapy should be the mainstay treatment of patients presenting with CRPS. It is important to obtain a baseline assessment of function including parameters such as dexterity, pain during activities of daily living, and range of motion. From this initial assessment, a care plan can be implemented to improve the overall function of the affected limb. Desensitization is often implemented first, followed by isometric stress loading and exercises aimed at improving range of motion and increasing overall strength. A slow and gradual increase in exercise is recommended, as CRPS patients who are put through aggressive rehabilitation schedules are often unable to tolerate physical therapy and fail to progress.[15] Land- and water-based therapies have both been found to be helpful in the rehabilitation of CRPS patients, with water-based exercises

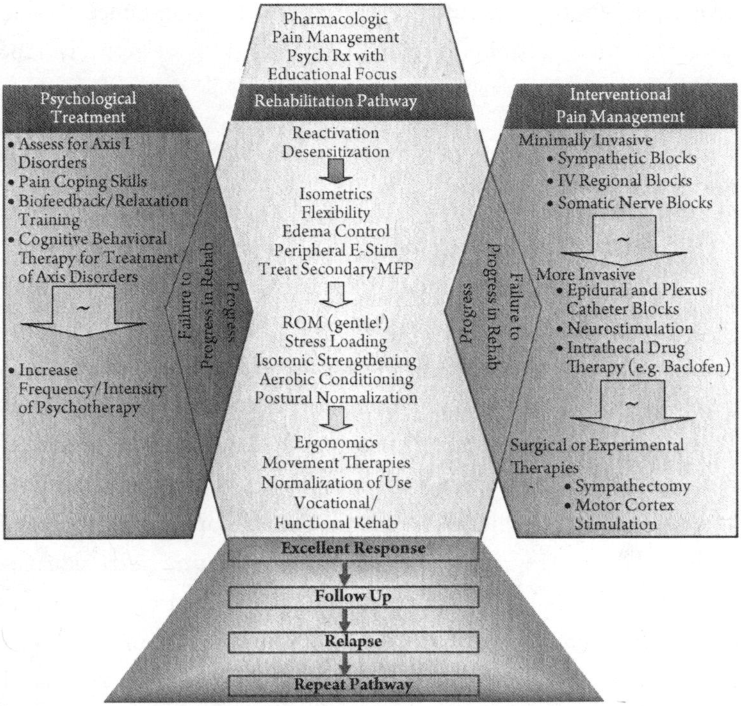

Figure 14.2. Modified diagram of proposed treatment algorithm for CRPS; rehabilitation remains at the core of treatment. ~, inadequate or partial response. MFP, myofascial pain; ROM, range of motion; e-stim, electrical stimulation. From Stanton-Hicks MB, Burton AW, Bruehl SP, et al. An updated interdisciplinary clinical pathway for CRPS: report of an expert panel. *Pain Pract.* 2002;2(1):1–16.

prescribed initially for patients with marked limb impairments. In those patients with features of deafferentation pain and altered body image, mirror therapy, which has been successfully used in patients with phantom limb pain, was found to be very helpful in the rehabilitation of CRPS-affected limbs. Using this modality, a CRPS patient can view the unaffected limb in a mirror while moving both limbs in synchrony. In early CRPS, visual input from a moving, unaffected limb re-establishes the pain-free relationship between sensory feedback and motor execution. The brain seeks congruence among motor intention, peripheral sensory input, and visual input. Mirror therapy "restores" this relationship.[23]

Pharmacotherapy

Pharmacotherapy is nearly always a part of the initial treatment plan. A majority of pain management practitioners (85 percent) will utilize medications as an initial treatment. However, there is a paucity of randomized controlled trials evaluating pharmacologic agents utilized in CRPS patients. Most of the studies that have been published are either small or uncontrolled. Despite the limitations in evidence, numerous medications are used to treat CRPS.[21]

Gabapentin is an anti-epileptic drug (AED) that is thought to work by modulating presynaptic calcium channels on nociceptive neurons in the dorsal horn. It has been found to be effective in the treatment of neuropathic pain in CRPS. In the largest placebo-controlled study evaluating gabapentin in CRPS patients (85 of the 305 studied patients had CRPS), a significant reduction in pain relative to placebo was demonstrated. Pregabalin, a newer AED, has a mechanism of action similar to that of gabapentin, but it has not been critically studied in CRPS patients. However, studies evaluating pregabalin in other neuropathic pain conditions such as diabetic neuropathy and postherpetic neuralgia have reported good outcomes. The main advantages of this medication over gabapentin are its more linear pharmacokinetic profile and less frequent dosing requirements; it has a side-effect profile similar to that of gabapentin.[21]

Sodium-channel-blocking AEDs have shown some promise in treating CRPS. Only carbamazepine has been studied in CRPS in a randomized controlled trial (7 of 38 neuropathic pain patients studied had CRPS). After 8 days of treatment, a significant reduction in pain relative to placebo was noted.[21,24] Other sodium-channel-blocking medications, such as intravenous lidocaine, have demonstrated efficacy in several studies for neuropathic pain and CRPS.[21] One uncontrolled study by Schwartzman and colleagues found that continuous intravenous lidocaine reduced spontaneous pain and specific characteristics of evoked pain in CRPS patients. The authors demonstrated a significant decrease in inflammation and mechanical and thermal allodynia for 3 months following a 5-day infusion, with minimal side effects.[25]

Tricyclic antidepressants (TCAs) have good evidence supporting their use in the treatment of neuropathic pain; however, there are few data on their use in the treatment of CRPS.[21] Their major mode of action might involve enhancement of the noradrenergic and serotonergic descending inhibitory pathways, along with several other possible mechanisms such as the blockade of *N*-methyl-D-aspartate (NMDA) receptors, sodium channels, and adenosine reuptake. Practitioners should be cautious when prescribing these medications because of their propensity for side effects in the elderly and their narrow therapeutic window.[21]

As with many other non-cancer-related pain conditions, there are few data to support the use of opioid medications as part of an effective long-term treatment regimen for CRPS. A randomized, placebo-controlled trial of opioids in CRPS patients showed no reduction in pain relative to placebo over an 8-day period.[15] Most important, the potential side effects of opioid medications are particularly problematic. Common side effects include nausea, constipation, somnolence, and cognitive impairment. More serious, opioids can depress respiration and lead to dependence and sometimes addiction.[21] CRPS patients will often require long-term treatment, and chronic opioid therapy can lead to problems such as tolerance, opioid-induced hyperalgesia, hormonal effects, and immune suppression. Therefore, chronic treatment with opioids might lead to more pain and dysfunction over the long term.[21]

Oral corticosteroids have shown promise in the treatment of acute CRPS. Small randomized controlled trials have shown that a short trial of steroids resulted in significantly better analgesia than placebo. This, again, highlights the inflammatory component of the disease.[1,21]

Bisphosphonates have been found to be effective for CRPS in multiple placebo-controlled studies.[26] Not only pain but also joint mobility and motor function might be improved following bisphosphonate therapy. Although uncertain, the mechanism of action is thought to involve the prevention of bone remodeling associated with CRPS. However, these agents might also possess analgesic properties that derive from central, as well as peripheral mechanisms.

One treatment that has generated intense interest in the pain medicine community is the use of ketamine infusions to treat CRPS and other chronic pain conditions. Ketamine exerts its pain-relieving effects via myriad mechanisms, but its main mechanism of action is the blockade of NMDA receptors, which are involved in central sensitization. There are currently two placebo-controlled studies[27,28] and several uncontrolled studies demonstrating modest benefit lasting at least 3 months in CRPS patients treated with continuous (4 to 10 days) intravenous infusions. The most concerning side effect of ketamine is the potential for psychomimetic effects, which can be reduced with the coadministration of benzodiazepines.

Interventional

Sympathetic blockade has become almost a standard early interventional modality for the treatment of patients with CRPS, despite limited clinical evidence. A recent randomized, double-blind, placebo-controlled trial in children with CRPS demonstrated the efficacy of lidocaine block of the sympathetic chain in reducing allodynia in response to brush, pinprick, and pinprick temporal summation, as well as for in verbal pain scores.[29] Recently, an evidence-based review on interventional procedures for the treatment of CRPS recommended sympathetic blockade as a first-line treatment.[30]

Spinal cord stimulation (SCS) is an established modality that can provide long-term benefit in the treatment of CRPS. SCS is achieved through electrical stimulation of the dorsal columns of the spinal cord. One prospective trial studied 29 patients with CRPS. These patients were followed for 35.6 ± 21 months, and implanted patients were found to have resolution of allodynia and improvement of deep pain.[31] In a randomized controlled study by Kemler et al., SCS combined with physical therapy provided significant improvements in pain scores and global perceived effect relative to physical therapy alone for at least 2 years.[32] After 5 years, the difference was not statistically significant using an intent-to-treat analysis; however, this might have been due to attrition in patient numbers. In general, SCS in patients with CRPS I might successfully provide long-term pain relief and improved quality of life, but large studies have not shown it to improve overall function.[1]

CRPS IN CHILDREN

There is little research published on the treatment of pediatric patients with CRPS. Approximately 90 percent of the pediatric cases are females between 8 and 16 years of age. Unlike in adults, lower extremity presentation is more common, and 97 percent of cases will go into remission with exercise therapy and behavioral management alone.[33] There are small studies that suggest the use of continuous nerve blocks, sympathetic nerve blockade, transcutaneous electrical nerve stimulation, or intravenous lidocaine infusions might provide additional benefit when added to exercise and behavioral management to help children with CRPS rehabilitate and regain function.[1]

PREVENTION

Because of the heterogeneity of this syndrome, prevention can be difficult. Individuals with a prior history of CRPS or other chronic pain conditions, female gender, ongoing psychopathology, and/or high levels of baseline pain and disability might be at greater risk of developing CRPS. Several double-blind, placebo-controlled studies have demonstrated that starting oral vitamin C (500 to 1000 mg/d for 50 days) might reduce the incidence of CRPS in cases of wrist and ankle fractures.[1] Although other preventive measures such as sympathetic blocks and adjuvant analgesic agents are often recommended, the evidence to support these therapies is anecdotal.

SUMMARY

In summary, CRPS is a complicated painful entity characterized by many unknown variables. Similar to other syndromes (e.g., irritable bowel syndrome and fibromyalgia) that comprise a constellation of signs and symptoms in the absence of well-defined causative mechanisms, the prognosis tends to be poorer than those seen with disease states distinguished by distinct pathophysiological mechanisms that can often be treated by specific pharmacological or interventional therapies that address these mechanisms. There are limited data supporting the use of a majority of therapeutic interventions, with treatment often guided empirically or based on anecdotal evidence. One should keep in mind that all the psychological, pharmacological, and interventional therapies are geared toward facilitating the main goal of CRPS treatment, namely, functional restoration (Fig. 14.2). Rapid strides are being made in elucidating the pathophysiologic processes behind CRPS. Hopefully, better studies will help identify specific interventions and multi-disciplinary treatment approaches that can improve pain and restore function in this difficult pain population.[15]

REFERENCES

1. Perez RS, Zollinger PE, Dijkstra PU, et al. Evidence based guidelines for complex regional pain syndrome type 1. *BMC Neurol.* 2010;10:1471–1485.
2. Turf RM, Bacardi BE. Causalgia: clarifications in terminology and a case presentation. *J Foot Surg.* 1986;25:284–295.
3. Evans JA. Reflex sympathetic dystrophy; report on 7 cases. *Ann Intern Med.* 1947;26:417–426.
4. Merskey H, Bogduk N. *Classification of Chronic Pain: Description of Chronic Pain Syndromes and Definition of Pain Terms.* IASP Press: Seattle, WA; 1994.
5. Huygen FJ, De Bruijn AG, De Bruin MT, Groeneweg JG, Klein J, Zijlstra FJ. Evidence for local inflammation in complex regional pain syndrome type 1. *Mediators Inflamm.* 2002;11:47–51.
6. Munnikes RJ, Muis C, Boersma M, Heijmans-Antonissen C, Zijlstra FJ, Huygen FJ. Intermediate stage complex regional pain syndrome type 1 is unrelated to proinflammatory cytokines. *Mediators Inflamm.* 2005;6:366–372.
7. Bruehl S, Chung OY. How common is complex regional pain syndrome Type I? *Pain.* 2007;129:1–2.
8. Kohr D, Singh P, Tschematsch M, et al. Autoimmunity against the B2 adrenergic receptor and muscarinic-2 receptor in complex regional pain syndrome. *Pain.* 2011;152:2690–2700.
9. de Mos M, de Bruijin AG, Huygen FJ, Dieleman JP, Stricker BH, Sturkenboom MC. The incidence of complex regional pain syndrome: a population-based study. *Pain.* 2007;128:12–20.
10. Sandroni P, Benrud-Larson LM, McClelland RL, Low PA. Complex regional pain syndrome type I: incidence and prevalence in Olmsted County, a population-based study. *Pain.* 2003;103:199–207.
11. Atkins RM, Duckworth T, Kanis JA. Algodystrophy following Colles' fracture. *J Hand Surg Br.* 1989;14:161–164.
12. Sarangi PP, Ward AJ, Smith EJ, Staddon GE, Atkins RM. Algodystrophy and osteoporosis after tibial fractures. *J Bone Joint Surg Br.* 1993;75:450–452.
13. Veldman PH, Reynen HM, Arntz IE, Goris RJ. Signs and symptoms of reflex sympathetic dystrophy: prosective study of 829 patients. *Lancet.* 1993;342:1012–1016.
14. Birklein F, Handwerker HO. Complex regional pain syndrome: how to resolve the complexity? *Pain.* 2001;94:1–6.

15. Harden RN. Complex regional pain syndrome. *Br J Anaes.* 2001; 87(1):99–106.
16. van Rijn MA, Marinus J, Putter H, Bosselaar SR, Moseley GL, van Hilten JJ. Spreading of complex regional pain syndrome: not a random process. *J Neural Transm.* 2011;118:1301–1309.
17. Bruehl S, Haden RN, Galer BS, et al. External validation of IASP diagnostic criteria for Complex Regional Pain Syndrome and proposed research diagnostic criteria. International Association for the Study of Pain. *Pain.* 1999;81:147–154.
18. Harden RN, Bruehl S, Perez RS, et al. Validation of proposed diagnostic criteria (the "Budapest Criteria") for Complex Regional Pain Syndrome. *Pain.* 2010;150:268–274.
19. Bruehl S, Harden RN, Galer BS, Saltz S, Backonja M, Stanton-Hicks M. Complex regional pain syndrome: are there distinct subtypes and sequential stages of the syndrome? *Pain.* 2002;95:119–124.
20. Vaneker M, Wilder-Smith OH, Schrombges P, de Man-Hermsen I, Oerlemans HM. Patients initially diagnosed as "warm" or "cold" CRPS 1 show differences in central sensory processing some eight years after diagnosis: a quantitative sensory testing study. *Pain.* 2005;115:204–211.
21. Mackey S, Feinberg S. Pharmacologic therapies for complex regional pain syndrome. *Curr Pain Headache Rep.* 2007;11:38–43.
22. Stanton-Hicks MB, Burton AW, Bruehl SP, et al. An updated interdisciplinary clincal pathway for CRPS: report of an expert panel. *Pain Pract.* 2002;2(1):1–16.
23. McCabe CS, Haigh RC, Ring EF, Halligan PW, Wall PD, Blake DR. A controlled pilot study of the utility of mirror visual feedback in the treatment of complex regional pain syndrome (type 1). *Rheumatology (Oxford).* 2003;42:97–101.
24. Harke H, Gretenkort P, Ladleif HU, Rahman S, Harke O. The response of neuropathic pain and pain in complex regional pain syndrome I to carbamazepine and sustained-release morphine in patients pretreated with spinal cord stimulation: a double-blinded randomized study. *Anesth Analg.* 2001;92:488–495.
25. Schwartzman RJ, Patel M, Grothusen JR, Alexander GM. Efficacy of 5-day continuous lidocaine infusion for the treatment of refractory complex regional pain syndrome. *Pain Med.* 2009;10:401–412.
26. Tran de QH, Duong S, Bertini P, Finlayson RJ. Treatment of complex regional pain syndrome: a review of the evidence. *Can J Anaesth.* 2010;57:149–166.
27. Schwartzman RJ, Alexander GM, Grothusen JR, et al. Outpatient intravenous ketamine for the treatment of complex regional pain syndrome: a double-blind placebo controlled study. *Pain.* 2009;147:107–115.
28. Sigtermans MJ, van Hilten JJ, Bauer MC, et al. Ketamine produces effective and long-term pain relief in patients with Complex Regional Pain Syndrome Type 1. *Pain.* 2009;145:304–311.

29. Meier PM, Zurakowski D, Berde CB, Sethna NF. Lumbar sympathetic blockade in children with complex regional pain syndromes: a double blind placebo-controlled crossover trial. *Anesthesiology*. 2009;111(2):372–380.
30. van Eijs F, Stanton-Hicks M, Van Zundert J, et al. Evidence-based interventional pain medicine according to clinical diagnoses. 16. Complex regional pain syndrome. *Pain Pract*. 2011;11:70–87.
31. Harke H, Gretenkort P, Ladleif HU, Rahman S. Spinal cord stimulation in sympathetically maintained complex regional pain syndrome type I with severe disability. A prospective clinical study. *Eur J Pain*. 2005;9:363–373.
32. Kemler MA, de Vet HC, Barendse GA, van de Wildenberg FA, van Kleef M. Spinal cord stimulation for chronic reflex sympathetic dystrophy—five year follow-up. *N Engl J Med*. 2006;354:2394–2396.
33. Stanton-Hicks MB. Plasiciticy of complex regional pain syndrome (CRPS) in children. *Pain Med*. 2010;11(8):1216–1223.

15

Primary Headache

WADE COOPER

Case Presentation

A 35-year-old male presents with a 5-year history of episodic headache lasting approximately 12 hours and occurring 8 days per month. He notes that the headaches might be related to work stressors. He describes a bilateral frontal headache of moderate to severe intensity that worsens when he climbs a flight of stairs. When it is severe, he experiences nausea. He denies any warning of headache escalation or visual changes.

Case Discussion

This case fulfills the International Headache Society (IHS) classifications[1] for episodic migraine with two characteristics (severe headache, worse with physical activity) and one associated symptom (nausea). This patient does not report aura, which is seen in only one-third of those with migraine. Having a severe, incapacitating headache excludes a diagnosis of tension type headache. The bilateral nature rules out cluster headache (CH). There are many treatment options to consider. In this case it is reasonable to start preventive therapy with magnesium glycinate and, if there is no improvement in 4 weeks, escalate to an alternative pharmacological therapy such as topiramate. Acute headache attacks may be abortively treated with a "triptan"-class medication, assuming no contraindications are present.

BACKGROUND

Headache is very common, with approximately 5 percent of the U.S. population seeking medical care for the condition annually. Careful history and subsequent clinical evaluation are keys to accurate diagnosis and effective management. Most recurrent headaches are symptoms of the primary headache disorder. Secondary structural causes of headache such as tumor or aneurysm are less commonly encountered and are beyond the scope of this chapter.

The IHS has published the IHS Headache Classifications,[1] which serves as a research tool for categorizing headache syndromes. Although the IHS Classifications were not intended to be a clinical tool, these classifications are commonly used in the clinical setting and are referred to throughout this chapter (Fig. 15.1).

MIGRAINE

Migraine is the most common headache diagnosis among those seeking care from physicians and other healthcare providers. More than 90 percent of patients presenting to a primary care physician for headache fulfill the diagnostic criteria of either migraine or probable migraine. Patients with migraine have an 80 percent likelihood that a

This flow chart is simplified to classify primary headache syndromes.
Confirmation of diagnosis with IHS criteria is required.

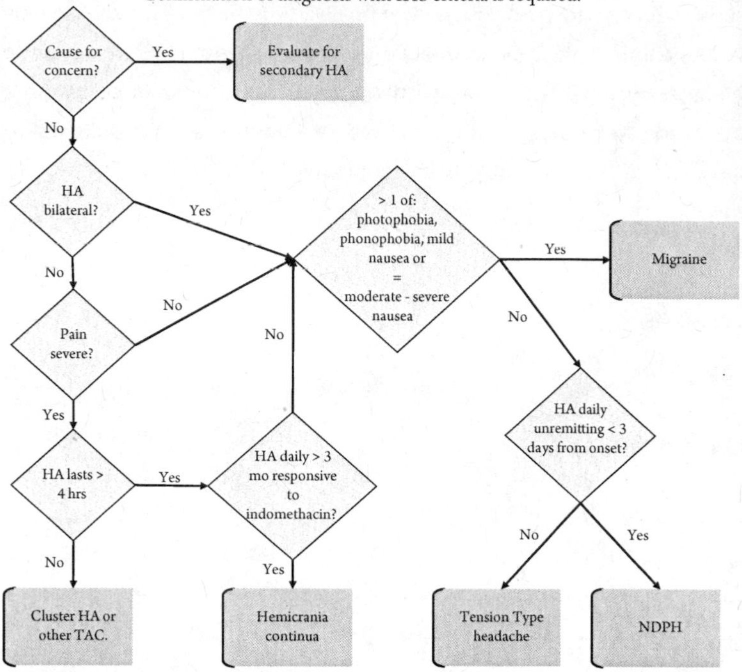

Figure 15.1. Headache diagnosis flow chart. HA, headache; NDPH, new persistent daily headache; TAC, trigeminal autonomic cephalgias.

first-degree relative also suffers from migraine, suggesting a substantial genetic component to this syndrome.[2]

The key anatomical components of migraine include meningeal vasculature, trigeminal nerves and the corresponding trigeminal nucleus caudalis, thalamus, hypothalamus, and other notable areas in the brain stem. When these areas are sensitized beyond their threshold, a migraine is triggered. This results in a positive feedback system between peripheral meninges and trigeminal nerves and the more central migraine components within the brain. It might take hours or days for a patient to return to his or her baseline state. Patients with frequent migraines (migraineurs) are known to have an increased sensitivity to external stimuli, also referred to as a hyperexcitable nervous system. Some of the most common triggers of migraine include poor sleep, stress, diet, and hormonal fluctuations, as commonly occur in menstruating women. The migraineur's brain is believed to have a low tolerance for these triggers, with exposure giving way to the experience of migraine symptoms. This threshold might fluctuate over time. A migraineur might develop migraines with minimal stimulation during one period of his or her life but be able to tolerate multiple triggers without migraines at another point in his or her lifetime.

Migraine aura is a transient neurologic phenomenon that occurs in approximately one-third of migraineurs, but it is also observed in other primary headache syndromes. In migraine aura, a wave of excitation followed by a relative inhibition spreads anteriorly across the cortex. It most commonly begins in the posterior occipital lobes, generating clinical descriptions such as "zigzags" and "sparkles" (hyperexcitable cortex), followed by visual scotoma (inhibited cortex) as it progresses anteriorly. When the parietal sensory cortex is involved, patients might experience paresthesias affecting the distal hand with progression to the face and tongue. This second most common aura follows the sensory homunculus, as evidenced by typical sparing of the abdomen and lower extremities because of the location of their relative sensory origins deep within the central sulcus. The clinical features of migraine aura typically progress over 30 minutes and last less than 2 hours. However, some prolonged aura events might last more than 24 hours. The presence of aura is not diagnostic of migraine, nor does the absence of aura exclude migraine.

It is important to recognize that every person has the capacity to exhibit migraine. Anyone placed in an environment with extreme stressors (which vary individually) such as alcohol intoxication or sleep deprivation can eventually develop the cardinal features of migraine. This may include headache, nausea, or light and/or sound sensitivity. Interestingly, individuals not prone to migraine who have experienced an alcohol-induced headache ("hangover headache") might respond to migraine-focused medications such as sumatriptan. A similar example may be seen in seizures. Those who have spontaneous seizures are diagnosed with epilepsy, but almost everyone can exhibit seizure activity if their serum glucose is rapidly reduced.

Episodic Migraine

Episodic migraine involves recurrent, self-limited attacks of headache and/or associated nervous system hypersensitivity that typically last between 4 hours and 48 hours. People with episodic migraine are commonly thought to function normally between episodes; however, multiple studies have shown that those with episodic migraine experience heightened levels of sensitivity to sensory input even in between attacks. This includes more sensitive senses of smell, vibration, sight, and visual processing during the time intervals when patients disclose no acute migraine symptoms.

The IHS criteria for Episodic Migraine require at least two of four characteristics and one of two accompanying symptoms (Fig. 15.2). For example, a patient who has more than 5 episodes of moderate headache that worsen with physical activity, and who prefers a dark, quiet room during the headache fulfills "episodic migraine" diagnostic criteria. Greater than 90% of patients with initial symptoms of only moderate to severe headache and nausea will fulfill diagnostic criteria for migraine after a more detailed history is taken. Many migraineurs report a "migraine prodrome" which involves diminished cognition and poor concentration during migraine, which returns to baseline towards the end of the attack. Other clinical features of episodic migraine include osmophobia (smell sensitivity), dizziness or true vertigo, scalp sensitivity (i.e., occipital nerve tenderness), and neck

A.	At least five attacks fulfilling criteria B-D
B.	Headache attacks lasting 4–72 h (untreated or unsuccessfully treated)
C.	Headache has ≥2 of the following characteristics: 1. unilateral location 2. pulsating quality 3. moderate or severe pain intensity 4. aggravation by or causing avoidance of routine physical activity (*e.g.*, walking, climbing stairs)
D.	During headache ≥1 of the following: 1. nausea and/or vomiting 2. photophobia and phonophobia
E.	Not attributed to another disorder

Figure 15.2. Migraine without aura.

Source: Headache Classifications Subcommittee of the American Headache Society. International Classifications of Headache Disorders. *Cephalalgia*. 2004;24(Suppl 1):1–160; Silberstein SD, Olesen J, Bousser M-G, et al. The International Classification of Headache Disorders, 2nd Edition (ICHD-II)—Revision of criteria for 8.2 *Medication-Overuse Headache*. *Cephalalgia*. 2005;25:460–465.

pain. Many patients with migraine will obtain at least partial relief with occipital nerve blocks.[3]

Chronic Migraine

Migraine is a continuum ranging from rare episodes of mild symptoms to constant daily symptoms of high intensity. Chronic migraine is defined as more than 15 headache days per month, with at least half of those days containing migraine features or involving symptoms that are relieved by migraine-targeted medications (Fig. 15.3). Episodic migraine might become more frequent and intense over time as a consequence of disease progression. In such cases, it is harder to identify triggers because of the frequent/constant symptoms. Chronic migraine has been associated with sleep disorders, obesity, mood disorders (especially depression and anxiety), and features of centralized pain. These disorders are thought to be initiated and/or exacerbated by the neurochemical basis for migraine, and not simply due to the impact of headache on the patient's quality of life. It should be the goal

A.	Headache fulfilling criteria C and D for Figure 15.2 (migraine without aura), for ≥ 15 d/mo for > 3 mo
B.	Not attributed to another disorder

Figure 15.3. Chronic migraine.

Source: Headache Classifications Subcommittee of the American Headache Society. International Classifications of Headache Disorders. *Cephalalgia*. 2004;24(Suppl 1):1–160; Silberstein SD, Olesen J, Bousser M-G, et al. The International Classification of Headache Disorders, 2nd Edition (ICHD-II)—Revision of criteria for 8.2 *Medication-Overuse Headache*. *Cephalalgia*. 2005;25:460–465.

of the treating provider to focus on prevention strategies and therapies to reduce the frequency and intensity of symptoms.

MEDICATION OVERUSE HEADACHE

Migraineurs are encouraged to treat migraine at the onset of first symptoms to reduce the impact and prevent progression. However, the frequent use of abortive treatments might result in increased migraine frequency, also known as medication overuse headache (MOH). MOH can be caused by both over-the-counter and prescription medications. The hallmark of MOH is escalation of the underlying pattern of migraine associated with the increased use of acute medication. Frequently, patients with MOH will worsen when trying to reduce or stop the offending abortive therapy; however, this is no longer part of the formal IHS criteria. Although the pathophysiology of MOH has not been well studied, it is thought to represent the remodeling of treatment-specific receptors, similar to what occurs in opioid-induced hyperalgesia. Interestingly, MOH appears to almost exclusively affect those with a previous history of migraine. In patients using daily analgesics for arthritis, only those with a history of migraine are at high risk of developing escalating headache symptoms. Clinical experience suggests that shorter-acting medications impart a greater risk for developing MOH, which prompts many headache specialists to consider relatively longer-acting treatments such as naproxen or buprenorphine as better treatments than drugs such as ibuprofen or hydrocodone, respectfully. It might take weeks or months from the point at which the offending therapy was stopped for the patient to return to his or her previous headache pattern. The presence of MOH in those with chronic migraine might limit the effectiveness of preventive therapies and should be identified and treated early. Preventive therapies that were not previously effective for migraine might prove to be effective once the MOH component has been eliminated. Patients who have a worsening headache pattern must be carefully monitored for MOH.

TENSION-TYPE HEADACHE

Tension-type headache (TTH) is the most prevalent primary head ache disorder across all populations and age groups. Because of its high prevalence, it carries a high socioeconomic cost related to absenteeism, presenteeism (i.e., working while sick), and medication treatment costs, including use of over-the-counter medications. TTH typically presents as a non-pulsating, constant, bilateral mild to moderate pain. It is often triggered by sleep disorders, environmental stressors, and menstruation. Despite the overlap in triggers, it is distinct from migraine in several ways, including that it does not typically involve nausea and is associated with minimal or absent photophobia and phonophobia (never both), as illustrated in IHS criteria (Fig. 15.4). It can be classified as either episodic (<180 days per year) or chronic (≥180 days per year) TTH, with further sub-categorization based on pericranial tenderness. The most pronounced clinical feature of TTH is increased myofascial tenderness involving the cranial and neck muscles that positively correlates with the intensity and frequency of headache. Pericranial tenderness may be present on days with or without headache. TTH by definition is never severe, although the constant nature of chronic TTH might have a substantial negative impact on quality of life. If a TTH patient reports

A. At least 10 episodes occurring on ≥1 but <15 d/mo for ≥3 mo (≥12 and <180 d/y) and fulfilling criteria B-D
B. Headache lasting from 30 min to 7 d
C. Headache has ≥2 of the following characteristics:
   1. bilateral location
   2. pressing/tightening (non-pulsating) quality
   3. mild or moderate intensity
   4. not aggravated by routine physical activity
D. Both of the following:
   1. no nausea or vomiting (anorexia may occur)
   2. no more than one of photophobia or phonophobia
E. Not attributed to another disorder

Figure 15.4. Frequent episodic tension-type headache.

Source: Headache Classifications Subcommittee of the American Headache Society. International Classifications of Headache Disorders. *Cephalalgia.* 2004;24(Suppl 1):1–160; Silberstein SD, Olesen J, Bousser M-G, et al. The International Classification of Headache Disorders, 2nd Edition (ICHD-II)—Revision of criteria for 8.2 *Medication-Overuse Headache. Cephalalgia.* 2005;25:460–465.

severe headaches, the clinician should reconsider the primary diagnosis. Because TTH contains many features of a secondary headache, a complete evaluation for other headache sources is warranted.

TRIGEMINAL AUTONOMIC CEPHALGIAS

Cluster Headache

Cluster Headache (CH) is a very severe primary headache syndrome and the best known of the trigeminal autonomic cephalgias (TACs). It has a one-year prevalence rate of 0.1 percent, affecting males more than females by a ratio of 5:1. CH consists of two subtypes: episodic CH (80 percent of patients), in which >1-month symptom-free intervals occur between cycles; and chronic CH (20 percent of patients), which does not involve spontaneous remission intervals. In episodic CH, the cycles are likely to begin in spring or fall and last for between 2 weeks and 3 months. Patients or providers frequently use the term "cluster headache" inappropriately to refer to migraine lasting weeks in duration with periods of improvement in between. An accurate diagnosis is based on the presenting symptoms in addition to the headache pattern (Fig. 15.5). CH presents with strictly unilateral symptoms and only rarely changes sides. It is never bilateral at the same time. CH has prominent trigeminal autonomic features ipsilateral to the headache including lid ptosis, rhinorrhea, tearing, conjunctival injection, and periorbital edema. Behaviors indicative of agitation such as pacing, rocking, vigorous rubbing of the eye, and striking the head are quite specific for CH and help differentiate CH from migraine. The attacks last between 30 minutes and 3 hours, and occur between once and 6 times per day. If a cluster headache occurs once per day, it invariably occurs within 2 hours into the sleep cycle. In between attacks, the patient is symptom-free, although episodes of mild aching or sensitivity might be reported. Similar to migraine, CH may have a preceding aura, have identifiable triggers such as alcohol or stress, and be accompanied by photophobia/phonophobia and/or nausea (more common in female patients). There is a strong association between CH and tobacco smoking. It is estimated that more than 90 percent of patients with CH

A. At least five attacks fulfilling criteria B-D
B. Severe or very severe unilateral orbital, supraorbital, and/or temporal pain lasting 15–180 min if untreated
C. Headache is accompanied by ≥1 of the following:
   1. ipsilateral conjunctival injection and/or lacrimation
   2. ipsilateral nasal congestion and/or rhinorrhoea
   3 .ipsilateral eyelid oedema
   4. ipsilateral forehead and facial sweating
   5. ipsilateral miosis and/or ptosis
   6. a sense of restlessness or agitation
D. Attacks have a frequency from 1–2 to 8/d
E. Not attributed to another disorder

Figure 15.5. Cluster headache.

Source: Headache Classifications Subcommittee of the American Headache Society. International Classifications of Headache Disorders. *Cephalalgia*. 2004;24(Suppl 1):1–160; Silberstein SD, Olesen J, Bousser M-G, et al. The International Classification of Headache Disorders, 2nd Edition (ICHD-II)—Revision of criteria for 8.2 *Medication-Overuse Headache*. *Cephalalgia*. 2005;25:460–465.

smoke tobacco, and those who do not smoke are more likely to have grown up in homes with environmental tobacco smoke exposure.

Hemicrania Continua

Hemicrania continua (HC) is a strictly one-sided headache that is daily and continuous from onset. Patients usually can remember the day their headache began. It presents with a continuous background, mild-intensity headache that escalates periodically for hours to days. During the headache escalation, trigeminal autonomic features of lacrimation, rhinorrhea, and lid ptosis are evident (Fig. 15.6). HC has the escalation pattern and female predominance observed in chronic migraine, combined with the hemicranial location and autonomic features of CH. Regional cerebral blood flow positron-emission tomography studies have shown brain activation patterns consistent with both classic migraine (ipsilateral pons) and CH (contralateral hypothalamus) occurring simultaneously. HC responds dramatically to indomethacin, such that clinical response to a trial of indomethacin is required in order to make the diagnosis. Other headache

A. Headache for >3 mo fulfilling criteria B-D
B. All of the following characteristics:
   1. unilateral pain without side-shift
   2. daily and continuous, without pain-free periods
   3. moderate intensity, with exacerbations of severe pain
C. At least one of the following autonomic features occurs during exacerbations, ipsilateral to the pain:
   1. conjunctival injection and/or lacrimation
   2. nasal congestion and/or rhinorrhoea
   3. ptosis and/or miosis
D. Complete response to therapeutic doses of indomethacin
E. Not attributed to another disorder

Figure 15.6. Hemicrania continua.

Source: Headache Classifications Subcommittee of the American Headache Society. International Classifications of Headache Disorders. *Cephalalgia*. 2004;24(Suppl 1):1–160; Silberstein SD, Olesen J, Bousser M-G, et al. The International Classification of Headache Disorders, 2nd Edition (ICHD-II)—Revision of criteria for 8.2 *Medication-Overuse Headache. Cephalalgia*. 2005;25:460–465.

syndromes that respond to indomethacin include paroxysmal HC, hypnic headache, cough headache, and primary stabbing headache.

HEADACHE TREATMENT

The impact of headache on quality of life can be substantial. Effective headache control can provide dramatic improvement in the quality of life of those with chronic or episodic headache. Effective treatment encompasses education, behavioral treatments, and pharmacologic therapy. As patients become educated and knowledgeable about the nature and mechanism of their primary headache syndrome, they become empowered and can actively participate in their individualized treatment program. Patients may keep a headache diary, which contributes to a better understanding of their headache pattern and provides a way to monitor clinical progress and improvement. A careful review of this diary at each visit aids the identification of possible headache triggers and facilitates discussion of treatment strategies. Simple behavioral strategies might be helpful, including sleep regulation, diet modification, and implementing a physical exercise program when appropriate. Several behavioral therapies have been shown to exert a positive effect on headache, including cognitive-behavioral therapy, stress management, relaxation training, and biofeedback therapy. The goal of headache treatment is to reduce the frequency, severity, and duration of the headache, along with associated features. It is helpful to separate headache therapy into acute treatments to stop an episode of headache and preventive treatments for reducing the frequency and severity of headache escalations.

Acute Headache Therapy

Patients' preferences for acute headache therapies include rapid onset, efficacy (i.e., complete or near-complete resolution of the headache and associated features such as nausea or light sensitivity without recurrence), reliability, and minimal side effects. Abortive treatment should be undertaken at the first sign of headache escalation. There are multiple options to consider for acute therapy (Table 15.1).

Table 15.1 RECOMMENDATIONS FOR ACUTE TREATMENT OF HEADACHE

Acute Treatment	*Typical Dosage*	*Frequency*	*Side Effects*
TRIPTANS			
Sumatriptan	100 g tablet or 6 oz SQ	One at start of HA; repeat in 2 hours if needed. Max 2 per day	Flushing/palpitation/transient paresthesias of scalp and extremities/adverse cardiovascular events in high-risk patients
Rizatriptan	10 g tablet		
Naratriptan	2.5 g tablet		
NSAIDS			
Naproxen sodium	500 g tablet	PO TID prn with food	GI irritation, bleeding, renal toxicity
Indomethacin	50 g capsule	PO TID prn with food	
Ketorolac	15 to 40 mg	IV q6h prn	Same as above
BARBITURATES			
Fioricet	50 mg butalbital, 325 mg acetaminophen, 40 mg caffeine	1–2 tablets q 4h prn	Sedation, light-headedness, nausea, vomiting, abdominal pain

(continued)

Table 15.1 *(CONTINUED)*

Acute Treatment	*Typical Dosage*	*Frequency*	*Side Effects*
NEUROLEPTICS			
Promethazine	25 g	PO TID prn	Fatigue, involuntary movements
ANTIEMETIC			
Ondansetron	4 g	PO TID prn	Fatigue, constipation

Source: Headache Classifications Subcommittee of the American Headache Society. International Classifications of Headache Disorders. *Cephalalgia*. 2004;24(Suppl 1):1–160; Silberstein SD, Olesen J, Bousser M-G, et al. The International Classification of Headache Disorders, 2nd Edition (ICHD-II)—Revision of criteria for 8.2 *Medication-Overuse Headache*. *Cephalalgia*. 2005;25:460–465.

HA, headache; GI, gastrointestinal.

Triptans

Triptans are commonly viewed as the most effective treatment for acute migraine. They are also effective in CH, TTH, and most other headache syndromes. Triptans function as selective serotonin 5-HT1B/1D agonists. Clinical efficacy is achieved via reduced signaling of trigeminal-mediated pain to the brainstem. Specifically, meningeal nociceptor signaling is reduced at the trigeminal nucleus caudalis. Triptans constrict meningeal blood vessels and reduce the release of inflammatory neuropeptides, which further inhibits migraine activation. Most patients experience no or minimal adverse effects with triptans. The most common side effects are transient and might include chest pressure, flushing, scalp parasthesia, fatigue, and nausea. Clinical concern about triptans causing cardiac ischemic events or stroke has not been demonstrated in large population studies. A large-scale epidemiological study involving over 60,000 migraine patients found that the use of triptans in those without cardiac risk factors does not appear to increase the risk of myocardial infarction or stroke relative to those not using triptans.[4] However, triptans are contraindicated in those with known cardiovascular, cerebrovascular, or peripheral vascular disease. There are currently seven triptans available in the United States. Sumatriptan and eletriptan are rapidly absorbed, resulting in fast onset and efficacy, whereas more slowly absorbed drugs such as naratriptan and frovatriptan demonstrate a better side-effect profile and longer duration of benefit. The second-generation "triptan" eletriptan has a unique metabolism profile that includes both 3A4 and P450 hepatic elimination, and according to some reports it is associated with a lower incidence of side effects than sumatriptan.

Non-steroidal Anti-inflammatory Drugs

Non-steroidal anti-inflammatory drugs (NSAIDs) have been used successfully for decades in treating acute migraine. Their clinical effects are centered on the inhibition of the enzyme cyclo-oxygenase, which results in decreased prostaglandin synthesis. Additionally, NSAIDS play a role in multiple other pathways of inflammation, including those involving neutrophils and mastocytes. Naproxen sodium is typically well tolerated, and its relatively long duration of action is well suited for headache treatment, as it may lower the risk of MOH relative to shorter-acting NSAIDs. The advent of liquid gel formulations provides for more rapid absorption and is tailor-made for acute headache management. Recent studies have shown a synergistic effect when naproxen is combined with sumatriptan.[5] Although indomethacin has better efficacy, it is associated with more adverse events. Ketorolac is a mainstay for abortive therapy when given intramuscularly or intravenously. A nasal preparation of ketorolac is now available in the United States and has shown some promise for the acute treatment of moderate to severe headache.

Neuroleptics and Anti-emetics

The migraine-associated symptoms of nausea and vomiting can be just as disabling as the headache itself. Neuroleptics not only target nausea but also have efficacy for migraine and CH. Promethazine is typically well tolerated and is commonly used in combination with other migraine treatments. Droperidol is very effective for status migrainosis when used intravenously; however, this requires cardiac monitoring in an inpatient setting. Ondansetron, a serotonin 5-HT_3 antagonist, is another very effective nausea treatment that is associated with minimal side effects.

Opioids and Barbituates

Opioid treatments are effective for the acute treatment of severe migraine or CH. However, because of the chronic nature of primary headaches and concerns regarding MOH, opioid-induced hyperalgesia, and aberrant behaviors, long-term therapy is relatively contraindicated for routine use in most patients.[6] In fact, some studies have found an association between chronic opioid use and negative treatment outcome.[7]

Butalbital-containing combinations have been used for decades in the treatment of headache. Butalbital has never been approved by the U.S. Food and Drug Administration for use in migraine and is viewed as a major contributor to MOH. Butalbital's tendency to cause rapid tolerance and reduce the efficacy of other treatments limits its clinical role, and it should be reserved for rare use in unique clinical scenarios.

Preventive Treatment

Preventive medication is taken daily to reduce the frequency, severity, and duration of headache escalations. Preventive therapy is considered in those individuals with recurrent headaches that significantly interfere with their daily routine; have poor response to abortive therapy for infrequent headaches; or headache frequency that exceeds 2 headaches per week. Headache prevention is focused on increasing headache threshold, and is typically achieved by stabilizing specific receptors in key headache pathways in the central and/or peripheral nervous system. Most medications are best titrated to effective doses over several weeks, and patients typically experience reduced frequency and severity within 2 weeks of being at their unique therapeutic dose. The selection of preventive medication(s) is based on tolerability, associated clinical features, and co-existing medical conditions and medication usage.

Topiramate

Topiramate has proven to be one of the most efficacious headache prevention therapies, especially for migraine and CH. It is considered first-line therapy at many headache clinics. Topiramate previously was thought to prevent migraine by blocking Na+ channels and augmenting activity of γ-aminobutyric acid (GABA) at certain GABA-A receptor subtypes; however, recent evidence demonstrates headache relief that stems from modulation of the glutamate-kainate receptors within the central nervous system.[8] Topiramate is excreted mostly unchanged in the urine and has a half-life of 21 hours. It is commonly started at 25 mg each night and is titrated to 50 mg twice a day (BID) or 100 mg at night over 3 weeks. Most patients respond to doses ranging between 50 and 200 mg/d, but many headache clinics commonly prescribe up to 400 mg/d, and some case reports have suggested added benefit at doses greater than 600 mg/d. Common side effects are typically mild and include dizziness, fatigue, and weight loss. Given that obesity is associated with headaches, this latter effect might afford additional benefit in overweight individuals. Rare cognitive side effects such as difficulty retrieving words might be reduced with once-nightly dosing and resolve once the medication is stopped.

Table 15.2 RECOMMENDATIONS FOR PREVENTATIVE TREATMENT OF HEADACHE

Preventive Treatment	*Starting Dosage*	*Effective Dose Range*	*Adverse Events*
Magnesium Glycinate	400 g/d	400–800 g/d	Diarrhea/bloating
Topiramate	25 g/qhs	50–200 g/qhs	Paresthesias Weight loss Cognitive changes Depression Renal stones
Valproic acid	250 g BID	250–500 g BID	Weight gain Dyspepsia Alopecia Hirsutism Tremor
Propranolol	60 g extended release	60–180 g	Weight gain Fatigue Lethargy Visual changes
Amitriptyline/ nortriptyline	25 g/qhs	25–150 g qhs	Weight gain Morning fatigue Tachycardia Dry mouth Cognitive changes Orthostatic hypotension

(continued)

Table 15.2 (CONTINUED)

Preventive Treatment	*Starting Dosage*	*Effective Dose Range*	*Adverse Events*
Verapamil	80 g TID	80–240 g TID	Edema Fatigue Constipation
Candesartan	8 g/d	16–32 g/d	Nausea Fatigue Blurred vision

Source: Headache Classifications Subcommittee of the American Headache Society. International Classifications of Headache Disorders. *Cephalalgia*. 2004;24(Suppl 1):1–160; Silberstein SD, Olesen J, Bousser M-G, et al. The International Classification of Headache Disorders, 2nd Edition (ICHD-II)—Revision of criteria for 8.2 *Medication-Overuse Headache*. *Cephalalgia*. 2005;25:460–465.

Parasthesias might occur during dose escalation and typically resolve after several days or with proper electrolyte maintenance (i.e., the use of electrolyte drinks).

Valproic Acid

Valproic acid and its sodium salt, sodium valproate, have proven to be effective in migraine prevention. At high doses, valproic acid is thought to increase GABA activity, and at low doses it stabilizes brainstem serotonin 5HT neurons to reduce migraine sensitivity. Typical dosing ranges from 250 mg/d to 1000 mg BID, with most patients responding to 500 mg BID. It has a half-life of between 8 and 17 hours, and extended-release capsules have shown no greater efficacy in migraine prevention. It is typically well tolerated, with common side effects including nausea, alopecia, tremor, and weight gain.[9] On rare occasions, valproic acid can be associated with pancreatitis and hepatitis, prompting the need for clinical monitoring with blood tests. Similar to other membrane stabilizing agents, it should be avoided in pregnancy. Smaller trials suggest a clinical benefit in CH.

Beta Blockers

Beta blocker medications are widely used for migraine prevention. Evidence consistently shows that these medications reduce the frequency and intensity of migraine. Beta blockers are thought to exert their primary effects within the central nervous system by blocking the actions of the endogenous catecholamines epinephrine and norepinephrine. The mechanisms by which they prevent headaches are not fully understood but might include direct inhibition of arterial dilatation, inhibiting the release of substances that result in vascular dilation and constriction, and central mechanisms. Propranolol is the most commonly used beta blocker and is typically started at a daily dose of 80 mg in extended-release formulation, with a range of 60–240 mg/d. Other well-studied beta blocker medications for prevention include metoprolol and timolol. The most common side effects of this class of drugs are fatigue, depression, nausea, and dizziness, which are all typically mild and dose-dependent.

Tricyclic Antidepressants

Several different classes of antidepressant medication have some migraine prevention benefit, with the tricyclic class being the best studied and most commonly prescribed. Antidepressant medications do not improve headache by treating depression. Although the mechanism for migraine prevention is not certain, they are thought to reduce β-adrenergic receptor activity and, to a lesser extent, increase GABA inhibition and antagonize histamine effects. Amitriptyline is the most extensively studied antidepressant for migraine prevention, with a therapeutic dose range of between 10 and 150 mg qhs—lower than the doses needed to treat depression. Patients over the age of

40 or with a history of cardiac disease should have a baseline electrocardiogram (ECG) before treatment is initiated. Side effects of amitriptyline include dry mouth, constipation, bladder retention, and tachycardia. Nortriptyline is less studied for headache prophylaxis but is also effective, with fewer cholinergic and sedative side effects. Protriptyline is considered more norepinephrine than serotonin selective and induces minimal fatigue.

Angiotensin Receptor Blockers

Candesartan has been found to be effective in migraine prevention in clinical trials. The mechanism of action is thought to be focused on angiotensin II receptors within the central nervous system. This class of medication is tolerated very well, with minimal side effects such as dizziness. Doses between 8 and 32 mg/d can be effective for refractory migraine.[10]

Calcium Channel Blockers

Migraine prevention studies with calcium channel blockers have demonstrated a possible benefit. In contrast, verapamil is considered as first-line therapy for CH prevention, with a large dosing range between 120 mg/d and >720 mg/d. Clinical benefit might result from inhibition of 5HT release and reduced neurovascular inflammation. Patients with CH are usually able to tolerate large doses of verapamil, with rare dose-dependent side effects such as constipation, fatigue, and palpitations. An ECG is advised after each dose increase beyond 500 mg/d because of verapamil's QTc prolongation effects.

Alternative Headache Preventives

Petasites (Butterbur) has shown clinical benefit in migraine prevention.[11] Its mechanism of action is uncertain, but it might involve the reduction of neurovascular inflammation surrounding the brain. The best efficacy is observed at doses of 75 mg BID, with minimal adverse events such as gastrointestinal effects and belching. Magnesium is thought to exhibit headache preventive benefits via its blockade of the N-methyl-D-aspartate receptor.[12] Magnesium also possesses muscle relaxation and peripheral vasodilatory effects. Side effects with magnesium are quite rare and include diarrhea without nausea due to poor absorption. Magnesium must penetrate the red blood cell membrane to be effective, and therefore magnesium glycinate 400 mg/d or magnesium oxide 500 mg/d is recommended.

CONCLUSIONS

Headache is one of the most common clinical conditions encountered in the outpatient setting. In most cases, an accurate diagnosis can be achieved through focused history and physical exam. Treatment options for headache are typically safe and lead to minimal adverse events. Clinicians are encouraged to discuss these options with their patients and initiate both acute and preventive therapy, when appropriate. Effective headache control can provide dramatic improvement in the quality of life for those with chronic or episodic headaches.

REFERENCES

1. Headache Classifications Subcommitte of the American Headache Society. International classifications of headache disorders. *Cephalalgia* 2004:24;1–160.
2. Lipton RB, Bigal ME, Diamond M, Freitag F, Reed ML, Stewart WF. The American Migraine Prevalence and Prevention Advisory Group. Migraine prevalence, disease burden, and the need for preventive therapy. *Neurology* 2007;68:343–349.
3. Young WB. Blocking the greater occipital nerve: Utility in headache management. *Curr Pain Headache Rep* 2010;14:404–408.

4. Hall GC, Brown MM, Mo J, MacRae KD. Triptans in Migraine: the risks of stroke, cardiovascular disease, and death in practice. *Neurology* 2004;64:563–568
5. Haberer LJ, Walls CM, Lener SE, Taylor DR, McDonald SA. Distinct pharmacokinetic profile and safety of a fixed-dose tablet of sumatriptan and naproxen sodium for the acute treatment of migraine.<http://www.ncbi.nlm.nih.gov/pubmed/20132340> *Headache* 2010;50:357–573.
6. Saper JR, Lake AE. Continuous opioid therapy (COT) is rarely advisable for refractory chronic daily headache: limited efficacy, risks, and proposed guidelines. *Headache* 2008;48:838–849.
7. Cohen SP, Plunkett AR, Wilkinson I, et al. Headaches during war: Analysis of presentation, treatment, and factors associated with outcome. *Cephalalgia* 2012;32:94–108.
8. Andreou AP, Goadsby PJ. Topiramate in the treatment of migraine: A kinate (glutamate) receptor antagonist within the trigeminothalamic pathway. *Cephalalgia* 2011;13:1343–1358.
9. Freitag F, Collins SD, Carlson HA, et al. A randomized trial of divalproex sodium extended-release tablets in migraine prophylaxis. *Neurology* 2002;58:1652–1659.
10. Tronvik E, Stovner LJ, Helde G, Sand T, Bovim G. Prophylactic treatment of migraine with angiotensin ii receptor blocker: A randomized control study. *JAMA* 2003;289:65–69.
11. Lipton RB, Gobel H, Einhaupl KM, Wilks K, Mauskop A. Petasites hybridus root (butterbur) is an effective preventive treatment for migraine. *Neurology* 2004;63 2240–2244.
12. Maizels M, Blumenfeld A, Burchette R. A combination of Ribofalvin, magnesium, and feverfew for migraine prophylaxis: A randomized Trial. *Headache* 2004;44:885–890.

16

Non-cardiac Chest Pain

SHARON X. H. HU AND GUY D. ESLICK

Case Presentation

A 57-year-old man with no prior cardiac history presents to his family physician with a 3-day history of intermittent left-sided chest pain. Five days ago he experienced 2 days of coryzal symptoms with a low-grade temperature of 37.3°C and a productive cough. These symptoms have since improved; however, he subsequently developed sharp, 8/10 severity, non-radiating, left-sided chest pain that occurs intermittently and lasts for a few minutes. The pain is sometimes exacerbated by movement and respiration but is not related to food intake.

He has a past history of gastroesophageal reflux but takes no regular medications and denies any allergies. He has a family history of cardiovascular disease.

On examination he was comfortable at rest with normal vital signs. Acute tenderness to palpation was elicited over the left sixth and seventh ribs in the anterior axillary line. No abnormalities were detected on cardiovascular, pulmonary, and abdominal examinations. Troponin levels and electrocardiogram (ECG) study were normal.

DIFFERENTIAL DIAGNOSIS

- Musculoskeletal chest pain
- Gastroesophageal reflux disease
- Cardiac chest pain
- Pulmonary disease
- Psychogenic chest pain

Based on the history and examination findings, this man's presentation is most consistent with musculoskeletal chest pain.

BACKGROUND

Chest pain is a common presentation in the primary care setting, and its diagnosis can prove challenging. Possible etiologies range from urgent and life-threatening, requiring immediate treatment, to benign and self-limiting, requiring only reassurance and patient education. Serious conditions must first be excluded prior to consideration of other diagnoses. A thorough history and physical examination in combination with the judicial use of diagnostic investigations are needed in order to determine the underlying cause.

WHAT CAUSES CHEST PAIN?

Chest pain may arise from any organ present in the chest cavity—namely, the heart, lungs, blood vessels, and esophagus—or the chest wall itself (Fig. 16.1). Pain arising from internal organs, such as the diaphragm, liver, or pancreas, might be confused with that arising

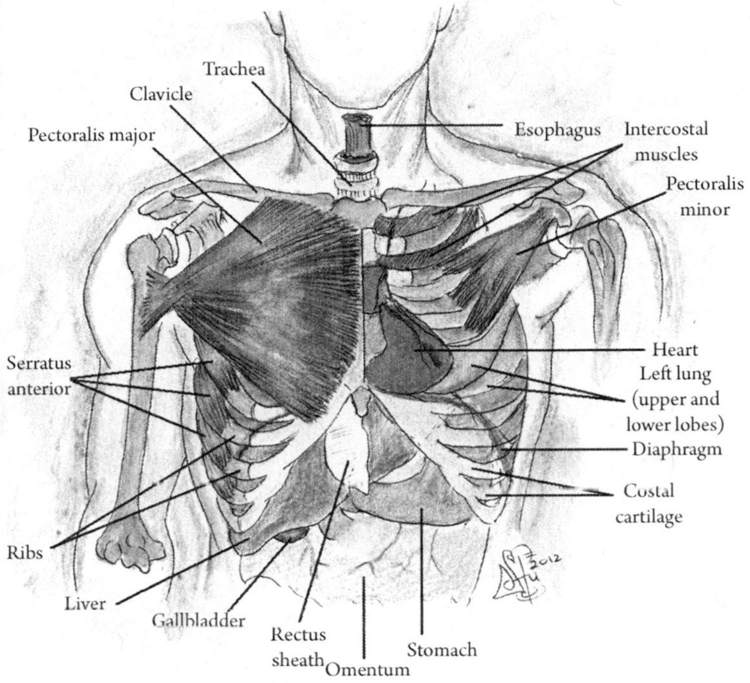

Figure 16.1. Anatomy of the chest wall and its organs. Organs which may cause chest pain in bold.

in the chest wall as a result of referred pain. Nerve endings involved in the experience of pain are present in both internal organs and the chest wall. Internal organs activate pain fibers during ischemia or stretching, whereas nerves in the chest wall, including the parietal pleura, the musculoskeletal wall, and skin, are sensitive to pin-prick sensation, pressure, and heat.

The differential diagnoses for chest pain is extensive, with the most serious cause being cardiac (Fig. 16.2). All patients presenting with chest pain should therefore be initially evaluated for possible cardiac causes. A detailed history, followed by a thorough examination, ECG, chest radiograph, and serial measurements of cardiac

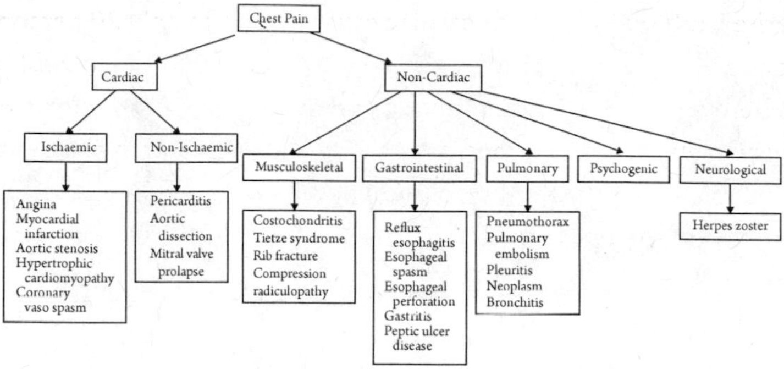

Figure 16.2. Classification of chest pain.

enzymes, should help the treating physician determine whether the pain is cardiac in nature.[1] If the patient is stable and the etiology remains unclear, referral for a cardiology consult, echocardiography, or exercise stress ECG is warranted.[1] Once a cardiac cause has been excluded, other diagnoses can be considered.

WHAT IS NON-CARDIAC CHEST PAIN?

Non-cardiac chest pain (NCCP) is defined as chest pain that has not been diagnosed as acute myocardial infarction or ischemic heart disease.[2] However, there is currently no standard classification for NCCP, with the condition generally diagnosed only after the exclusion of other conditions. The majority of NCCP cases arise from musculoskeletal, gastrointestinal, psychiatric, and pulmonary conditions.[3]

HOW COMMON IS NCCP?

The complaint of chest pain leads to more than 6 million hospital admissions and more than $8 billion in healthcare costs annually in the United States,[4] with cardiac causes found in only 20 percent of admissions.[5] One study estimated healthcare costs for NCCP to be over $315 million annually, including costs for doctor and hospital visits and for medication. Even after excluding patients with known cardiac disease, a population-based study in Australia revealed that 33 percent of individuals experienced NCCP at some point in their lives.[4]

CAUSES OF NCCP

NCCP has many causes, and possible diagnoses often overlap. Potential causes of NCCP include musculoskeletal, gastrointestinal, psychogenic, and pulmonary illness (Table 16.1). The remainder of this chapter focuses primarily on musculoskeletal etiologies; the other causes are briefly addressed.

MUSCULOSKELETAL CAUSES OF CHEST PAIN

Musculoskeletal chest pain includes all causes of chest pain that arise from structures in the chest wall, including the muscles, ribs, costal cartilages, spine, and intercostal nerves. Herpes zoster infection can also be associated with a prodrome of severe unilateral chest pain that radiates along a dermatome (see Chapter 13).

Costochondritis

A common cause of anterior chest pain is costochondritis, also known as costosternal syndrome, parasternal chondrodynia, and anterior chest wall syndrome.[6] Costochondritis is defined as inflammation of costochondral junctions of the ribs or chondrosternal joints, usually

Table 16.1 HOSPITAL OR POPULATION STUDIES THAT HAVE CLASSIFIED NON-CARDIAC CHEST PAIN INTO CLINICAL GROUPS

Study	*Design*	*Ischaemic Heart Disease, %*	*GERD, %*	*Psychiatric Disorders, %*	*Musculoskeletal Disorders, %*	*Microvascular Disease, %*	*Others, %*
Cannon et al.[a] ($n = 87$)	Hospital-based	–#	–*	–*	–*	73	27^
Janssens et al.[b] ($n = 60$)	Hospital-based	–#	88	–*	–*	–*	12
Rouan et al.[c] ($n = 772$)	Outpatient clinic	8	9	1	23	–*	59^
Katon et al.[d] ($n = 74$)	Hospital-based	–#	–*	79	–*	–*	21
Wise et al.[e] ($n = 100$)	Hospital-based	–#	–*	–*	16	–*	84^
Fruergaard et al.[f] ($n = 204$)	Hospital-based	31	42	–*	28	–*	12

Eslick et al.[g] ($n = 672$)	Population-based	7	54	24	11	*	12

Notes: GERD, gastrointestinal reflux disease; IHD, ischaemic heart disease.

[a]Cannon RO 3rd, Bonow RO, Bacharach SL, et al. Left ventricular dysfunction in patients with angina pectoris, normal epicardial coronary arteries, and abnormal vasodilator reserve. *Circulation.* 1985;71(2):218–226.

[#]Already excluded.

[*]Not considered.

[^]Unstable angina, unknown causes.

[b]Janssens J, Vantrappen G, Ghillebert G. 24-hour recording of esophageal pressure and pH in patients with noncardiac chest pain. *Gastroenterology.* 1986;90(6):1978–1984.

[c]Rouan GW, Hedges JR, Toltzis R, et al. A chest pain clinic to improve the follow-up of patients released from an urban university teaching hospital emergency department. *Ann Emerg Med.* 1987;16(10):1145–1150.

[d]Katon W, Hall ML, Russo J, et al. Chest pain: relationship of psychiatric illness to coronary arteriographic results. *Am J Med.* 1988;84(1):1–9.

[e]Wise CM, Semble EL, Dalton CB. Musculoskeletal chest wall syndromes in patients with noncardiac chest pain: a study of 100 patients. *Arch Phys Med Rehabil.* 1992;73(2):147–149.

[f]Fruergaard P, Launbjerg J, Hesse B, et al. The diagnoses of patients admitted with acute chest pain but without myocardial infarction. *Eur Heart J.* 1996;17(7):1028–1034.

[g]Eslick GD, Jones MP, Talley NJ. Non-cardiac chest pain: prevalence, risk factors, impact and consulting—a population-based study. *Aliment Pharmacol Ther.* 2003;17(9):1115–1124.

Adapted with permission from Eslick GD, Coulshed DS, Talley NJ. Review article: the burden of illness of non-cardiac chest pain. *Aliment Pharmacol Ther.* 2002;16(7):1217–1223.

at multiple levels and lacking swelling or induration. It is a self-limited condition.

Pain involving the costochondral and chondrosternal regions is the main presenting complaint. Pain reproduced by palpation of the affected segments suggests costochondritis but depends on the exclusion of other underlying causes (Table 16.2). Multiple lesions are present in 90 percent of costochondritis cases, with the second to fifth costal cartilages being the most frequently affected. Costochondritis is present in 13 percent to 36 percent of adults with acute chest pain symptoms, depending on the study and patient setting.[7]

Patients with other respiratory findings such as fever, cough, or chest wall swelling should undergo chest radiography. Computed tomography (CT) can delineate pathology in costal cartilages and rule out underlying pathology, such as tumors. CT imaging should be reserved for cases in which there is high suspicion of infectious or neoplastic processes. Routine laboratory testing is not necessary in patients with suspected costochondritis unless the diagnosis is uncertain or fever or inflammation is present.

There have been no clinical trials evaluating treatment for costochondritis. Therapy usually consists of symptom-based treatment with acetaminophen, non-steroidal anti-inflammatory drugs (NSAIDs), or other analgesics. Heat compresses can be beneficial, particularly with muscle overuse. Minimizing activities that provoke symptoms, such as work or lifestyle modification and the use of cough suppressants, might also relieve symptoms.[8] Physical therapy has also been used for musculoskeletal chest pain.[9] Refractory cases can be treated with local injections of combined lidocaine/corticosteroid.[8]

The prognosis for costochondritis is excellent. Symptoms typically last from weeks to months, but they usually abate within one year. Patients should be educated and reassured about the fact that this is a benign condition that should eventually resolve.

Table 16.2 DIFFERENTIAL DIAGNOSIS AND TREATMENT OF CHEST WALL CONDITIONS

Condition	*Diagnostic Considerations*	*Treatment Principles*
Arthritis of sternoclavicular, sternomanubrial, or shoulder joints	Tenderness to palpation of specific joints of the sternum; evidence of joint sclerosis on radiography	Analgesics, intra-articular corticosteroid injections, physiotherapy
Costochondritis	Tenderness to palpation of costochondral junctions; palpation reproduces patient's pain; usually multiple sites on same side of chest	Simple analgesics, heat, or ice; rarely, local anesthetic and steroid injections
Destruction of costal cartilage by infections or neoplasm	Bacterial or fungal infections or metastatic neoplasms to costal cartilages; infections seen post-surgery or in intravenous drug users; chest computed tomography imaging useful to show alteration or destruction of cartilage and extension of masses to chest wall; gallium scanning might be helpful in patients with infection	Antibiotics or antifungal drugs; surgical resection of affected costal cartilage; treatment of neoplasm based on tissue type

(continued)

Table 16.2 (CONTINUED)

Condition	*Diagnostic Considerations*	*Treatment Principles*
Fibromyalgia	Based on self-report of widespread pain and co-morbid symptomatology (trouble thinking, remembering, headache, depression)	Graded exercise is beneficial; cyclobenzaprine, antidepressants, and pregabalin might be effective
Herpes zoster of thorax	Clusters of vesicles on red bases that follow one or two dermatomes and do not cross the midline; usually preceded by a prodrome of pain; postherpetic neuralgia is common	Oral antiviral agents (e.g., acyclovir, famciclovir, valvacyclovir); analgesics may include antidepressants, membrane stabilizers, and opioids; topical lidocaine patches helpful with evoked pain
Painful xiphoid syndrome	Tenderness at sternoxiphoid joint or over xiphoid process with palpation	Usually self-limited unless associated with congenital deformity; analgesics; rarely, corticosteroid injections

Slipping rib syndrome	Tenderness and hypermobility of anterior ends of lower costal cartilages causing pain at lower anterior chest wall or upper abdomen; diagnosis by "hooking maneuver" (curving fingers under costal margin and gently pulling anteriorly)—a "click" and movement are felt that reproduce patient's pain	Rest, physiotherapy, intercostal nerve blocks; or, if chronic and severe, surgical removal of hypermobile cartilage segment
Tietze's syndrome	A single tender and swollen but non-suppurative costochondral junction, usually at ribs two or three	Simple analgesics; usually self-limiting; rarely, corticosteroid injections
Traumatic muscle pain and overuse myalgia	History of trauma to chest or recent new onset of strenuous exercise to upper body (e.g., rowing); may be bilateral and affect multiple costochondral areas; muscles might also be tender to palpation	Simple analgesics; refrain or reduce strenuous activities that provoke pain

Adapted from Fam AG, Smythe HA. Musculoskeletal chest wall pain. *CMAJ*. 1985;133(5):379–389.

Tietze Syndrome

A rare and self-limited disorder, Tietze syndrome is a benign condition characterized by painful, non-suppurative swelling of the cartilaginous articulations of the anterior chest wall. The cause is unknown. Diagnosis is made on clinical grounds after exclusion of other conditions affecting the costal cartilages, such as rheumatoid arthritis, pyogenic arthritis, tumors, and relapsing polychondritis.

Tietze syndrome is an inflammatory process causing visible enlargement of the costochondral junction. It occurs in a single rib 70 percent of the time, usually affecting the costal cartilages of the second and third ribs (predominantly in rib two).[7] Costochondritis is often confused with Tietze syndrome (Table 16.3), but unlike in

Table 16.3 COMPARISON OF TIETZE'S SYNDROME AND COSTOCHONDRITIS

Feature	*Tietze's Syndrome*	*Costochondritis*
Frequency	Rare	More common
Age group	<40 years	≥40 years
Number of sites affected	1 (in 70 percent of patients)	≥1 (in 90 percent of patients)
Costochondral junctions commonly involved	Second and third	Second through fifth
Local swelling	Present	Absent
Associated conditions	Respiratory tract infections	Cervical strain syndrome, coronary heart disease, "fibrositis" syndrome

Tietze syndrome, the pain and tenderness in costochondritis is not associated with notable swelling.

The disorder runs a self-limiting course with remissions and exacerbations. Pain might cease spontaneously within weeks or months, although cartilaginous swelling might persist for longer periods. Magnetic resonance imaging (MRI) is an excellent technique for investigating primary Tietze's syndrome because of its high sensitivity, diagnostic reliability, and lack of radiation exposure.[10] MRI findings can include enlarged cartilage at the sites of complaint, focal or widespread increased signal intensities of affected cartilage on T2-weighted images, and gadolinium uptake in areas of thickened cartilage.[10] However, the high costs associated with MRI prohibit its routine use.

Treatment consists of reassurance, local application of heat, and the use of salicylates or NSAIDs. Local infiltration of the involved costal cartilage with steroids and local anesthetic, or intercostal nerve blocks, is indicated in refractory cases.

Slipping Rib Syndrome

Slipping rib syndrome is a less widely known cause of mechanical rib pain. It is characterized by intense pain in the lower chest or upper abdominal area caused by subluxation of the tips of the lower (8th–10th) ribs from their cartilages. Because these ribs attach to each other via a cartilaginous cap or fibrous band rather than to the sternum directly, they are more mobile and prone to trauma than other ribs. Loosening of the fibrous attachments binding the lower costal cartilages allows a rib tip to curl upward and override the inner aspect of the rib above, causing impingement on the intercostal nerves.[7]

The condition has been variously described as slipping rib cartilages, clicking ribs, lower rib pain syndrome, and rib-tip syndrome. The disorder is thought to be traumatic in origin, though not all patients recall an inciting event. The onset is insidious, with intermittent unilateral pain in the anterior lower costal cartilages. Occasionally, severe, sharp pain is felt in the anterior costal margin and abdominal wall.

Pain associated with a clicking sound is sometimes felt over the tip of the involved costal cartilage with certain movements. The involved costal cartilage is tender and moves more freely than normal. The pain may be reproduced by the "hooking maneuver," in which the examiner places his fingers under the anterior costal margin and pulls the rib cage anteriorly. Occasionally, a clicking sound accompanies the pain during this maneuver. Treatment is by reassurance or local intercostal nerve block for pain relief.[11] Surgery is occasionally required.

Muscle Strain and Trauma

Muscular tenderness of the intercostal and pectoral muscles might be one of the commonest causes of musculoskeletal chest pain.[12] Muscle or joint pain from the shoulders or spine can also be referred to the chest. A history of non-routine or excessive activity, such as lifting, painting a ceiling, or chopping wood, is often elicited in pectoral muscle fatigue. Anxiety might also produce excessive muscular tension. Onset of pain may be either gradual or sudden, with patients reporting localized pain and tenderness over the strained muscles. Treatment is avoidance of the offending stress.

Fractures of any of the bones of the thoracic wall can cause chest pain, as can trauma to the rib cage. Even seemingly inconsequential trauma such as sporting activities or a bout of coughing might result in rib pain.[13] Pain is exacerbated by deep breathing and movement with point tenderness at the site of trauma. Radiographs will reveal 50 percent to 66 percent of all rib fractures. When a fracture line is not seen, a healing callus might appear some weeks later.[7]

Painful chest walls or stress rib fractures might be secondary to other disease processes such as rheumatoid arthritis, osteoporosis, osteomalacia, and Paget's disease of the bone.[7] Rib tumors, presenting either as painful rib swelling or a pathologic fracture, can arise from cartilage, bone, and chondrosarcomas.[14]

Precordial Catch Syndrome

Precordial catch syndrome (PCS), also known as Texidor's twinge, is a self-limiting disorder characterized by the sudden onset of intense sharp, stabbing, non-radiating pain, typically on the left side of the chest. The pain usually lasts between 30 seconds and 3 minutes. The intensity of pain can vary from a dull and annoying pain to pain so intense as to cause momentary vision loss. The etiology of PCS is unknown, but intercostal muscle spasm has been postulated as a cause.[15]

Respiration intensifies pain in PCS, such that sufferers might need to adopt shallow breathing until the episode passes. Paradoxically, some individuals find that forcing themselves to breathe as deeply as possible will result in a "popping" or "ripping" sensation that can actually resolve the PCS episode. The frequency of episodes varies among different individuals and might range from several times per day to years between episodes.

Because PCS is not inherently dangerous, the worst part might be the sufferer's fearful association of his or her chest pain with a heart attack. Correctly identifying PCS subsequently relieves these fears. Because PCS occurs intermittently, medications are rarely indicated.

HISTORY AND PHYSICAL EXAMINATION

The diagnosis of musculoskeletal chest wall syndromes rests upon a detailed clinical history and physical examination. A thorough pain history should be taken, and cardiac risk factors should be ascertained. Any history of trauma or of new or excessive physical activity is important. Relevant past history includes rheumatic diseases such as rheumatoid arthritis, spondyloarthropathies, and fibromyalgia.[16] A history of cough or dyspnea could indicate chest pain from intercostal muscle strain. It is important to identify systemic features associated with serious medical conditions, such as fevers, night sweats, and weight loss.

The physical examination begins with inspection of the chest wall to identify deformities, inflammation, or a rash that might suggest herpes zoster or psoriatic arthritis. One hallmark of musculoskeletal chest pain is that it is reproducible with palpation or movements of the joints and musculature of the affected area. The cervical and thoracic spine should be palpated, and its range of motion tested. Specific pain syndromes such as costochondritis and Tietze's syndrome usually occur in conjunction with multiple tender costosternal joints.

DIAGNOSIS

Chest pain is likely to be musculoskeletal in origin if palpation or movements reproduce the pain (Fig. 16.3). In patients without cardiac risk factors or a history suggestive of fractures or systemic illness, no further investigations are usually necessary. Chest radiographs are cost-effective ways to identify solid tumors, whereas CT can be useful in visualizing sternoclavicular structures and soft tissue swelling.[17] In cases of suspected joint infection, a blood count and culture should be performed. Erythrocyte sedimentation rate is nonspecific and might be elevated in patients with any rheumatic process. Further tests such as antinuclear antibody tests are indicated only if the clinical picture warrants it.

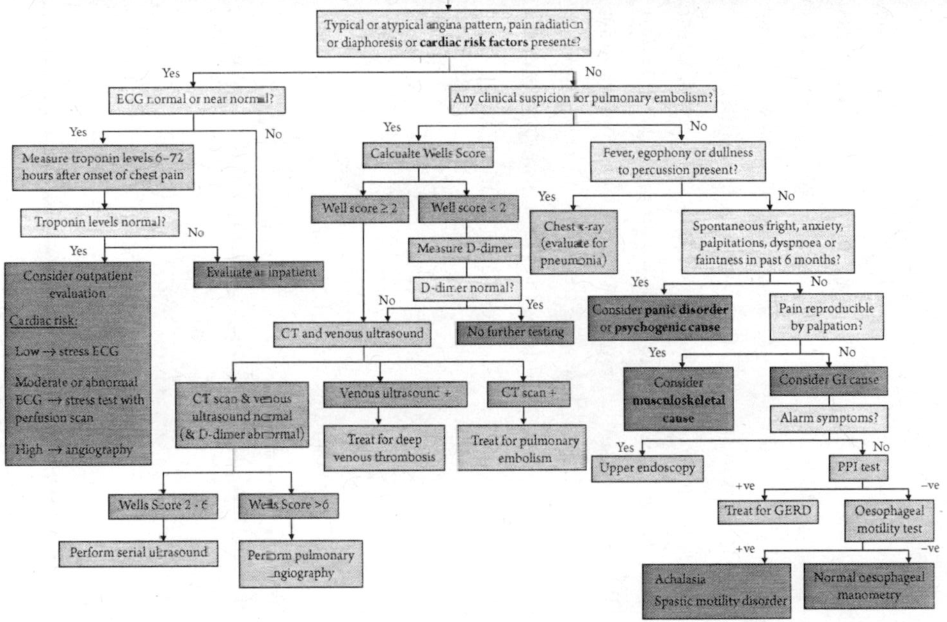

Figure 16.3. Treatment algorithm for patients presenting with chest pain. Legend: red = initial symptom; blue = questions to ask; purple = investigation; orange = investigation result; green = diagnosis or further evaluation. ECG = electrocardiography; CT = computed tomography; PPI = proton pump inhibitor.

TREATMENT

The first-line treatments for most patients with musculoskeletal chest pain are education and reassurance. Activities that exacerbate the pain should be suspended or limited. Generally, a gradual resolution of symptoms over time is expected. NSAIDs are useful for managing pain and reducing inflammation. Short-term use of opioids such as oxycodone or hydrocodone can be used for more severe, acute causes of musculoskeletal chest pain, such as a rib fracture. Inflammatory diseases such as costochondritis or Tietze syndrome can be safely treated with joint injections containing steroids and local anesthetic.[7,18] Tricyclic antidepressants may also be employed in treating generalized pain and have shown particular efficacy for neurogenic pain, such as that arising from herpes zoster.[19] In addition, herpes zoster should be treated with an antiviral agent within 72 hours to limit the outbreak's duration (see Chapter 13 for more details).

GASTROINTESTINAL CAUSES OF CHEST PAIN

Several esophageal abnormalities have been identified in patients suffering from NCCP.[20] Conditions such as esophageal perforation, bolus obstruction, or hiatal hernia strangulation might be suspected based on a careful history and examination. These emergencies require immediate evaluation with the aid of imaging or other specialized studies. Non-urgent conditions include gastroesophageal reflux disease (GERD), which is the most common cause of gastrointestinal-associated chest pain; esophageal dysmotility; autonomic dysregulation; and abnormal mechanophysical properties of the esophagus.[21] Less common esophageal abnormalities are Mallory-Weiss tears and Zenker's diverticulum. Cholecystitis and pancreatitis can also present with chest pain and left shoulder discomfort because of diaphragmatic or phrenic nerve irritation.

History and Physical Examination

Asking questions that pertain to GERD diagnosis is important because GERD is the most common cause of gastrointestinal-associated chest pain. Salient features on history include heartburn, dysphagia, acid regurgitation, pain associated with recumbent positions, and pain occurring post-prandially or after eating spicy or fatty foods.[4]

A history of dysphagia can indicate esophageal dysfunction or, if it occurs in association with late regurgitation, Zenker's diverticulum.[22] Mallory-Weiss tears are characterized by an abrupt onset of chest pain during vomiting or coughing, with subsequent hematemesis.

Physical examination is somewhat limited in chest pain with a gastrointestinal source. A thorough abdominal examination noting tender points, especially along the epigastrium, could indicate peptic ulcer disease or pancreatitis. A positive Murphy's sign suggests gallbladder disease. A digital rectal examination and stool guaiac test can help determine whether gastrointestinal bleeding is present.[17]

Diagnosis

The most common gastrointestinal cause of NCCP is GERD.[23] A 2-week course of moderate to high doses of a proton pump inhibitor (PPI) is a cost-effective test for the condition, with reported sensitivity and specificity rates of 71 percent to 90 percent and 67 percent to 88 percent, respectively.[24,25] If pain is reduced with a PPI, then the likely cause is GERD (Fig. 16.3). If pain persists, esophageal motility testing is advised. For patients exhibiting alarm symptoms such as odynophagia or dysphagia, upper endoscopy is indicated (Fig. 16.3). Barium swallows should be used only when other tests are non-diagnostic or when Mallory-Weiss tears or Zenker's diverticulum is suspected. Ambulatory 24-hour esophageal *p*H monitoring can identify GERD-associated chest pain with sensitivity of 60 percent to 90 percent and specificity of 85 percent to 100 percent.[22] However, this investigation is expensive, invasive, and not always available.

Treatment

Therapeutic modalities for gastrointestinal causes of NCCP should be targeted toward the underlying mechanism(s) (Table 16.4). Patients with GERD-related NCCP should receive high-dose PPIs for 4 to 8 weeks, such as esomeprazole 40 mg twice daily.[17] Selective serotonin reuptake inhibitors (SSRIs), such as sertraline, and the serotonin-norepinephrine reuptake inhibitor venlafaxine have been shown to be efficacious in relieving NCCP in patients without evidence of GERD or esophageal motility disorders.[26] Patients with coexisting psychological morbidity or those not responding to medical therapy should be considered for psychological interventions.

PSYCHOGENIC REGIONAL PAIN SYNDROME

A relationship exists between certain psychological disorders and NCCP. Among patients with NCCP, between 15 percent and 60 percent have associated panic disorder.[11,27,28] Generalized anxiety disorder, obsessive-compulsive disorder, and major depressive disorder have also been implicated as contributors to NCCP, but to a lesser degree.[28]

Although the exact mechanisms behind the physiology of psychiatric NCCP are not known, several studies have shown a relationship between hyperventilation and esophageal spasms.[17] Hypersensitivity to visceral pain, particularly esophageal, could trigger the classic panic vicious cycle of anxiety leading to worsening symptoms, resulting in increased anxiety, leading to even more symptoms.[27]

Table 16.4 TREATMENT OPTIONS FOR GASTROINTESTINAL NON-CARDIAC CHEST PAIN ACCORDING TO UNDERLYING MECHANISM

Gastroesophageal reflux disease
Reassurance
Lifestyle and dietary modifications
Proton pump inhibitors
Histamine-2 receptor antagonists
Esophageal dysmotility
Nitrates
Phosphodiesterase 5 inhibitors
Cimetropium/ipratropium bromide
Calcium channel blockers
Benzodiazepines
Botulinum toxin
Surgery
Esophageal hypersensitivity
Tricyclic antidepressants
Trazodone
Selective serotonin reuptake inhibitors
Serotonin-norepinephrine reuptake inhibitors
Adenosine antagonists
Cognitive-behavioral therapy

Adapted from Hershcovici T, Achem SR, Jha LK, et al. Systematic review: the treatment of noncardiac chest pain. *Aliment Pharmacol Ther*. 2012;35:5–14.

History and Physical Examination

After assurance that the cardiovascular system is not causing the pain, direct, specific questions should be asked about the symptoms of panic disorder: intense feelings of doom, profuse sweating, dizziness, palpitations, dyspnea, paresthesias, or a sensation of choking. Questions about recent stressors such as job loss, divorce, or the death of a loved one can be helpful in assessing a patient's current psychological state.[27] Restlessness, lack of energy, muscle tension, sleep disturbances, and irritability point toward generalized anxiety disorder.[17] Inquiring about other psychiatric illnesses and the family history of psychiatric illnesses can also be helpful. A complete physical examination, although necessary, is generally not helpful in diagnosing psychiatric causes of chest pain.

Diagnosis

Questionnaires, such as the Hospital Anxiety and Depression Scale and the Patient Health Questionnaire, serve as screening tools. Even a simple screening question such as whether the patient has ever experienced a sudden feeling of anxiety or panic has high sensitivity (93 percent) and is probably the most efficient screening tool.[17] If a patient exhibits severe psychiatric symptoms or if the provider is uncomfortable managing these issues, the patient should be referred to a psychiatrist.

Treatment

When a patient's chest pain has a psychiatric cause, reassurance and encouragement are vital. Many patients require education about their condition, gentle persuasion, and reassurance that effective treatments exist in order to accept recommendations. Effective treatments for these disorders include antidepressants, anxiolytics, or cognitive-behavioral therapy (see Chapter 4).[27] Recommended medications include trazodone 25 to 50 mg at bedtime, imipramine 25 mg, and SSRIs, which have a better side-effect profile than benzodiazepines.[26] Nonetheless, benzodiazepines have been shown to be safe and well tolerated when administered alone or in combination with other medications for NCCP, with minimal risk of dependence when prescribed on a short-term basis.[29]

PULMONARY CAUSES OF CHEST PAIN

Chest pain as a result of lung disease is usually due to pleuritis. Pleural inflammation may occur in pneumonia, pulmonary embolism (PE), or lung cancer or as an isolated phenomenon.

History and Physical Examination

Pulmonary chest pain usually presents acutely. Symptoms suggestive of pulmonary involvement include cough, sputum, hemoptysis, dyspnea, tachycardia, anxiety, and feeling light-headed. Pneumothorax can present with acute chest pain and shortness of breath. Night sweats and weight loss should raise suspicions of malignancy.

Diagnosis

Following a detailed history and examination, a chest x-ray can provide valuable diagnostic information when pulmonary causes are suspected (Fig. 16.3). No individual signs or symptoms can reliably identify a PE, but the simplified Wells scoring system (Table 16.5) is well validated for determining whether patients have a low, moderate, or high likelihood of PE.

Table 16.5 WELLS MODEL FOR CLINICAL DIAGNOSIS OF PULMONARY EMBOLISM

Clinical Finding[a]	*Points*
Clinical signs and symptoms of DVT (objectively measured leg swelling or pain with palpation of deep leg veins)	3.0
PE as likely or more likely than an alternative diagnosis	3.0
Heart rate > 100 beats per minute	1.5
Immobilization (i.e., bedrest except for bathroom access for at least 3 consecutive days) or surgery in the past 4 weeks	1.5
Previous objectively diagnosed DVT or PE	1.5
Hemoptysis	1.0
Malignancy (treatment for cancer that is ongoing, within the past 6 months, or palliative)	1.0

Total Points	*Risk of PE*	*LR+*	*Probability of PE, %*
<2	Low	0.13	1–28
2–6	Moderate	1.82	28–40
>6	High	6.75	38–91

Notes: DVT, deep venous thrombosis; PE, pulmonary embolism; LR+, positive likelihood ratio.

[a]Findings are listed in order of clinical importance.

Adapted from Wells PS, Anderson DR, Rodger M, et al. Derivation of a simple clinical model to categorize patients probability of pulmonary embolism: increasing the models utility with the SimpliRED D-dimer. *Thromb Haemost.* 2000;83:418.

D-dimer testing and CT pulmonary angiography are often required in order to diagnose PE. Venous ultrasound, together with D-dimer testing, is required in order to investigate suspected cases of deep venous thrombosis.

Treatment

Treatment for pulmonary causes of chest pain depends on the etiology. Treatment for pneumothorax is determined by symptom severity, indicators of acute illness, presence of underlying lung disease, estimated size of the pneumothorax on chest x-ray, and, in some instances, the patient's personal preference. Air travel is discouraged until a spontaneous pneumothorax has completely resolved. In traumatic pneumothorax, chest tubes are usually inserted, whereas tension pneumothorax should be treated with urgent needle decompression. Conservative management is recommended for small spontaneous pneumothoraces, defined as <50 percent of the lung field, no breathlessness, and an absence of underlying lung disease.

For pneumonia, oral antibiotics, rest, simple analgesics, and fluids are usually sufficient.[30] The elderly or patients with concomitant illnesses or significant trouble breathing require more advanced care and hospitalization. The CURB-65 score is useful for determining the need for hospital admission in adults. Children who display respiratory distress or <90 percent oxygen saturation should be hospitalized.

In most cases, anticoagulant therapy is the mainstay of treatment for PE. Heparin, low-molecular weight heparin, or fondaparinux is administered initially, while warfarin, acenocoumarol, or phenprocoumon therapy is commenced. If anticoagulant therapy is contraindicated and/or ineffective, an inferior vena cava filter may be implanted surgically. Thrombolysis is indicated in cases of massive PE in which hemodynamic instability is present.

CONCLUSIONS

Pain in the chest can be the presenting feature of a diverse number of disorders, many of which are non-cardiac in origin.[31–36] The most common causes of NCCP are musculoskeletal, gastrointestinal,[37] psychological, or pulmonary[38] in origin. Careful analysis of the history, physical findings, and results of rational investigations is essential for precise diagnosis, effective treatment, and optimal management. Support and reassurance are important cornerstones in the management of NCCP.

REFERENCES

1. Panju AA, Hemmelgarn BR, Guyatt GH, et al. The rational clinical examination. Is this patient having a myocardial infarction? *JAMA*. 1998;280(14):1256–1263.
2. Eslick GD, Talley NJ. Non-cardiac chest pain: predictors of health care seeking, the types of health care professional consulted, work absenteeism and interruption of daily activities. *Aliment Pharmacol Ther*. 2004;20(8):909–915.
3. Klinkman MS, Stevens D, Gorenflo DW. Episodes of care for chest pain: a preliminary report from MIRNET. Michigan Research Network. *J Fam Pract*. 1994;38(4):345–352.
4. Eslick GD, Jones MP, Talley NJ. Non-cardiac chest pain: prevalence, risk factors, impact and consulting—a population-based study. *Aliment Pharmacol Ther*. 2003;17(9):1115–1124.
5. Eslick GD, Coulshed DS, Talley NJ. Review article: the burden of illness of non-cardiac chest pain. *Aliment Pharmacol Ther*. 2002;16(7):1217–1223.
6. Proulx AM, Zryd TW. Costochondritis: diagnosis and treatment. *Am Fam Physician*. 2009;80(6):617–620.
7. Fam AG, Smythe HA. Musculoskeletal chest wall pain. *CMAJ*. 1985;133(5):379–389.
8. How J, Volz G, Doe S, et al. The causes of musculoskeletal chest pain in patients admitted to hospital with suspected myocardial infarction. *Eur J Intern Med*. 2005;16(6):432–436.
9. Spalding L, Reay E, Kelly C. Cause and outcome of atypical chest pain in patients admitted to hospital. *J R Soc Med*. 2003;96(3):122–125.
10. Volterrani L, Mazzei MA, Giordano N, et al. Magnetic resonance imaging in Tietze's syndrome. *Clin Exp Rheumatol*. 2008;26(5):848–853.

11. Huffman JC, Pollack MH. Predicting panic disorder among patients with chest pain: an analysis of the literature. *Psychosomatics.* 2003;44(3):222–236.
12. Stochkendahl MJ, Christensen HW. Chest pain in focal musculoskeletal disorders. *Med Clin North Am.* 2010;94(2):259–273.
13. Hanak V, Hartman TE, Ryu JH. Cough-induced rib fractures. *Mayo Clin Proc.* 2005;80(7):879–882.
14. Andrianopoulos E, Lautidis G, Kormas P, et al. Tumours of the ribs: experience with 47 cases. *Eur J Cardiothorac Surg.* 1999;15:615–620.
15. Gumbiner CH. Precordial catch syndrome. *South Med J.* 2003;96(1):38–41.
16. Almansa C, Wang B, Achem SR. Noncardiac chest pain and fibromyalgia. *Med Clin North Am.* 2010;94(2):275–289.
17. Watson GS. Noncardiac chest pain: a rational approach to a common complaint. *JAAPA.* 2006;19(1):20–25.
18. Kamel M, Kotob H. Ultrasonographic assessment of local steroid injection in Tietze's syndrome. *Br J Rheumatol.* 1997;36(5):547–550.
19. O'Malley PG, Jackson JL, Santoro J, et al. Antidepressant therapy for unexplained symptoms and symptom syndromes. *J Fam Pract.* 1999;48(12):980–990.
20. Fass R, Achem SR. Noncardiac chest pain: epidemiology, natural course and pathogenesis. *J Neurogastroenterol Motil.* 2011;17(2):110–123.
21. Achem SR. Treatment of non-cardiac chest pain. *Dis Mon.* 2008;54(9):642–670.
22. Faybush EM, Fass R. Gastroesophageal reflux disease in noncardiac chest pain. *Gastroenterol Clin North Am.* 2004;33(1):41–54.
23. Dickman R, Mattek N, Holub J, et al. Prevalence of upper gastrointestinal tract findings in patients with noncardiac chest pain versus those with gastroesophageal reflux disease (GERD)-related symptoms: results from a national endoscopic database. *Am J Gastroenterol.* 2007;102(6):1173–1179.
24. Cremonini F, Wise J, Moayyedi P, et al. Diagnostic and therapeutic use of proton pump inhibitors in non-cardiac chest pain: a metaanalysis. *Am J Gastroenterol.* 2005;100(6):1226–1232.
25. Wang WH, Huang JQ, Zheng GF, et al. Is proton pump inhibitor testing an effective approach to diagnose gastroesophageal reflux disease in patients with noncardiac chest pain?: a meta-analysis. *Arch Intern Med.* 2005;165(11):1222–1228.
26. Nguyen TMT, Eslick GD. Systematic review: the treatment of noncardiac chest pain with antidepressants. *Aliment Pharmacol Ther.* 2012;35:493–500.
27. Fleet RP, Beitman BD. Unexplained chest pain: when is it panic disorder? *Clin Cardiol.* 1997;20(3):187–194.
28. Ho KY, Kang JY, Yeo B, et al. Non-cardiac, non-oesophageal chest pain: the relevance of psychological factors. *Gut.* 1998;43(1):105–110.
29. Huffman JC, Stern TA. The use of benzodiazepines in the treatment of chest pain: a review of the literature. *J Emerg Med.* 2003;25(4):427–437.
30. Lim WS, Baudouin SV, George RC, et al. BTS guidelines for the management of community acquired pneumonia in adults: update 2009. *Thorax.* 2009;64(Suppl 3):iii1–iii55.

31. Cannon RO 3rd, Bonow RO, Bacharach SL, et al. Left ventricular dysfunction in patients with angina pectoris, normal epicardial coronary arteries, and abnormal vasodilator reserve. *Circulation*. 1985;71(2):218–226.
32. Janssens J, Vantrappen G, Ghillebert G. 24-hour recording of esophageal pressure and pH in patients with noncardiac chest pain. *Gastroenterology*. 1986;90(6):1978–1984.
33. Rouan GW, Hedges JR, Toltzis R, et al. A chest pain clinic to improve the follow-up of patients released from an urban university teaching hospital emergency department. *Ann Emerg Med*. 1987;16(10):1145–1150.
34. Katon W, Hall ML, Russo J, et al. Chest pain: relationship of psychiatric illness to coronary arteriographic results. *Am J Med*. 1988;84(1):1–9.
35. Wise CM, Semble EL, Dalton CB. Musculoskeletal chest wall syndromes in patients with noncardiac chest pain: a study of 100 patients. *Arch Phys Med Rehabil*. 1992;73(2):147–149.
36. Fruergaard P, Launbjerg J, Hesse B, et al. The diagnoses of patients admitted with acute chest pain but without myocardial infarction. *Eur Heart J*. 1996;17(7):1028–1034.
37. Hershcovici T, Achem SR, Jha LK, et al. Systematic review: the treatment of noncardiac chest pain. *Aliment Pharmacol Ther*. 2012;35:5–14.
38. Wells PS, Anderson DR, Rodger M, et al. Derivation of a simple clinical model to categorize patients probability of pulmonary embolism: increasing the models utility with the SimpliRED D-dimer. *Thromb Haemost*. 2000;83:418.

17

Chronic Functional Abdominal Pain

ROY DEKEL AND AMI D. SPERBER

Case Presentation

RJ is a 45-year-old woman who has had severe chronic abdominal pain for years. The pain has become dramatically worse over the past 6 months. It is diffuse and described as a dull ache compounded by daily episodes of severe burning pain that last from minutes to hours. There is no clear association between the pain and eating. She denies any connection between the pain and stress or tension. In fact, she believes that any stress she might have is due to the pain, and that if the pain would only go away she would no longer be stressed.

RJ denies constipation, diarrhea, or excessive straining. She also denies fever, rectal bleeding, or significant weight loss, and her family history is unremarkable for malignancy or gastrointestinal (GI) disease. Her past medical history includes a laparoscopic cholecystectomy performed 4 years ago after she experinced right upper quadrant abdominal pain and a laparoscopic hysterectomy performed 2 years ago for pelvic pain. Not only did these operations fail to improve her symptoms, but after her hysterectomy the pain got worse, and her gynecologist attributed this to adhesions. She has recurrent headaches and was diagnosed in the past with fibromyalgia. She frequently takes over-the-counter painkillers that help her deal with her pain.

RJ has undergone an extensive work-up including blood tests, abdominal computed tomography (CT), upper endoscopy and colonoscopy (×3), a fecal calprotectin test, and a capsule video-endoscopy, all without pathological findings.

On physical examination she is a somewhat distressed and anxious well-nourished woman. Physical examination is unremarkable, except for diffuse abdominal tenderness and a positive Carnett's sign, manifested by increased abdominal pain when she tenses the abdominal wall muscles by raising her upper body from the waist in a supine position against resistance.

At the end of the first appointment, RJ bursts into tears and tells you that the pain is ruining her life, she cannot go on living like this, and she knows that you, her last remaining hope, will make it go away.

BACKGROUND

Chronic abdominal pain is a common symptom frequently seen in primary care, gastroenterology, and surgery clinics. Although a common symptom, it can stem from a large number of potential causes, so a systematic work-up is the optimal way to reach a definitive diagnosis. The etiology of abdominal pain, like that of any other symptom, can be divided into chronic versus acute conditions and then further subdivided into structural versus functional disorders (Fig. 17.1). The physician's primary concern should be to rule out serious, potentially life-threatening structural conditions. The list in Table 17.1, which

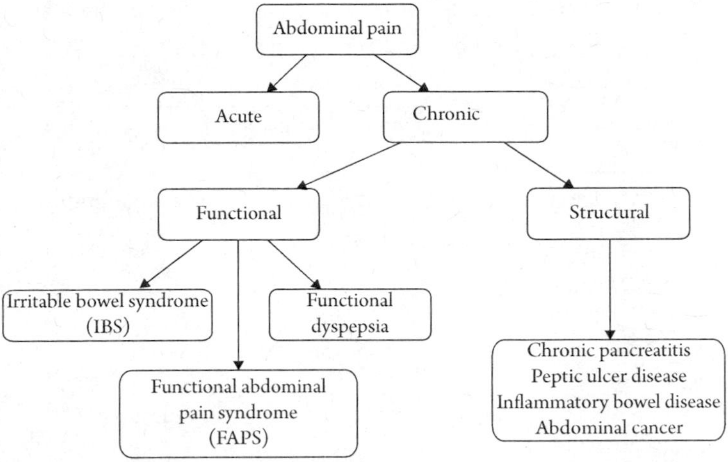

Figure 17.1. A flow diagram showing the place of FAPS in the domain of abdominal pain.

shows some of the common causes of chronic abdominal pain, indicates that a practical approach using relatively simple and generally accessible tools can rule out most, if not all, of the possible causes. However, after excluding structural causes, clinicians need to consider a broad range of functional GI disorders (FGIDs) that manifest as abdominal pain, including functional dyspepsia, irritable bowel syndrome (IBS), and functional abdominal pain syndrome (FAPS).

Patients suffering from FAPS are hard to diagnose and even more difficult to treat. In fact, FAPS patients are among the most challenging patients encountered in primary care and in tertiary clinics. Consequently, physicians seeing and treating these patients should know how to make a confident, expedient diagnosis of FAPS with the minimum possible work-up, as well as how to provide optimal treatment.

In this chapter we review the presentation, epidemiology, and pathophysiology of FAPS and outline a practical approach to the diagnosis and management of FAPS patients, based on the typical case of the patient presented above.

Table 17.1 MAJOR CAUSES OF CHRONIC STRUCTURAL ABDOMINAL PAIN (ARRANGED BY ALPHABETICAL ORDER)

Diagnosis	*Clinical Clues*	*Diagnostic Approach*
Abdominal angina	• Elderly patients • Diffuse atherosclerotic disease • Post-prandial pain—sitophobia	• CT angiography
Abdominal neoplasm	• Constant pain • Progressive clinical coarse • Weight loss • Nocturnal pain	• Abdominal CT
Abdominal wall pain syndromes	• Pain localized to a specific point • Exacerbation during abdominal muscle contraction • Surgical scars	• Abdominal ultrasound • Abdominal CT
Chronic pancreatitis	• Alcohol abuse • Steatorrhea	• Abdominal CT
Chronic pelvic inflammatory disease (PID)	• Prior PID • Dysmenorrhea • Dyspareunia	• Gynecological referral
Endometriosis	• Dysmenorrhea • Exacerbation during menstruation	• Gynecological referral • Empirical hormone Rx • Laparoscopy

(continued)

Table 17.1 (CONTINUED)

Diagnosis	*Clinical Clues*	*Diagnostic Approach*
Functional dyspepsia	• Epigastric pain exacerbated by eating/ stress, bloating, nausea and vomiting, heartburn	• Symptom-based Rome criteria
IBS	• Pain associated with: • change in bowel frequency/consistency • relieved by defecation • exacerbated by eating, bloating	• Symptom-based Rome criteria
Inflammatory bowel disease	• Diarrhea, fever, rectal bleeding, right lower quadrant pain/ inflammatory mass	• Colonoscopy, abdominal CT
Intestinal obstruction	• Previous surgery • Abdominal distension • Episodic colicky pain relieved by vomiting • Weight loss	• Abdominal CT
Peptic ulcer disease	• Long-standing episodic pain	• Gastroscopy

WHICH IS THE CORRECT DIAGNOSIS: IBS OR FAPS?

Many physicians would diagnosis RJ with IBS, using IBS as a generic term to describe chronic functional abdominal pain. Although IBS and FAPS are related in many ways, they are not the same disorder and should be distinguished to optimize patient management. In IBS, the abdominal pain or discomfort is frequently relieved by a bowel movement and is associated with a change in the frequency or consistency of the stool. In FAPS patients, pain is the hallmark. It is moderate to severe and not associated with the triggers seen in IBS patients, such as eating. The Rome III diagnostic criteria for FAPS are presented in Table 17.2. The Rome Foundation also published a clinical diagnostic algorithm that serves as a framework for the diagnosis and work-up of these patients[1] (Fig. 17.2).

Table 17.2 ROME III DIAGNOSTIC CRITERIA FOR FUNCTIONAL ABDOMINAL PAIN SYNDROME

Must include *all* of the following:
1. Continuous or nearly continuous abdominal pain
2. No or only occasional relationship of pain with physiological events (e.g., eating, defecation, or menses)
3. Some loss of daily functioning
4. The pain is not feigned (e.g., malingering)
5. Insufficient symptoms to meet criteria for another functional gastrointestinal disorder that would explain the pain

Note: Criterion fulfilled for the past 3 months with symptom onset at least 6 months prior to diagnosis.

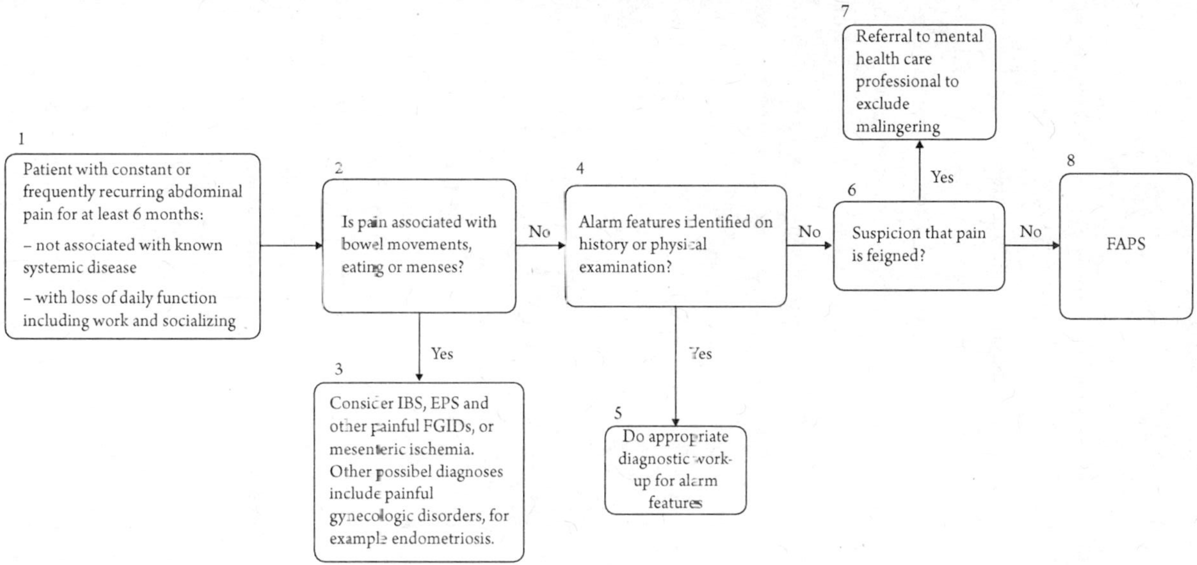

Figure 17.2. Clinical algorithm for the diagnosis of FAPS. From the *American Journal of Gastroenterology*.[1]

FAPS: DEFINITION, EPIDEMIOLOGY, AND PATHOPHYSIOLOGY

The Rome classification for FGIDs defines FAPS as chronic (at least 6 months per the definition, but usually longer in clinical practice) constant, nearly constant, or frequently recurring abdominal pain in the absence of any organic cause. The pain is not associated with physiologic events such as eating or defecation. The criteria also require that the pain be associated with loss of daily function, such as work and socializing. As in other functional disorders, the diagnosis is based on subjective patient report, and there are no specific objective test findings that can confirm it.

The prevalence rate is estimated at 1 percent of the adult population.[2,3] As in other functional conditions, most FAPS patients are female, with an estimated ratio around 2:1. In spite of its relatively low overall prevalence, its relative weight in primary care and GI clinics is considerably greater.[4] This can be attributed to the chronic nature of the condition and the high utilization rate of healthcare resources seen in FAPS patients. Moreover, the absence of effective treatment leads to recurrent consultations with different doctors and additional testing in search of a solution.

IBS has a spectrum of severity, and FAPS is close in presentation and pathophysiology to severe IBS. In both cases, symptoms are attributed mainly to central sensitization to and processing of visceral afferent signals and are amplified by psychopathology such as anxiety, depression, and somatization. In contrast, in mild and moderate IBS, which affect the vast majority of IBS patients, the symptoms are related more to peripheral (visceral) hypersensitivity and as such are frequently associated with eating and bowel movements. Thus, a considerable degree of overlap might exist between severe IBS and FAPS, making differentiation difficult at times. However, in most clinical scenarios, drawing an exact line between the two disorders also might be unnecessary.

WHAT IS THE PATHOPHYSIOLOGY OF FAPS?

Data regarding the pathophysiology of FAPS are scarce, as they are for other aspects of the syndrome, so many of the data in the following section are based on studies of severe IBS.

The central nervous system can up-regulate peripheral signals so that normal physiological or mildly pathological input is perceived as an extremely painful event. Central factors such as anxiety, depression, and somatization are probably involved in this process. Some clinical evidence reinforces the validity of this theory. The only predictor for the development of chronic pelvic pain after a gynecological operation for non-painful indications was the psychological profile of the patient. Patients anticipating difficulty preoperatively and those with lower scores on a scale of coping skills were more likely to develop pain postoperatively.[5] Another example is the development of IBS after an episode of gastroenteritis. Here again, patients with higher levels of anxiety were more likely to develop IBS after bacterial gastroenteritis than patients without.[6]

Whereas in cases of acute pain, as well as in some cases of chronic pain, it is clear that the peripheral component is predominant, in functional syndromes the central component is dominant. Abdominal pain syndromes such as IBS and FAPS have a spectrum of severity. In most IBS patients with mild to moderate severity, the peripheral component is dominant, so pain is connected to physiologic events such as eating or defecation. As the syndrome worsens, the central component becomes more and more pivotal, and the peripheral component becomes less important. Finally, at the extreme end of the severity spectrum, where most FAPS patients are, the pain is mainly due to central disinhibition and is unrelated to physiologic events[7] (Fig. 17.3).

A small physiological study showed that FAPS patients were not hypersensitive to balloon distention like IBS patients and did not report pain at low balloon distention, implying that the pain reported by FAPS patients is due not to rectal (i.e., peripheral) hypersensitivity but to other (i.e., central) mechanisms.[8,9]

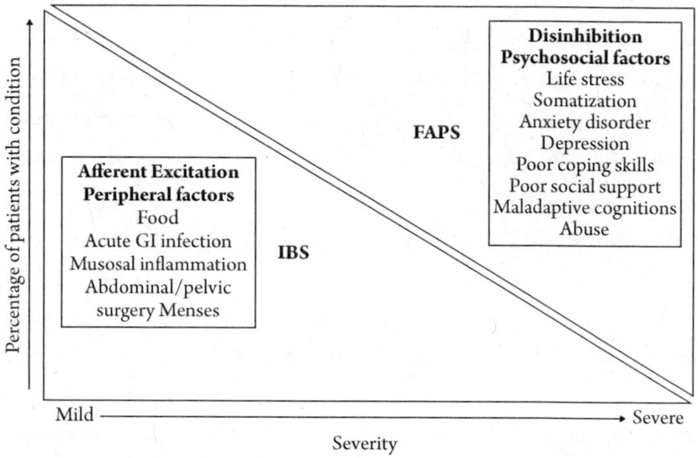

Figure 17.3. A conceptual model showing IBS and FAPS symptom severity as a function of the interaction between peripheral sensory initiating factors and central processing variables (psychosocial variables). Impaired central processing of the afferent signals leads to disinhibition and more severe symptoms. It is modulated by the presence of psychosocial co-morbidity. The *y*-axis represents the percentage of patients with each (central or peripheral) contribution. The opposing triangle shapes demonstrate that most IBS patients have mild or moderate symptoms and more peripheral (visceral) activity, with a minority having more severe symptoms (and increasingly impaired central processing), whereas most FAPS patients have more severe symptoms with a major component of impaired central processing and psychosocial modulation. Reprinted with permission of Blackwell Publishing Ltd., publishers of *Alimentary Pharmacology and Therapeutics*.[7]

PRACTICAL CLINICAL APPROACH AND WORK-UP

The differential diagnosis for chronic abdominal pain is extensive and includes almost any inflammatory or neoplastic process within the abdominal cavity (Table 17.1). At first it can appear to be overwhelming; however, the majority of possible diagnoses can, and should, be ruled out by means of good clinical judgment and a few simple diagnostic tests. As always, taking the patient's history and conducting a thorough physical examination are essential to the diagnostic process.

The Rome diagnostic criteria should be kept in mind while taking the history. If the patient's pain improves with defecation and is associated with a change in the form and/or frequency of stool, IBS is more likely than FAPS. If the patient's pain is localized and changes with movement or exercise, an abdominal wall origin should be suspected. If it is localized to the right upper quadrant (RUQ), and especially if there are liver enzyme abnormalities, rare causes such as sphincter of Oddi dysfunction or functional gallbladder disorder should be considered. If eating exacerbates the pain, especially in an older patient with diffuse atherosclerotic disease, vascular ischemia would be another possibility. Whenever pain is associated with menses, one should look for causes such as endometriosis. In general, it is good practice for women with lower abdominal pain, which might be hard to distinguish from pelvic pain, to have a gynecological consultation. If the pain is associated with menses or vaginal bleeding, such a consult becomes mandatory.

One should always look for alarm signs such as weight loss, fever, rectal bleeding, nocturnal pain, or a positive family history of other GI-related conditions. In these cases, as well as in cases of recent-onset pain, a more comprehensive work-up is recommended.

None of these are the case for RJ, who has a long history of abdominal complaints, a clinically benign course, and no alarm signs that might suggest other conditions. In addition, functional conditions tend to cluster, and our patient has been diagnosed with fibromyalgia and chronic headache.

In a previous study conducted by one of the authors (A.D.S.), fibromyalgia was diagnosed in 31.6 percent of IBS patients, compared to 4.2 percent of controls. Correspondingly, IBS was diagnosed in 32 percent of women with known fibromyalgia.[10] In all clinical and health-related variables assessed, including global feeling of well-being, sleep disturbances, relation of stress to symptoms, physician visits, concerns about illness, and psychological distress, patients with both IBS and fibromyalgia had more severe disorders than those with IBS only. The same pattern held true for the Sense of Coherence Index (a measure of coping ability)[11] and the Functional Bowel Disorder Severity Index.[12] Although these associations have not been studied to the same extent in FAPS, it is reasonable to assume that similar associations do exist.

The various functional disorders have important characteristics in common, including epidemiology (female predominance), pathophysiology (inflammation, hypersensitivity, impaired central processing of afferent sensory information, role of serotonin, psychological distress and somatization, the role of stress and life events), diagnosis (symptom-based), the central role of the patient–physician relationship in therapy, and common therapeutic modalities.[13]

Inasmuch as the functional disorders overlap significantly and have similarities in terms of patient characteristics, impact of illness on quality of life, psychological co-morbidity, and treatment, it has been suggested that they might represent a group of illnesses sharing a common pathogenesis.[14–16] In fact, they are so similar in many respects that some authorities have suggested that their classification into separate entities is artificial[17] and a result of the division of modern medicine into medical sub-specialties.

We find it very beneficial to emphasize that fact to the patient. Some of the patients believe that they are very ill because they have so many symptoms and different medical diagnoses, a belief that further impairs their quality of life and coping skills. By providing patients with a unifying paradigm that connects different, apparently unrelated symptoms to one disorder (i.e., central sensitization), we can alleviate many of their fears and concerns.

A good patient history frequently can elicit longstanding "IBS-like" symptoms that are related to stress. Another sensitive issue is a history of sexual, physical, or emotional abuse, which is common in these patients.[18] Addressing these issues is a delicate matter and should be done with sensitivity and empathy. Although many doctors do not feel comfortable discussing these subjects with their patients, it is very important to identify and discuss them as much as possible.

Because concomitant psychopathology (e.g., anxiety, depression, somatization) is common in FAPS patients, experienced clinicians should always look for it. Clues to this might appear naturally during the course of the conversation, but if they do not, the clinician should be proactive and use direct questions such as "how would you describe your mental state" or "how does your situation make you feel" or look for evidence for prior use of psychoactive drugs.

There are scant "positive findings" in the physical examination of a patient with FAPS. It is conducted mainly to look for evidence of malnourishment, an abdominal mass, localized tenderness, hepatosplenomegaly, or blood in the stool. However, one can still get useful clues from the physical examination that point to a functional diagnosis. FAPS patients often look anxious, distressed, or depressed, with a discrepancy between their report about their condition and their affect and general "benign" appearance. During palpitation of the abdomen, patients often manifest diffuse tenderness without any sign of localized peritoneal irritation. Distracting the patient by talking with him or her might reduce pain reporting and behavior. Other subtle findings on physical examination are the "open eyes sign" and the "stethoscope sign." In the former, the patient closes his or her eyes during abdominal examination, in contrast to the normal behavior of a patient with organic pain who leaves his or her eyes open in anticipation of pain. The latter can be elicited when using the stethoscope for abdominal palpation. In patients with organic pain, any contact with the abdomen exacerbates the pain, whereas in FAPS patients palpation with the stethoscope seems to diminish pain behavior. A positive Carnett's sign, whereby abdominal pain increases when the muscles of the abdominal wall are tensed, might be elicited. Although this sign's main purpose is to differentiate between pain arising from the abdominal wall and visceral pain, it is frequently seen in FAPS patients without abdominal wall pain, most likely signifying central hypersensitivity and hypervigilance more than an abdominal wall etiology.

A complete blood count and chemistry panel, upper and lower endoscopy, and an abdominal CT scan virtually rule out most of the organic causes of chronic abdominal pain, but they should be used with clinician discretion, as they are not always indicated. In current practice, most patients undergo these procedures, which are relatively safe. This is particularly true in the climate of medical liability in which most clinicians work. Nevertheless, it is preferable to refrain from the excessive work-up that many of these patients undergo, including repeated imaging studies and endoscopies.

TREATMENT

Many physicians are reluctant to treat patients with FAPS, as doing so is perceived as energy- and time-consuming on the one hand and having a small chance for success on the other. This perception can become a self-fulfilling prophecy that leads to a feeling of frustration among doctors and patients alike and contributes to an unsuccessful therapeutic outcome. Indeed, treating FAPS patients is a challenging process that demands commitment and devotion on the part of both the doctor and the patient. If physicians do not believe that they can commit to such a process, they should consider referring the patient to the care of someone who can. However, treating FAPS patients can be very rewarding. In fact, there are many options in the therapeutic armamentarium, so doctors should not feel overwhelmed and helpless when considering the care of FAPS patients.

The Doctor–Patient Relationship

The basis for a successful therapeutic outcome is a good doctor–patient relationship. This is especially true when treating patients with chronic pain syndromes. As mentioned above, both parties should be willing to commit to an extended therapeutic process and partnership. The doctor should use patience and empathy and acknowledge that the patient's symptoms and distress are real. It is also important to identify and address the patient's fears and concerns, such as the fear of cancer or other life-threatening diseases.[19]

Confidence in the diagnosis is one of the cornerstones of a successful treatment. The doctor should explain in detail the nature of functional disorders and should aim to have the patient both understand and accept the diagnosis. One other extremely important issue is setting realistic goals for treatment. Unrealistic goals such as a "quick fix" or "cure" can lead to frustration and failure. This can be addressed in a constructive manner with a statement such as, "If I were treating patients with hypertension or diabetes, they would not expect me to have a cure; instead they would expect that I could help them get it under control. That should also be the case for a chronic disorder such as FAPS. I am willing, in partnership with you, to develop a treatment strategy that could lead to reduced pain and improved quality of life over the course of the coming months. How do you feel about that?" Many patients who have suffered past disappointments when unrealistic goals were set would gain confidence in their doctors based on this sincerity and dedication and would gladly accept these therapeutic goals and "sign up" for the partnership.

Medical Treatment

The options for the medical treatment of FAPS patients are summarized in Table 17.3. Because FAPS is a pain syndrome, the therapeutic goal should be the alleviation of pain. Although narcotics are the most potent analgesics available, their use should be avoided in FAPS. However, many physicians prescribe opiates to these patients either because the patient demands it or because they are not familiar with other options. In contradiction to this approach, the results of studies have shown that patients with centralized pain states have lower opioid-receptor availability, possibly making opioids a less effective therapy.[20] Moreover, these drugs can result ultimately in the development of narcotic bowel syndrome.[21]

Antidepressants should be the cornerstone of medical therapy in FAPS for two reasons. First, they have a direct analgesic effect and are used in various pain syndromes, with or without concomitant depression, to elevate pain thresholds via central and peripheral effects. Second, many FAPS patients have psychological co-morbidities, and they can gain direct benefit from these drugs. A recent meta-analysis found all classes of antidepressants to be effective in IBS with a number-needed-to-treat as low as 4.[22] Because tricyclic antidepressants (TCAs) and serotonin-norepinephrine reuptake inhibitors (SNRIs) have an independent indication in other pain syndromes such as neuropathic pain and fibromyalgia, they are the drugs of

Table 17.3 COMMON INTERVENTIONS USED IN FUNCTIONAL ABDOMINAL PAIN SYNDROME

Drug	*Drug (Daily Dose Range, mg)*	*Comments*
Tricyclic antidepressants	• Desipramine (25–150) • Nortriptyline (25–150) • Amitriptyline (25–150)	• Begin with low doses and titrate according to response • Allow 4 to 8 weeks for maximal response
Selective serotonin reuptake inhibitors	• Paroxetine (20–60) • Escitalopram (10–20)	• Begin with low doses and titrate according to response
Serotonin-norepineprhine reuptake inhibitors	• Venlafaxine (25–150) • Duloxetine (20–80)	• Psychological and analgesic effects
Gabapentinoids	• Gabapentin (300–1800) • Pregabalin (150–450)	• Gradual dose increase • Preliminary reports
Atypical antipsychotics	• Quetiapine (25–100)	• Preliminary reports
Hypnosis	• Non-pharmacological Rx	• Should be "gut-directed"
Cognitive-behavioral treatment	• Non-pharmacological Rx	• Identifies and helps to manage maladaptive thoughts, behaviors, and concerns

Note: For optimal results, these interventions can be used in combination ("augmentation" therapy). The use of more than one drug in a low dose can augment the therapeutic response to and minimize the side effects of others.

choice. The choice between them is often based on the therapeutic profile of the drugs, including potential adverse effects. For example, TCAs tend to be more constipating and have fewer anxiolytic properties, so an SNRI would be a preferred option in a patient with constipation or prominent anxiety. However, in most cases a combination of two drugs or more is necessary, and the use of a combination of two or more drugs from different classes (e.g., a TCA and an SNRI or selective serotonin reuptake inhibitor [SSRI]) is recommended. Furthermore, this "augmentation therapy" enables the use of lower doses, thus minimizing adverse effects, to which patients with FGIDs are prone.[23] When combining multiple antidepressants, care should be taken to account for the total dosing to avoid serotonin syndrome or excessive norepinephrine effects.

There are two main barriers that clinicians face when trying to treat FAPS patients with antidepressants. The first is the general reluctance of these patients to take "chemical" and "mind altering" agents. The second is patients' tendency to underestimate the psychological component of their symptoms. A thorough explanation regarding the mechanisms of the pain (visceral hypersensitivity modulated by central mechanisms) and the drug's independent analgesic properties is enough in many cases. In our experience, the adherence rate for drug therapy increases if the physician is available to address, in real time, early adverse effects and other concerns that otherwise might lead the patient to discontinue therapy on his or her own.

Drugs can and should be combined not only with other drugs but also with non-pharmacological treatment. The use of psychological interventions such as cognitive-behavioral therapy (CBT) and hypnosis has been shown to be effective in the treatment of different pain syndromes, including IBS.[24,25] CBT can help patients recognize misperceptions and maladaptive thoughts regarding their symptoms and help them enhance their coping abilities. Hypnosis has been shown to be effective in IBS patients in both the short and long term. Further details about CBT can be found in Chapter 4.

CONCLUSIONS

In summary, FAPS is a serious medical problem that, though not life threatening, can have a tremendous impact on patients' quality of life and result in disability and considerable loss of daily function. The diagnosis should be made with a parsimonious work-up and be presented to the patient in detail and with confidence. Doctors should not be "afraid" of treating these challenging patients, because treatment options are available and the results can be very rewarding for both the patient and the physician.

REFERENCES

1. Sperber AD, Drossman DA. Functional abdominal pain syndrome: constant or frequently recurring abdominal pain. *Am J Gastroenterol.* 2010;105:770–774.
2. Drossman DA, Li Z, Andruzzi E, et al. U.S. householder survey of functional GI disorders: prevalence, sociodemography and health impact. *Dig Dis Sci.* 1993;38:1569–1580.
3. Thompson WG, Irvine EJ, Pare P, Ferrazzi S, Rance L. Functional gastrointestinal disorders in Canada: first population-based survey using Rome II criteria with suggestions for improving the questionnaire. *Dig Dis Sci.* 2002;47:225–235.
4. Longstreth GF, Drossman DA. Severe irritable bowel and functional abdominal pain syndromes: managing the patient and health care costs. *Clin Gastroenterol Hepatol.* 2005;3:397–400.
5. Sperber AD, Blank Morris C, Greemberg L, et al. Development of abdominal pain and IBS following gynecological surgery: a prospective, controlled study. *Gastroenterology.* 2008;134:75–84.
6. Dai C, Jiang M. The incidence and risk factors of post-infectious irritable bowel syndrome: a meta-analysis. *Hepatogastroenterology.* 2012;59:67–72.
7. Sperber AD, Drossman DA. Review article: the functional abdominal pain syndrome. *Aliment Pharmacol Ther.* 2011;33:514–524.

8. Nozu T, Kudaira M. Altered rectal sensory response induced by balloon distention in patients with functional abdominal pain syndrome. *Biopsychosoc Med.* 2009;3:13.
9. Nozu T, Okumura T. Visceral sensation and irritable bowel syndrome; with special reference to comparison with functional abdominal pain syndrome. *J Gastroenterol Hepatol.* 2011;26(Suppl 3):122–127.
10. Sperber AD, Atzmon Y, Neumann L, et al. Fibromyalgia in the irritable bowel syndrome: studies of prevalence and clinical implications. *Am J Gastroenterol.* 1999;94:3541–3546.
11. Sperber AD, Carmel S, Atzmon Y, et al. The sense of coherence index and the irritable bowel syndrome. A cross-sectional comparison among irritable bowel syndrome patients with and without coexisting fibromyalgia, irritable bowel syndrome non-patients, and controls. *Scand J Gastroenterol.* 1999;34:259–263.
12. Sperber AD, Carmel S, Atzmon Y, et al. Use of the Functional Bowel Disorder Severity Index (FBDSI) in a study of patients with the irritable bowel syndrome and fibromyalgia. *Am J Gastroenterol.* 2000;95:995–998.
13. Sperber AD, Dekel R. Irritable bowel syndrome and co-morbid gastrointestinal and extra-gastrointestinal functional syndromes. *J Neurogastroenterol Motil.* 2010;16:113–119.
14. Veale D, Kavanagh G, Fielding JF, Fitzgerald O. Primary fibromyalgia and the irritable bowel syndrome: different expressions of a common pathogenetic process. *Br J Rheumatol.* 1991;30:220–222.
15. Gruber AJ, Hudson JI, Pope HGJ. The management of treatment-resistant depression in disorders on the interface of psychiatry and medicine. *Psychiatr Clin N Amer.* 1996;19:351–369.
16. Hudson JI, Goldenberg DL, Pope HGJ, Keck PEJ, Schlesinger L. Comorbidity of fibromyalgia with medical and psychiatric disorders. *Am J Med.* 1992;92:363–367.
17. Wessely S, Nimnuan C, Sharpe M. Functional somatic syndromes: one or many? *Lancet.* 1999;354:936–939.
18. Drossman DA. Abuse, trauma, and GI illness: is there a link? *Am J Gastroenterol.* 2011;106:14–25.
19. Drossman DA. Psychological sound bites: exercises in the patient-doctor relationship. *Am J Gastroenterol.* 1997;92:1418–1423.
20. Harris RE, Clauw DJ, Scott DJ, McLean SA, Gracely RH, Zubieta JK. Decreased central mu-opioid receptor availability in fibromyalgia. *J Neurosci.* 2007;27:10000–10006.
21. Grunkemeier DM, Cassara JE, Dalton CB, Drossman DA. The narcotic bowel syndrome: clinical features, pathophysiology, and management. *Clin Gastroenterol Hepatol.* 2007;5:1126–1139.
22. Ford AC, Talley NJ, Schoenfeld PS, Quigley EMM, Moayyedi P. Efficacy of antidepressants and psychological therapies in irritable bowel syndrome: systematic review and meta-analysis. *Gut.* 2009;58:367–378.

23. Drossman DA. Beyond tricyclics: new ideas for treating patients with painful and refractory functional gastrointestinal symptoms. *Am J Gastroenterol.* 2009;104:2897–2902.
24. Drossman DA, Toner BB, Whitehead WE, et al. Cognitive-behavioral therapy versus education and desipramine versus placebo for moderate to severe functional bowel disorders. *Gastroenterology.* 2003;125:19–31.
25. Miller V, Whorwell PJ. Hypnotherapy for functional gastrointestinal disorders: a review. *International J Clin Exper Hyp.* 2009;57:279–292.

18

Pelvic Pain

SAWSAN AS-SANIE, MARK HOFFMAN,
AND DEVON SHUCHMAN

Case Presentation

JL is a 26-year-old nulligravid female who presents with increasing bilateral lower quadrant pain of 2-year duration. She describes her pain as a throbbing ache, with occasional stabbing pain that radiates to her back and thighs. The pain occurs daily but worsens shortly before and during her menses. She recalls having severe menstrual cramping since menarche, but these pain symptoms have progressed and are no longer controlled with non-steroidal anti-inflammatory drugs (NSAIDs).

BACKGROUND

Chronic pelvic pain (CPP) is defined by the American College of Obstetricians and Gynecologists as "non-cyclic pain of 6 or more months" duration that localizes to the anatomic pelvis, anterior abdominal wall at or below the umbilicus, lumbosacral back, or buttocks and is of sufficient severity to cause functional disability or lead to medical care.[1] CPP is estimated to affect between 15 percent and 20 percent of women in the

United States, with direct healthcare costs approaching $2.8 billion per year.[1,2] It is the primary indication for 10 percent of all outpatient gynecology visits, 40 percent of all diagnostic laparoscopies, and 12 percent to 17 percent of all hysterectomies performed each year.[3,4]

CPP represents a constellation of symptoms and is not a single disease entity. Its evaluation and management usually entail a complex process because there are many organ systems within the pelvis that can contribute to these symptoms. In addition to the female reproductive organs, the pelvis contains the bladder and distal ureters, the distal gastrointestinal tract, muscle, bone, and nerves. Many of these can act as pain generators, and it is not always clear which, if any, are contributing to a patient's symptoms. Occasionally, there is a single, easily identified cause of pain, such as a persistent, large ovarian cyst or degenerating uterine fibroid, and treatment is singular and curative. More often than not, the pain is associated with several diagnoses arising from multiple organ systems, and treatment is multimodal but not curative. Table 18.1 summarizes common conditions that might act as pain generators in

Table 18.1 COMMON CONDITIONS THAT MIGHT BE PAIN GENERATORS IN WOMEN WITH CHRONIC PELVIC PAIN

GYNECOLOGIC
• Endometriosis*
• Ovarian remnant syndrome*
• Pelvic congestion syndrome*
• Pelvic inflammatory disease*
• Gynecologic cancer*
• Adenomyosis
• Uterine fibroids
• Pelvic adhesive disease

(*continued*)

Table 18.1 *(CONTINUED)*

UROLOGIC

- Interstitial cystitis/painful bladder syndrome*
- Radiation cystitis*
- Bladder cancer*
- Urethral syndrome
- Recurrent cystitis
- Recurrent/chronic urolithiasis

GASTROENTEROLOGIC

- Irritable bowel syndrome*
- Inflammatory bowel disease*
- Chronic constipation*
- Colorectal carcinoma*
- Celiac disease
- Abdominal/pelvic hernias

MUSCULOSKELETAL

- Abdominal wall myofascial pain (including trigger points)*
- Pelvic floor tension myalgia*
- Fibromyalgia*
- Coccygodynia*
- Piriformis syndrome

NEUROLOGIC

- Abdominal wall cutaneous nerve entrapment (ilioinguinal and iliohypogastric)*
- Pudendal neuralgia

*Conditions with level A evidence of a causal relationship to chronic pelvic pain.
Adapted from Howard F. Chronic pelvic pain. *Obstet Gynecol.* 2003;101(3):594–611.

women with CPP and highlights those conditions for which there is high-level evidence of a causal relationship with CPP.[5]

The primary care physician is ideally positioned to oversee the care of women with CPP. Establishing a supportive and open relationship while setting reasonable goals and expectations at the first visit is of utmost importance. The identification of a definitive diagnosis is not likely following a single visit, and a thoughtful and directed evaluation by a primary care provider can efficiently guide a patient through the most appropriate diagnostic and treatment approaches.

DIAGNOSTIC APPROACH

The history and physical exam are the most informative diagnostic tools for the clinician evaluating a woman with CPP, and appreciation of the complex nature of CPP should encourage the use of a multidisciplinary approach. There is much value not only in the accurate diagnosis of the various pain generators contributing to a patient's pelvic pain, but also in addressing co-morbid medical conditions and psychosocial stressors that might exacerbate a patient's pain and reduce her quality of life.

HISTORY

Pain Characteristics

Describing the experience of pelvic pain can be challenging for a patient. To assist in the evaluation, the provider should obtain specific subjective details to guide the examination and differential diagnosis. Pelvic pain can be located in the low back, abdomen, hips, groin, buttock, or legs, in addition to the vagina, urethra, and/or rectum.

A complete pain history must also address the onset, duration, intensity, frequency, and quality of the pelvic pain, as well as exacerbating and alleviating factors. As with the patient described above, symptoms suggesting cyclic pain associated with menses should be identified, as well as symptoms related to urination, defecation, and intercourse. Table 18.2 provides a sample list of questions that should be included in a history for a patient complaining of pelvic pain.[5]

Table 18.2 QUESTIONS TO ASK DURING INITIAL PELVIC PAIN HISTORY

CHARACTERISTICS OF PAIN SYMPTOMS
• Where does it hurt? • How did your pain start, and has it changed since then? • Is your pain constant or intermittent? • On average, how many days of pain do you have per month? • What is your average, least, and maximum pain level (0–10)? • What is the quality or character of your pain? (e.g., cramping, stabbing, pulling, burning) • Does your pain change before, during, or after your menstrual period? • What makes your pain better or worse?
ASSOCIATED SYMPTOMS
• Do you have any urinary symptoms such as pain with urination, pain with a full bladder, frequent urge to urinate, blood in your urine, or urine leakage? • Do you have any bowel symptoms such as pain associated with constipation, diarrhea, blood or mucus in your stool, or abdominal bloating? • Do you have any associated weakness, numbness, or tingling in your pelvis, buttocks, vulva, or legs? • Do you have pain during sexual intercourse? If so, is it with initial entry, with deep penetration, or both? Does it continue afterward?

(continued)

Table 18.2 *(CONTINUED)*

ASSOCIATED MEDICAL CONDITIONS AND PRIOR TREATMENTS

- Do you have any other pain symptoms? (e.g., headaches, back pain, etc.)
- What other medical problems do you have?
- Have you ever been diagnosed with or treated for a sexually transmitted disease or pelvic inflammatory disease?
- Have you undergone any surgeries? Were any of these for the evaluation or treatment of pain?
- What prior evaluations or treatment have you had for your pain? Have any of these treatments been helpful, and if so, how much?
- Have you ever used any form of birth control? If so, have any been helpful for your pelvic pain?

MENTAL HEALTH AND SOCIAL STRESSORS

- How has the pain affected your quality of life?
- Do you feel depressed or anxious?
- Do you have trouble falling or staying asleep? Do you feel well rested in the morning?
- Are you taking any non-prescription drugs?
- Have you been or are you now being abused verbally, physically, or sexually? Are you now safe?

PATIENT-CENTERED GOALS

- What do you believe is the cause of your pain?
- What are *you* worried about?
- What are your goals for this visit? What are your long-term goals?

Adapted from Howard F. Chronic pelvic pain. *Obstet Gynecol.* 2003;101(3):594–611.

Medical History

The evaluation of a patient with pelvic pain should include consideration of reproductive, gastrointestinal, urologic, musculoskeletal, and neurologic conditions. Spine disorders, hip dysplasia, joint replacements, and leg length discrepancies are relevant to the diagnosis of secondary biomechanical dysfunctions. Additional chronic pain disorders, such as irritable bowel syndrome (IBS), interstitial cystitis, and fibromyalgia, are common in women with CPP. If present, prior treatment outcomes and their relationship to current pelvic pain symptoms should be explored.

Many patients have been seen by other physicians before their first visit with a new primary care provider. In such a scenario, a complete history of other prior diagnostic studies or interventions performed, treatments attempted, and results of those treatments is also necessary. Treatment history may include prior surgeries, interventional procedures, skilled therapies (i.e., physical therapy), acupuncture, chiropractic care, pharmacologic agents, psychiatric care, and psychological treatment.

Psychological History

Associated symptoms of depressed mood, disordered sleep, and disordered eating can be seen in patients presenting with any chronic pain condition. Given the high prevalence of psychological, physical, and/or sexual abuse in women with CPP, one should perform a careful history related to abuse.[6,7] This aspect of the patient's history should be obtained in a private setting without others present. Questions should include an assessment of a current safe environment and social support.

Social History

A thorough assessment of how pain might be functionally impairing self-care, school, work, or leisure activities should be obtained. Inquiry should also be made regarding the use of tobacco, alcohol, and illegal drugs. Patients often "self-medicate" when standard medical therapies have been ineffective.

PHYSICAL EXAMINATION

The physical exam, which is often painful and emotionally stressful for the patient, is essential in the evaluation of pelvic pain and should be performed with a systematic and gentle approach. The primary goal is to identify the anatomic locations and structures that reproduce the patient's pain. The exam should be interactive, and the examiner should maintain eye contact with the patient, eliciting feedback regarding whether each maneuver elicits the same pain experienced by the patient.

Table 18.3 provides a summary of the physical exam. After reviewing vital signs and making an overall assessment of the patient's demeanor and posture, the examination begins with the back while the patient is sitting. The exam should include the sacrum, coccyx, sacroiliac joints, and paraspinal muscles. Spinal curvature or abnormal posture or gait suggests a musculoskeletal component of the patient's pain.

The abdominal exam is then performed while the patient lies supine. The patient should first point to *all* the areas of pain and then the area of *maximal* pain. A cotton swab or light touch can be used to detect allodynia (pain with light touch), which might suggest a possible neuropathy. Single-digit deep palpation is performed by pressing firmly and systematically across and down the abdominal wall. The examiner should differentiate diffuse lower abdominal pain from focal pain associated with a taught band of muscle, or trigger point, by applying pressure to the abdominal wall in the area of maximal pain while the patient flexes her abdominal

Table 18.3 OVERVIEW OF PHYSICAL EXAMINATION OF FEMALE PATIENT WITH CHRONIC PELVIC PAIN

GENERAL
• Vital signs
• General appearance, mood, affect, or emotional state
• Gait, posture
BACK, PATIENT SITTING
• Spine curvature, evidence of previous injury or surgery
• Spinal (including sacrum and coccyx), paraspinal, and sacroiliac joint tenderness
ABDOMINAL, PATIENT SUPINE
• Appearance: fat distribution, scars or evidence of previous trauma or surgery
• Evidence of masses, hernia, inguinal adenopathy, pubic symphysis pain
• Light palpation or stroking (evaluate for allodynia)
• Single-digit deep palpation: differentiate focal vs. diffuse pain, trigger points (focal, taught muscle band, pain worsens with abdominal wall flexion)
EXTREMITY, PATIENT SUPINE
• Hip flexion, extension, internal and external rotation, abduction and adduction to evaluate for range of motion
• Muscle strength, tone, spasticity, or asymmetry

(continued)

Table 18.3 *(CONTINUED)*

PELVIC (PATIENT LITHOTOMY) • External genitalia: lesions, abrasions, ulcerations, erythema, or edema of clitoris, urethral meatus, vulva, and/or vestibule (Q-tip exam if patient has dyspareunia and/or vulvar pain) • Single-digit vaginal exam: tenderness or spasticity of pelvic floor muscles (pubococcygeus, obturator internus, piriformis), urethra, bladder, cervix, lower uterine segment, and vaginal fornices • Bimanual exam: uterine size, mobility, adnexal masses, and tenderness • Rectovaginal exam: tenderness and/or nodularity of rectovaginal septum and uterosacral ligaments • Speculum exam: lesions, ulcerations, or erythema of vaginal mucosa, cervix, and posterior vaginal fornix; cervical and/or vaginal cultures if purulent or malodorous discharge noted

wall during palpation. Worsened pain during flexion, a "positive Carnett's sign," is more likely a result of pain in the abdominal wall, whereas improved pain during flexion suggests an underlying visceral etiology.

The exam should include palpation of the pubic symphysis, as well as of the inguinal area to evaluate for a possible hernia. Reproductive organs are *not* normally palpable above the pelvic brim, and any palpable mass noted on abdominal exam should be considered abnormal and deserving of further evaluation.

The lower extremities and hips can be examined while the patient is still supine. Passive and active range of motion and muscle strength should be tested, including hip flexion, extension, internal and external rotation, abduction, and adduction. An evaluation of resting muscle tone or spasticity should be included, and bilateral examination allows for the identification of subtle asymmetries.

Pelvic Examination

As with all pelvic examinations, a chaperone should be present throughout the assessment. The pelvic exam is typically performed in the lithotomy position. Vulvar scars, lesions, skin changes, swelling, cysts, or asymmetries in the pelvic floor at rest should be noted. A mirror can be used to explain the findings.

The cotton swab (or Q-tip) test is suggested specifically for women with vulvar pain or symptoms of painful intercourse (dyspareunia). The moistened soft end of a cotton swab should be used to press lightly, beginning at the lateral thighs and moving medially to include evaluation at the 1, 4, 6, 8, and 11 o'clock locations of the vestibule. Vestibulodynia, a subtype of vulvodynia, is characterized by exquisite tenderness in the vulvar vestibule and is a common cause of dyspareunia.

The internal single-digit pelvic exam should begin with the placement of a well-lubricated finger into the vagina. In addition to noting whether this produces pain, the examiner should note whether the pelvic floor muscles feel spastic or contracted. The single-digit exam is then used to identify specific areas that reproduce the patient's pain. Muscles to be assessed include the levator ani (three to five o'clock and seven to nine o'clock positions), internal transverse perineal, and obturator internus (three and nine o'clock) muscles. Provocative examination techniques that reproduce or exacerbate the patient's typical pain must be differentiated from those techniques or tests that produce a "new" pain, or pain that is not familiar to the patient. The bladder, urethra, and rectum should be palpated independently with a single digit to assess for tenderness, followed by the cervix, posterior lower uterine segment, adnexa, and lateral vaginal fornices.

This is helpful in distinguishing uterine, cervical, or adnexal pain from abdominal wall or bladder pain noted on the traditional bimanual exam.

The bimanual exam is then performed by placing two fingers in the vagina and examining for uterine size and mobility and adnexal masses or tenderness. Alternating pressure between the abdominal hand and the vaginal hand while asking the patient which areas are most tender will help distinguish pain arising from the pelvic floor, bladder, uterus, or adnexa (vaginal fingers) from that originating in the abdominal wall. Rectovaginal examination should be performed to identify rectovaginal septum or uterosacral nodularity or tenderness, which might occur with deeply infiltrating endometriosis.

The speculum exam should occur after the bimanual examination and should be performed with the smallest speculum that allows adequate visualization of the cervix, posterior fornix, and vaginal walls. Cervical and possibly vaginal cultures should be obtained if there is concern about cervicitis, vaginitis, or pelvic inflammatory disease. Careful inspection of the posterior fornix is particularly important if the patient has symptoms of endometriosis, as endometriosis lesions can occasionally be seen in this area.

ADDITIONAL TESTING

Chronic or recurrent urinary tract infections can lead to significant bladder irritation and spasm. If there is any concern, urine should be sent for complete urinalysis and culture. When hematuria is found, urine cytology should be performed for women over 40 years of age or for those with a history of cigarette smoking to evaluate for an underlying urinary tract malignancy.[8]

A pelvic ultrasound should be considered when pelvic exam findings suggest an enlarged uterus or ovarian mass or in a patient with additional symptoms of heavy or irregular bleeding. Uterine fibroids or ovarian masses can occasionally present with symptoms of pelvic pain. A complex adnexal mass can be a clue to the existence of endometriosis, although a normal ultrasound does not rule out endometriosis involving the peritoneal surface. In addition, a complex pelvic mass could represent an ovarian malignancy and warrants a referral to a gynecologist for evaluation.

EVALUATION AND TREATMENT OF SPECIFIC CONDITIONS

Although CPP can be caused by any number of disorders in several organ systems, the most common conditions identified include endometriosis, interstitial cystitis, IBS, and musculoskeletal disorders. Figures 18.1 and 18.2 provide algorithms that can be helpful in the initial management of CPP.

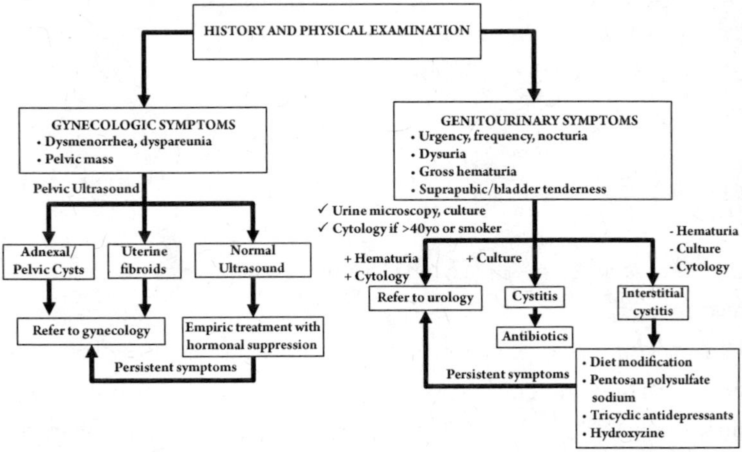

Figure 18.1. Algorithm for the evaluation and treatment of chronic pelvic pain: gynecologic and genitourinary symptoms. Modified from Wang K, As-Sanie S. Chronic pelvic pain. *Female Patient (Parsippany)*. 2007;32:1–3.

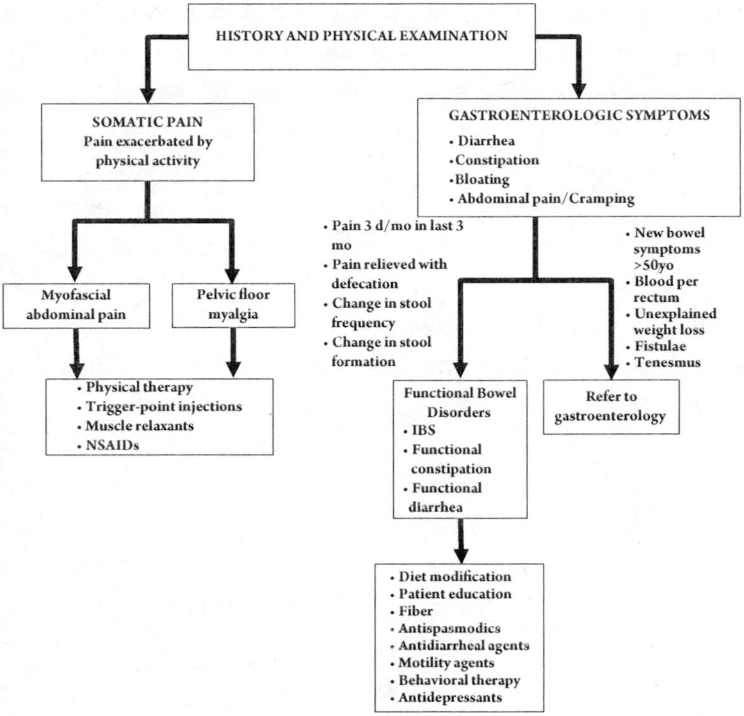

Figure 18.2. Algorithm for the evaluation and treatment of chronic pelvic pain: somatic and gastroenterologic symptoms. Modified from Wang K, As-Sanie S. Chronic pelvic pain. *Female Patient (Parsippany)*. 2007;32:1–3.

Common Gynecologic Causes

Dysmenorrhea, or pain associated with the menstrual cycle, is a common symptom in women of reproductive age. Many women with CPP report a history of dysmenorrhea prior to the onset of daily pelvic pain, and their CPP is often still exacerbated by menstruation. Primary dysmenorrhea is defined as cramping pain in the lower abdomen around the time of menstrual bleeding in the absence of any identifiable pelvic disease, whereas secondary dysmenorrhea is painful menses associated with a known pelvic disease. Numerous gynecologic conditions can cause painful menses and can be associated with either secondary dysmenorrhea or CPP (e.g., adenomyosis, uterine fibroids, pelvic congestion syndrome), but endometriosis is the most common.

Endometriosis is defined as the presence of endometrial glands and stroma in locations other than the endometrium. Although a constellation of symptoms (dysmenorrhea, dyspareunia) and physical exam findings (uterosacral nodularity) can point to the diagnosis, the diagnosis can be confirmed only via surgical biopsy. In patients with dysmenorrhea or symptoms suggestive of endometriosis, empiric medical treatment can be initiated without a definitive surgical diagnosis.

NSAIDs such as ibuprofen and naproxen can be very effective in the treatment of CPP, including endometriosis-related pain. They can be used around the clock in large, but safe and monitored, doses around the time of cyclic bleeding.[9] In patients with regular menstrual cycles, it is best to schedule the initiation of the medication for 1 to 2 days prior to the onset of bleeding, which can help improve pain control, as well as reduce menstrual flow.

Hormonal suppression is routinely a first-line treatment of endometriosis-related pain and any other cause of pelvic pain with menstrual exacerbation.[9] Hormonal options in the form of combined estrogen and progesterone therapy (pills, vaginal ring insert, or transdermal patch) or progesterone-only options (pills and intramuscular depo-medroxyprogesterone) are low-cost and safe options with overall low side-effect profiles. In addition, the levonorgestrel-containing intrauterine device is also effective in treating primary dysmenorrhea and pelvic pain related to endometriosis, and it has the added benefit of reducing heavy menstrual bleeding. These can be placed in the clinic by a trained provider and left in place for up to 5 years. These hormonal treatment options have been shown to be equally effective in several comparative randomized controlled trials for the treatment of endometriosis-related pelvic pain, and practitioners should select treatment options based on cost, side effects, and prior success in an individual patient.[10]

Other medications that suppress hormones, such as gonadotropin-releasing hormone agonists and aromatase inhibitors, are being studied in the treatment of endometriosis, but their use can lead to significant side effects including irreversible bone loss and diffuse joint pain.[5] Their use should be reserved for specialists familiar with treating complex gynecologic pain. Pain associated with adnexal or uterine masses or pain refractory to an empiric trial of hormonal suppression should warrant a referral to a gynecologist for further evaluation and management.

Common Urologic Causes

Interstitial cystitis/painful bladder syndrome (IC/PBS) is a chronic bladder disorder characterized by pelvic pain and irritative voiding symptoms, such as urinary urgency, frequency, and/or nocturia. It is the most commonly identified urologic source of chronic pain, but it is considered a diagnosis of exclusion. The precise etiology of IC/PBS remains unknown, but it is likely multifactorial, involving defective bladder urothelium, neurogenic inflammation, mast cell activation, and central pain amplification.[8,11] It occurs up to 10 times more frequently in women than in men, and it is commonly diagnosed in women with other gynecologic pain disorders such as endometriosis and vulvodynia. The diagnosis of interstitial cystitis is based on clinical symptoms and the exclusion of other etiologies of pain, such as infection and malignancy.[12] Standardized screening questionnaires, such as the Pelvic Pain and Urgency/Frequency Symptom Scale[13] and the O'Leary-Sant Interstitial Cystitis Problem Index,[14] can be useful screening tools. Invasive tests, such as the potassium sensitivity test and cystoscopy, are not required for diagnosis, but cystoscopy might be necessary in order to rule out other bladder pathology.

Treatment for interstitial cystitis should be initiated in patients who have been excluded for other sources of bladder pain. Recommendations for treatment include diet modifications, including eliminating bladder irritants from the diet.[15] Pentosan polysulfate sodium has been shown to be an effective oral treatment for interstitial cystitis and is the only treatment approved by the U.S. Food and Drug Administration for this condition. If the treatment is effective, patients should continue it for 6 months, followed by use as needed. Other medications, such as tricyclic antidepressants, anticonvulsants, hydroxyzine, and intravesical instillation of dimethylsulfoxide or heparin and alkanized lidocaine, can also provide relief of pain symptoms.[8,16] Patients with hematuria, severe pain, or symptoms refractory to conservative treatment should be referred to a urologist for further evaluation.

Gastroenterologic Causes

Complaints of pelvic pain associated with meals or bowel movements suggest gastrointestinal etiology. Functional gastrointestinal disorders are very common in women with pelvic pain, and IBS affects up to 15 percent of adults.[17] IBS is twice as common in women as in men and is present in as many as 50 percent of women with CPP.[5] The evaluation and treatment of IBS and chronic abdominal pain are reviewed in Chapter 17.

In women found to have endometriosis at the time of surgery, approximately 5 percent will have involvement of the bowel, though most lesions are superficial and asymptomatic.[18] Invasion of endometriosis through the bowel wall, resulting in cyclical rectal bleeding, pelvic pain, and/or bowel obstruction, is rare. Bowel symptoms in women with endometriosis, such as abdominal pain, bloating, and constipation or diarrhea, are far more likely to be a symptom of a concomitant functional bowel disorder than of endometriosis itself. Thus, it is very important that a history of endometriosis not delay the treatment of a functional bowel disorder or the referral of a patient with concerning bowel symptoms to a gastroenterologist for further evaluation.[18]

Neurologic Causes

Neuropathic pain related to peripheral nerve injury has been described in women with CPP. The pelvis contains a large number of nerves and nerve plexi, both somatic and visceral, and injury can lead to chronic pain. Previous surgery, trauma, and/or repetitive use injury might result in ilioinguinal, iliohypogastric, femoral, sciatic, or pudendal neuropathies. For example, ilioinguinal-iliohypogastric neuropathy should be considered in a woman with persistent abdominal pain and localized hyperalgesia following cesarean section or low transverse abdominal incision. Pudendal neuralgia has been described in patients with repetitive movements that compress the pudendal nerve (such as cyclists and equestrians) and in women following pelvic surgeries for prolapse and/or incontinence. A careful neurologic examination mapping areas of hyperalgesia might point to an underlying neuropathy. Patients with suspected motor deficits should be referred to neurology for further evaluation. In the absence of motor loss, initial treatments may include anesthetic injections and/or neuromodulatory medications (e.g., gabapentin, amitriptyline). Refractory cases often require referral to an interventional pain specialist and possibly a neurosurgeon.

In addition to the peripheral nervous system, the central nervous system also plays an important role in the etiology of CPP. Although much of this chapter is devoted to the evaluation of various "peripheral" pain generators, it is also important to recognize that there is increasing evidence that the initiation and maintenance of CPP might be partly related to central nervous system modulation of pain processing, even when peripheral pathology is also present.[19,20] This process of central pain modulation (amplification or inhibition of peripheral pain signals) could explain why some women suffer from pelvic pain but do not have an identifiable peripheral nociceptive input, while other women with severe pelvic pathology experience little if any pain. Although more research is desperately needed in this area, the use of neuromodulatory medications (e.g., gabapentin, amitriptyline) could be considered in women with CPP when other traditional therapies have failed.

Musculoskeletal Causes

Pelvic pain can present as a direct result of biomechanical/musculoskeletal dysfunction or as a secondary etiology of neuropathic or visceral dysfunction. In either case, this aspect of the patient's pain must be acknowledged and addressed appropriately. Disorders of the spine, such as lumbar or sacral radiculopathy by innervation of the pelvis and pelvic floor, can cause painful neuropathic and somatic symptoms. Other likely etiologies of pelvic pain are more easily localized, such as pubic symphysitis, coccydynia, and intra-articular hip disorders. Asymmetries in resting muscle tone, which can be found in primary neurologic dysfunction or result from biomechanical strain or dysfunction, can cause pain in structurally related joints. Even a seemingly benign leg length discrepancy can lead to asymmetry in hip and sacroiliac joint motion, which can then cause painful dysfunction. Referral to a physical medicine and rehabilitation physician can help diagnose dysfunction in the spine, pelvis, or lower extremities that can be contributing factors in the patient's pain profile.

Referral to physical therapy is an appropriate strategy when clinical examination suggests musculoskeletal etiology. Definitive diagnosis is not always required, as skilled therapists are trained in the evaluation and treatment of musculoskeletal dysfunction. Pelvic floor physical therapy focuses on muscle motor control, using biofeedback, manual therapy, acupressure, muscle energy, and mobilization techniques. Therapy often includes internal (vaginal) treatment and focuses on core muscle strength for support of the pelvis and spine. This type of treatment does require additional training and is not available at all physical therapy facilities. Any new neurologic deficit, involving either sensory or motor function, warrants referral and evaluation by an appropriate medical specialist.

Interventions

Injections can be diagnostic and/or therapeutic, often with a local anesthetic with or without steroid. There are a number of minimally invasive interventions that can benefit select patients.[21] Patients can be referred to a pain specialist for evaluation if needed.

CONCLUSION

CPP represents a constellation of symptoms and is not a single disease entity. The importance of primary care providers in the initial evaluation, as well as the continued support and management of women with CPP, should not be understated. Understanding which patients can be managed conservatively in a primary care setting, which require evaluation by a specialist, and which have signs or symptoms indicative of a more serious diagnosis can help a practitioner avoid unnecessary steps and subsequent delays in providing the appropriate care. As with all other chronic pain disorders, the diagnosis and treatment of CPP can be complex, long term, and not curative. The goals of the treatment must be realistic and should help the patient focus on improving function and quality of life.

REFERENCES

1. ACOG Practice Bulletin No. 51. Chronic pelvic pain. *Obstet Gynecol.* 2004;103(3):589–605.
2. Mathias SD, Kuppermann M. Chronic pelvic pain: prevalence, health-related quality of life, and economic correlates. *Obstet Gynecol.* 1996;87(3):321–327.
3. Whiteman MK, Hillis SD, Jamieson DJ, et al. Inpatient hysterectomy surveillance in the United States, 2000–2004. *Am J Obstet Gynecol.* 2008;198(1):34.e31–34.e37.
4. Howard FM. The role of laparoscopy in chronic pelvic pain: promise and pitfalls. *Obstet Gynecol Surv.* 1993;48(6):357–387.
5. Howard F. Chronic pelvic pain. *Obstet Gynecol.* 2003;101(3):594–611.
6. Paras ML, Murad MH, Chen LP, et al. Sexual abuse and lifetime diagnosis of somatic disorders. *JAMA.* 2009;302(5):550–561.
7. Committee opinion no. 498: adult manifestations of childhood sexual abuse. *Obstet Gynecol.* 2011;118:392–395.
8. Butrick CW, Howard FM, Sand PK. Diagnosis and treatment of interstitial cystitis/painful bladder syndrome: a review. *J Womens Health (Larchmt).* 2010;19(6):1185–1193.
9. Jarrell JF, Vilos GA, Allaire C, et al. SOGC clinical practice guidelines: consensus guidelines for the management of chronic pelvic pain. *J Obstet Gynaecol Can.* 2005(164):869–887.
10. Falcone T, Lebovic DI. Clinical management of endometriosis. *Obstet Gynecol.* 2011;118(3):691–705.
11. Bogart LM, Berry SH, Clemens JQ. Symptoms of interstitial cystitis, painful bladder syndrome and similar diseases in women: a systematic review. *J Urol.* 2007;177(2):450–456.
12. Hanno PM, Burks DA, Clemens JQ, et al. AUA guideline for the diagnosis and treatment of interstitial cystitis/bladder pain syndrome. *J Urol.* 2011;185(6):2162–2170.
13. Parsons CL, Dell J, Stanford EJ, et al. Increased prevalence of interstitial cystitis: gynecologic cases identified using a new symptom questionnaire and intravesical potassium sensitivity. *Urology.* 2002;60:573–578.
14. O'Leary MP, Sant GR, Fowler FJ, et al. The interstitial cystitis symptom index and problem index. *Urology.* 1997;49(Suppl 5A):58–63.

15. Marinkovic SP, Moldwin R, Gillen LM, Stanton SL. The management of interstitial cystitis or painful bladder syndrome in women. *BMJ*. 2009;339(2):b2707–b2707.
16. Dimitrakov J, Kroenke K, Steers WD, et al. Pharmacologic management of painful bladder syndrome/interstitial cystitis: a systematic review. *Arch Intern Med*. 2007;167(18):1922–1929.
17. Mayer EA. Irritable bowel Syndrome. *N Engl J Med*. 2008;358(16):1692–1699.
18. Remorgida V, Ferrero S, Fulcheri E, Ragni N, Martin DC. Bowel endometriosis: presentation, diagnosis, and treatment. *Obstet Gynecol Surv*. 2007;62(7):461–470.
19. Howard FM. Endometriosis and mechanisms of pelvic pain. *J Minim Invasive Gynecol*. 2009;16(5):540–550.
20. Stratton P, Berkley KJ. Chronic pelvic pain and endometriosis: translational evidence of the relationship and implications. *Hum Reprod Update*. 2011;17(3):327–346.
21. Tu FF, As-Sanie S, Steege JF. Musculoskeletal causes of chronic pelvic pain: a systematic review of diagnosis: part I. *Obstet Gynecol Surv*. 2005;60(6):379–385.

19

Central Pain Syndromes

BRIAN G. WILHELMI AND SRINIVASA N. RAJA

Case Presentation

Mr. Smith is a 75-year-old Caucasian with a 6-year history of atrial fibrillation. Despite being treated with warfarin, Mr. Smith suffers an embolic stroke that affects the left ventroposterior thalamus. Following several months of rehabilitation, Mr. Smith presents with complaints of constant burning pain and parasthesias over the right forearm and hand. The pain is reported as being moderate to severe in intensity and ranging from 5–7 on a 0–10 numerical rating scale. He indicates that the continuous pain affects his sleep and has interfered significantly with his quality of life. On examination, there is mild motor weakness and loss of temperature sensation in the distal right upper extremity. He has been taking several acetaminophen tablets a day with minimal relief and seeks your help in controlling his pain.

INTRODUCTION AND DESCRIPTION

Central pain syndrome (CPS) is a painful constellation of symptoms initiated or caused by a primary lesion in the central nervous system

(CNS).[1] The diagnosis of CPS is one of exclusion, as CPS patients often have pains attributable to other causes (musculoskeletal, nociceptive, psychogenic, etc.) and no one feature is pathognomonic of central pain.[2] The personal experience of pain varies from individual to individual because of the heterogeneous etiologies, localization, and pathology of injuries leading to this syndrome. Common CPS causes include stroke, brain or spinal cord tumors, epilepsy, brain or spinal cord trauma, syringomyelia, phantom limb pain, and Parkinson's disease.[3] Despite variable presentations, unifying traits characterizing this syndrome have been described. Descriptions of the nature of the pain might include sensations such as "burning," "pricking," or "pressing," with exacerbations typified by descriptors such as "shooting" and "lancinating." The pain is typically constant and often lifelong. It is generally of moderate to severe intensity, with evoked dysesthsias, allodynia, or hyperalgesia arising from touch, movement, emotions, and temperature changes (usually cold temperatures). In addition, patients frequently experience spontaneous, unprovoked pain. There is considerable variation in the onset of symptoms, which ranges from immediately post-insult to months or years later. Patients also frequently report negative symptoms such as deficits in sensations of light touch or temperature (especially cold) over similar distributions.

PATHOPHYSIOLOGY

Several theories have been advanced to explain the mechanism of CPS. "Central sensitization" is theorized to occur when an injury to the CNS leads to anatomic, neurochemical, excitotoxic, and inflammatory changes. These changes can lead to an increase in neuronal excitability at various sites in the pain signaling pathway. The end result is a lowering of action potential thresholds, increased responses to suprathreshold stimuli, and the generation of ectopic pain signals within the CNS. This "*facilitation*" theory is supported by the presence of both spontaneous and evoked pain, and by the efficacy of anti-epileptic medications, which decrease neuronal excitability and the intensity of pain. A second theory is that altered excitability or injury to the spinothalamic tract is necessary for the development of CPS. CPS patients display sensory alterations specific to the spinothalamic tract, including altered sensitivity to fine touch and temperature (particularly cold) in addition to pain. Although not all patients with an injury to the spinothalamic tract demonstrate CPS, injuries to the dorsal column alone are even less likely to result in central pain. An imbalance between excitatory and inhibitory oscillatory signaling in thalamocortical loop pathways has been advanced as another theoretical explanation for CPS.[4] This "*disinhibition*" theory is based on the finding that CPS occurs more frequently in patients with CNS injuries in areas where inhibitory neurons are commonly found, such as the lateral thalamus. As a result of disruption of the normal balance of excitatory and inhibitory signals, pain pathways might become over-excited. Cortical reorganization has also been postulated to explain CPS.[5] Supporting this are studies evaluating functional magnetic resonance imaging (MRI) changes in CPS patients with ongoing central neuropathic pain resulting from amputation or spinal cord injuries (SCIs) that demonstrate a correlation between pain intensity and the amount of reorganization. Imaging studies conducted in individuals with SCI have revealed a large portion of the somatosensory cortex being activated by afferent pain signals from the affected regions.

DIAGNOSIS

The diagnosis of central pain is attained through cosideration of medical history, physical examination findings, and selected diagnostic test results that are consistent with a pattern of CNS injury and CPS symptoms, as well as the exclusion of other causes of chronic pain.

Given that central pain is by definition a sequela of prior injury, a focused discussion of a patient's medical history provides a wealth of information vital to the diagnosis. Providers should elicit a comprehensive pain history including temporally related injuries or surgeries; a family history of autoimmune, neurological, or neoplastic disease; a social history of risk factors for the development of specific illnesses; psychiatric elements of pain; and the presence of autonomic symptoms. The use of written worksheets that allow patients to focus the description of their pain and its temporal evolution and identify the regions of the body affected by pain can aid in this process.

The physical examination should focus on delineating the neurologic distribution of pain and associated autonomic symptoms. Defining a pattern of localization via objective exam might reveal a peripheral nerve distribution, dermatomal distribution, spinal level, or central causative injury. Findings on physical examination suggestive of CPS include the presence of alterations in the sensation of temperature, as well as dysesthesias, paresthesias, allodynia, and hyperalgesia in the affected region. A good physical exam can also discern associated complaints that frequently accompany central pain such as musculoskeletal, spastic, and visceral pain.

The use of selected diagnostic studies can identify a specific lesion of the brain or spinal cord that correlates with the distribution of pain elicited by the medical history and physical examination. Imaging studies such as MRI or computed tomography of the CNS can provide visual evidence of a stroke, traumatic injury, tumor, syrinx formation, or white matter lesion. Functional MRI has been employed to demonstrate a remodeling effect of central sensorimotor processing functions. Functional studies such as sensorimotor evoked potentials can illustrate injury to the functional transmission of neurological signals that might result from CNS lesions. An electroencephalogram can demonstrate changes in neurologic activity consistent with functional reorganization of the brain. Electromyography and nerve conduction studies might be beneficial in differentiating CNS dysfunction from peripheral nervous system or myogenic processes.

Various quantitative studies of sensory function involving graded physiological stimuli such as thermal, pressure, pinprick, and vibration have been used in research to document sensory abnormalities in CPS. Despite the potential diagnostic value of quantitative sensory testing, such tests are not typically used as part of the routine work-up because of the time and expense involved and their limited ability to influence the development of a treatment plan.[6] In the future, such testing might be used to clarify the extent of injury or the potential benefit of therapeutic interventions.

ETIOLOGIES

Traumatic Brain Injury

Traumatic brain injury (TBI) occurs when a sudden blunt or penetrating trauma causes damage to the brain. It is estimated that 1.4 million Americans suffer from TBI each year. Among these individuals, approximately 58 percent will develop chronic headache, and 52 percent will develop chronic pains in other regions of the body.[7] The severity of CPS experienced by patients with TBI has been found to be worse in patients with mild TBI. Confounding symptoms in TBI patients include orthopedic and peripheral nerve injuries, postural-control deficits, and diffuse musculoskeletal pain (i.e., neck and back pain), as well as behavioral problems and cognitive dysfunction from injuries suffered concurrently (Fig. 19.1).

Table 19.1 COMPONENTS OF A CENTRAL PAIN SYNDROME EVALUATION

Medical History	*Physical Exam*	*Diagnostic Testing*
Pain History – Location, temporal profile, nature, intensity, aggravating factors, alleviating factors, treatments attempted – Hyperalgesia, allodynia, spontaneous pain *Neurological History* – Alterations in fine touch, temperature, proprioception, pressure – Paresthesias *Past Medical History* – Surgeries – Injuries – Cancer – Arteriovenous malformation – Seizures *Family History* – Autoimmune, neurological, or neoplastic disease	*Nervous System Exam* – Posture and gait examination – Cranial nerve exam – Motor nerve exam –Muscle strength –Deep motor reflexes –Motor tone – Spasticity – Cog-wheel rigidity – Flaccidity – Sensory nerve exam – Constant/spontaneous pain –Evoked pain • Allodynia • Hyperalgesia • Paresthesia –Temperature –Proprioception –Pressure –Vibration – Autonomic examination	*Laboratory Studies* – Metabolic derangements – Cell count abnormalities *Physiological Studies* – Sensorimotor evoked potentials – Electroencephalogram – Nerve conduction studies – Electromyography *Imaging Studies* – Magnetic resonance imaging (MRI) – Computed tomography – Functional MRI

(continued)

Table 19.1 (CONTINUED)

Medical History	*Physical Exam*	*Diagnostic Testing*
Social History – Exposures, risk factors, psychiatric health (depression)	– Sweating – Flushing – Piloerection – Hypo-/hyperthermia	*Quantitative Sensory Testing* – Laser evoked thermal sensory testing
Autonomic Symptoms – Increased/decreased sweating – Hyper-/hypothermia – Flushing – Raynaud's phenomena	–Raynaud's phenomena	– Monofilament pressure testing

Phantom Limb Pain

Phantom limb pain (PLP) is the perception of a painful, unpleasant sensation in the distribution of a missing or deafferented body part.[8] Common causes of amputation leading to PLP are vascular disease, cancer, and trauma. Estimates of the lifetime prevalence of PLP in major limb amputees range as high as 80 percent. The pathophysiology of PLP likely involves both peripheral and central neurological components. Central neurological symptoms result from the deafferentation of dorsal column sensory tracts of the spinal cord. Deafferentation leads to structural, neurochemical, and physiologic changes that result in autonomous pain signals propagated through the CNS. In addition to increased signaling, there is a loss of inhibitory

Table 19.2 THE CHARACTERISTICS OF CENTRAL PAIN SYNDROME

Etiology	– Traumatic brain injury – Ischemic or hemorrhagic stroke – Neoplasm – Abscess – Myelitis – Epilepsy – Parkinson's disease – Multiple sclerosis – Syringomyelia – Traumatic spinal cord injury
Temporal Profile	–*Onset:* Varies from immediately post-injury to several years after injury – *Daily duration of pain:* Usually constant pain with additional evoked or spontaneous pains; a subset of patients describe intermittent pain-free periods or only evoked or spontaneous pain. – *Cessation:* Usually a lifelong pain; rare resolution reported following further central nervous system injury or lesions
Intensity	– Varies from mild to severe – *Includes:* – Allodynia (pain from otherwise non-painful stimuli); – Hyperalgesia (increased pain from otherwise painful stimuli); – Paresthesias (abnormal, non-painful sensations); and – Dysesthesias (unpleasant, but not necessarily painful, abnormal sensations) – Extremely troubling to the patient; even mild pains can be disabling because of their unrelenting nature

(continued)

Table 19.2 *(CONTINUED)*

Location	– *Variability:* Generally correlated with location of injury such as a dermatome or spinal level, but injuries to the brain have more variability in their presentation (e.g., hemibody vs. single hand) – *Specific presentations:* –*Spinal cord injury:* Both at level and below level of spinal injury pains – *Stroke:* Wallenberg syndrome (medullary stroke) ipsilateral face and contralateral body, and hemi-body; ipsilateral eye – *Syringomyelia:* Cape-like distribution, intrascapular – *Parkinson's:* Often associated with hypertonia or dystonia – *Epilepsy:* Headache; arm, leg, or hemi-body; abdominal/visceral – *Multiple sclerosis:* Peri-orbital, trigeminal neuralgia, Lhermitte's sign	
Characteristic Nature	– Burning – Pins and needles – Unrelenting	– Band-like pressure – Sharp/shooting – Lancinating
Stimuli Affecting central pain syndrome	– Cutaneous stimuli – Temperature changes – Body movements	– Visceral stimuli (urination, defecation, orgasm) – Emotions
Concomitant Findings	Pure somatosensory changes in pain (allodynia, hyperalgesia) and temperature sensation (hyposensitivity or allodynia from temperature stimuli) are independent of abnormalities in muscle function, coordination, vision, hearing, vestibular function, and other higher cortical functions	

signaling observed from regions such as the brainstem reticular areas. CPS might also result from neuroplastic reorganization of the brain following amputation, which alters the cortical somatosensory representation such that painful and non-painful phantom sensations are experienced following peripheral somatosensory input originating on disparate regions of the body (i.e., a brush on the face eliciting PLP "from" an amputated arm).

Spinal Cord Injury

Approximately 30 percent to 40 percent of patients with spinal cord injury (SCI) will suffer from CPS.[9] SCI patients experience both "at level" mixed peripheral and central neuropathic pain found at the dermatome level corresponding to the SCI, as well as "below level" central neuropathic pain, which is localized to areas on the body distal to the level of the injury.[10] Central pain experienced by SCI patients has been linked to spinothalamic tract injury by MRI imaging and can be reproduced by hot or cold stimuli applied to below-injury body areas. As do those with other forms of CPS, SCI patients often experience a diffuse and intense burning pain, but they can also describe a band-like pressure sensation at below-injury levels. Autonomic dysreflexia results in hemodynamic instability and extreme heart rate variation following sensory inputs.

Stroke

Central post-stroke pain (CPSP), or central pain following a cerebrovascular accident, is common among stroke survivors and was one of the first central pain conditions described by clinicians.[11] Chronic pain affects between 11 percent and 55 percent of stroke survivors, and among those individuals it is estimated that approximately 1 percent to 12 percent will suffer from CPSP. Both hemorrhagic and ischemic stroke can induce central pain.[12] CPSP can occur following lesions in any part of the somatosensory pathways of the brain, but lesions to the lateral medulla or ventroposterior thalamus are most strongly correlated with CPSP. Pain is classified as CPSP when pain and sensory abnormalities correspond to areas of the brain injured by the cerebrovascular accident. The area of the body affected may be discrete (i.e., a single hand) or large (ipsilateral face and contralateral hemi-body [Wallenberg's syndrome]). The onset of pain can vary from immediately following the stroke to many months thereafter, but generally it will not appear until some sensation has returned.

Parkinson's Disease

Parkinson's disease (PD) is a neurological disease primarily defined by motor dysfunction; however, between 40 percent and 85 percent of PD patients experience chronic pain.[13] Central pain associated with PD is estimated to occur in 1 percent to 4.5 percent of patients.[14] To diagnose CPS in PD patients, the provider must distinguish CPS from more common PD pains including musculoskeletal pain, dystonic pain, peripheral neuropathic pain, and akathitic discomfort. Specific regions in which CPS is more clearly differentiated from musculoskeletal or dystonic pain include the face, head, pharynx, epigastrium, abdomen, pelvis, rectum, and genitalia. In PD, CPS symptoms have been improved by appropriate dopamine repletion therapy.

Multiple Sclerosis

Multiple sclerosis (MS) is a chronic progressive inflammatory disease that results in the demyelination of white matter tracts and neuronal degeneration within the CNS.[15] Central pain is common in patients with MS (up to 28 percent lifetime incidence), and its incidence and severity increase with the severity of disease. Sites of neuronal inflammation known as plaques within the brain and spinal cord have been shown to correlate with the distribution of pain. CPS is more common in the primary progressive or progressive-relapsing subtypes of MS than in the relapsing-remitting subtype. Pain in MS can manifest as Lhermitte's sign (brief, shock-like painful sensations with bilateral radiation from neck flexion), dysesthetic pain, and trigeminal neuralgia.

Epilepsy

Epilepsy is a disease defined by the presence of abnormal or excessive synchronous neuronal activity in the brain. Although tremulous activity and alterations in consciousness are more common, pain has been documented to occur in a small subset (<5 percent) of epilepsy patients in the peri-ictal period.[16] Pain associated with seizures typically presents in one of three forms: (1) headache; (2) unilateral "central" dysethetic pain of the face, facet arm, leg, and/or trunk; and (3) visceral abdominal pain. The timing of the onset of epileptic central pain varies among the pre-ictal aura, ictal, and post-ictal periods.[17] Therapy for all epilepsy-related central pain is based upon algorithmic treatment with anti-seizure medications and, for medically intractable cases, surgical resection of the epileptogenic foci if anatomically discrete.

Syringomyelia

Syringomyelia is a chronic disease caused by the creation of a fluid-filled cavity within the spinal cord caused by etiologies such trauma or Arnold-Chiari malformations.[18] It is estimated that 50 percent to 90 percent of patients with syringomyelia experience radicular-type pain symptoms that are often described as "sharp and shooting." Approximately 40 percent of patients might also

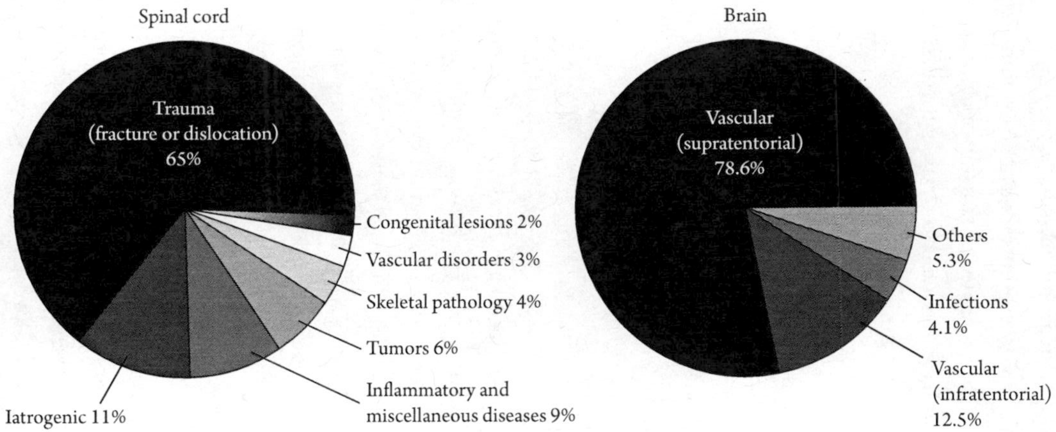

Figure 19.1. Etiology of central pain states. Reproduced from Brummett CM, Raja SN. Central pain states. In: Benzon HT, Raja SN, Liu SS, et al., eds. *Essentials of Pain Medicine*. 3rd ed. Philadelphia, PA: Elsevier-Saunders; 2011.

experience dysesthetic pain that is "burning, prickling, or stretching" in nature. This central pain is classically described as having a cape-like distribution, but it might also be interscapular or dermatomal in pattern. Pain is commonly accompanied by trophic changes such as hyperhidrosis, glossy skin, coldness, and paleness. Surgical decompression or evacuation of the syrinx is effective in relieving the dysesthetic pain in a majority of patients; however, a minority might experience a worsening of such symptoms with surgical correction. CPS symptoms gradually subside in those patients in whom surgery is effective. Residual CPS symptoms have been effectively treated with sympathectomy in a subpopulation of patients (Fig. 19.1).

TREATMENT

The treatment of patients with CPS is often challenging to both patient and clinician alike, as central pain is typically recalcitrant to clinical treatment methods. A core component of "success" is therefore based upon establishing rapport with patients through frequent and ongoing discussion of realistic treatment goals and the tolerability of side effects of available therapies. The treatments available for CPS involve six general categories that are frequently offered concurrently or sequentially as part of a multimodal algorithm: psychological, conservative/alternative, pharmacological, neuromodulation, intrathecal, and ablative.

Psychological therapy of chronic pain recognizes the affective component of pain and uses strategies to restructure beliefs and behaviors surrounding the "pain experience." Cognitive-behavioral therapy (CBT) is among the most commonly employed psychological therapy methods. Systematic reviews evaluating psychological therapies for chronic pain have concluded that CBT results in modest improvements in pain and mood but has minimal effects on disability or long-term outcomes.

Physical and alternative therapies that have been studied in neuropathic pain include transcranial magnetic stimulation (TMS), transcutaneous electrical nerve stimulation (TENS), and acupuncture.[19,20] The mechanism of action of TMS is unclear, but it is postulated that creating a magnetic field around the brain induces neurons to discharge with a frequency that can be influenced by the operator. The results of meta-analyses evaluating TMS are mixed, with some suggesting pain-relieving benefits and others concluding that it offers little to no benefit for neuropathic pain.[21] TENS is the application to the skin of electrical stimulation of varying frequency, intensity, and pulse duration for the purpose of pain relief. As with TMS, randomized trials evaluating TENS for central pain have failed to adhere to appropriate scientific rigor; consequently, conclusions regarding its efficacy remain uncertain. Acupuncture has been studied in patients with SCI in several small clinical trials. One study conducted in 17 wheelchair-bound SCI patients found no significant differences between true and sham acupuncture for chronic musculoskeletal pain.[22] In a more recent comparative-effectiveness study conducted in 30 patients with SCI, both acupuncture and massage therapy were found to alleviate neuropathic pain, with no differences noted between groups.[23]

The pharmacological treatment of CPS is based upon the trial of medications either alone or in combination in accordance with a limited body of scientific evidence and expert opinion.[24,25] Despite the recognized prevalence of CPS, the scientific study of pharmacologic therapy thus far has consisted of few prospective clinical studies with relatively low power and short-term follow-up.

Tricyclic antidepressants, such as amytriptyline, nortriptyline, and clomipramine, which block the reuptake of both norepinephrine and serotonin, have been shown to reduce global central pain ratings in prospective clinical trials performed in patients with CPSP, MS, PLP, and SCI.[25,26] Randomized comparative-effectiveness studies performed in SCI and CPSP patients found amitriptyline to provide superior benefit relative to gabapentin and carbamazepine. Tricyclic antidepressants have also proven effective in reducing global pain for peripheral neuropathic pain conditions, including diabetic polyneuropathy and postherpetic neuralgia. Currently, tricyclic antidepressants are generally considered first-line pharmacological therapy for CPS.

Gabapentin and pregabalin are calcium channel antagonists that block the release of the excitatory neurotransmitter glutamate. In small prospective trials, gabapentin has shown benefit in reducing average pain in SCI patients. Pregabalin has demonstrated reduction in mean pain ratings in one large and one small prospective trial on SCI patients, as well as in a placebo-controlled trial performed in CPSP, TBI, and SCI patients. Both gabapentin and pregabalin have also been shown to provide significant pain relief in the peripheral neuropathic pain population. Gabapentin and pregabalin are currently first-line therapies for PLP and SCI-related central pain.

Studies involving selective serotonin reuptake inhibitors and selective norepinephrine reuptake inhibitors have yielded mixed results; consequently, these drug classes are not indicated for CPS.[26] Mixed serotonin-norepinephrine reuptake inhibitors, such as venlafaxine and duloxetine, have not been studied in CPS; however, they have demonstrated benefit in peripheral neuropathic pain conditions such diabetic neuropathy, and generally they are associated with a more favorable side-effect profile than tricyclic antidepressants. Mixed serotonin-norepinephrine reuptake inhibitors are considered second-line therapy in CPS but are sometimes used as first-line treatments in the elderly.

Lamotrigine is an anti-epileptic drug that blocks sodium channels and inhibits the release of the excitatory neurotransmitter glutamate. In the CPSP population, it has been shown to be effective in reducing pain intensity and cold allodynia. In SCI, one randomized study found that lamotrigine did not significantly improve pain in the entire study sample, though subgroup analysis showed benefit in patients with incomplete SCI. Another double-blind study evaluating add-on therapy to gabapentin, tricyclic antidepressants, or other non-opioid analgesics in patients with peripheral and central neuropathic pain (MS, SCI, traumatic nerve injury) found that the use of lamotrigine as adjunctive pain therapy provided no additional benefit. Lamotrigine has had mixed results in studies on peripheral neuropathic pain. Lamotrigine is currently a second-line therapy for CPSP pain and a third-line therapy for SCI-related central pain.

Most, but not all, studies have found that intravenous lidocaine provides transient benefit in relieving SCI and other forms of central pain; however, its oral analogue, mexiletine, which is sometimes used after a positive temporary response to lidocaine, has not been found to be effective for central pain. At present, neither lidocaine nor mexilitine is recommended for the treatment of central pain.

The use of opioids for the treatment of neuropathic pain in general, and particularly in central pain, remains controversial. Opioids with pure opioid receptor agonism that have been trialed in CPS patients have failed to demonstrate significant, clinically meaningful pain relief. Morphine was found to provide superior relief in a controlled trial relative to mexilitine and placebo for PLP, but it was associated with low overall efficacy and significant side effects. In contrast, the potent oral opioid levorphanol, which exhibits opioid receptor agonism and weak *N*-methyl-D-aspartate (NMDA)-receptor antagonism, has demonstrated efficacy in reducing pain intensity among a limited number of patients with central pain secondary to stroke, SCI, or MS. Tramadol, which in addition to possessing weak μ-agonist properties inhibits the reuptake of serotonin and norepinephrine, was shown to be effective in a small trial performed in SCI patients.

Currently, opioids should be considered second- or third-line therapy for central pain.

Cannabinoids are cannabis derivatives that play a role in inhibiting synaptic transmission and controlling synaptic plasticity in pain pathways. Studied oral formulations include dronnabinol and δ-9 tetrahydrocannabinol/cannabidiol. In clinical trials, cannabinoids have demonstrated statistically significant improvement in pain scores and spasticity in patients with MS.

The parenteral NMDA receptor antagonist ketamine has been shown in randomized studies to provide significant short-term pain relief in patients with PLP, SCI, and chronic posttraumatic neuropathic pain. However, its use in an outpatient setting is impractical because of its poor side-effect profile, short half-life, and lack of a readily available oral formulation. In a majority of controlled studies performed in individuals with PLP, memantine has proven no more effective than placebo (see Table 19.3).

Intrathecal pumps, neuromodulation techniques, and ablative neurosurgical procedures all might provide some benefit in the CPS population.[27] Intrathecal pumps deliver medications such as baclofen, morphine, midazolam, or ziconotide directly to the spinal cord, where they affect the neurotransmission of afferent pain signals. The use of intrathecal therapy is perhaps most frequently employed in patients who experience significant pain relief with systemic opioids but suffer from limiting side effects. Neuromodulation or neurostimulation has been used at three locations: epidurally over the spinal cord, epidurally over the motor cortex, and with deep brain stimulation to the thalamus or periaqueductal or periventricular gray matter. Neuromodulation creates electrical interference with afferent pain transmission. Instead of perceiving pain, patients feel a more palatable "tingling or vibration" sensation in the affected area(s). Whereas the results of spinal cord and deep brain stimulation have been largely disappointing, motor cortex stimulation has

Table 19.3 PHARMACOLOGICAL RESULTS FOR THE TREATMENT OF CENTRAL PAIN

Medication	*Level of Evidence*	*Suggested Dosage Range/Minimum-Maximum*
Tricyclic antidepressants		
• Amitriptyline	SCI, CPSP moderate pos.	10–150 mg/d
• Imipramine	CPSP neg.	75–200 mg/d
• Nortriptyline	PLP weak pos.	10–150 mg/d
Selective serotonin reuptake inhibitors		
• Citalopram	CPSP neg.	10–40 mg/d
• Clomipramine	CPSP conflicting	25–250 mg/d
• Fluoxetine	CPSP weak pos.	25–125 mg/d
• Trazodone	SCI neg.	150–400 mg/d
Selective norepinephrine reuptake inhibitors	CPSP neg.	2–10 mg/d
• Duloxetine		
Other	CPSP, SCI conflicting	60–120 mg/d
• Trazodone		
Anticonvulsants (Na^+ channel)		
• Lamotrigine	CPSP weak pos.	25–400 mg/d
• Carbamazepine	MS weak pos.	100–1400 mg/d
• Topiramate	CPSP neg.	50–600 mg/d
Anticonvulsants (Ca^{2+} channel)		
• Gabapentin	SCI, PLP weak pos.	100–3600 mg/d
• Pregabalin	SCI moderate pos.	25–600 mg/d
• Phenytoin	CPSP conflicting	150–300 mg/d

(continued)

Table 19.3 (CONTINUED)

Medication	*Level of Evidence*	*Suggested Dosage Range/Minimum-Maximum*
Opioids		
• Levorphanol	CPSP, SCI, MS moderate pos.	2.5–9.0 mg/d
• Tramadol	SCI weak pos.	50–400 mg/d
• Morphine	CPSP conflicting, PLP moderate pos.	1–300 mg/d (oral)
NMDA receptor antagonists		
• Ketamine	SCI, PLP weak pos.	0.4 mg/kg/40 min
• Dextromethorphan	CPSP neg., PLP weak pos.	120–180 mg/d
• Memantine	PLP neg.	30 mg/d
Local anesthetics		
• Lidocaine	SCI, CPSP, PLP moderate pos.	2.5–5 mg/kg/30 min
• Mexilitine	CPSP neg.	150–800 mg/d
Cannabinoids		
• Tetrahydrocannabinol	MS moderate pos.	2.5–40 mg/d

Notes: neg. = negative, pos. = positive, NMDA = *N*-methyl-D-aspartate.

Adapted from Wasner G. Central pain syndromes. *Curr Pain Headache Rep*. 2010;14:489–496. & Frese A, Husstedt IW, Ringlestein EB, Evers S. Pharmacologic treatment of central post-stroke pain. *Clin J Pain*. 2006;22:252–260.

been successfully utilized around the world to treat CPSP, SCI, MS, PLP, and other forms of central pain.

Ablative techniques alleviate pain by directly severing afferent pain pathways through surgical resection, chemical neurolysis, or radiofrequency lesioning. Spinal cord ablative techniques (i.e., dorsal root entry zone lesions) have relieved evoked and paroxysmal pain in patients with central pain, but concomitant morbidity has limited their usefulness. Ablative techniques applied to the brain are mostly of historical interest at this point in time. All three techniques (intrathecal, neuromodulation, and ablative) have only retrospective data or limited prospective data to support their efficacy (because of difficulties in designing randomized controlled trials), but the data that do exist suggest some efficacy in patients with severe and medically intractable pain. Experts have suggested referral for these modalities after 6 months of documented conservative medical treatment failure (see Table 19.4).

Table 19.4 OVERVIEW OF TREATMENTS FOR CENTRAL PAIN SYNDROME

PSYCHOLOGICAL
– *Cognitive-behavioral therapy*
– *Relaxation*
– *Biofeedback*
– *Cognitive restructuring*
– *Hypnosis*
CONSERVATIVE-ALTERNATIVE
– *Transcranial magnetic stimulation*
– *Transcutaneous electrical nerve stimulation*
– *Acupuncture*

(continued)

Table 19.4 (CONTINUED)

MEDICATIONS

Antidepressants	*Anticonvulsants*	*Opioids*	*Cannabinoids*	*Other*
–Amytriptyline	*–Gabapentin*	*–Levorphanol*	*–δ4-THC*	*–Lidocaine*
–Clomipramine	*–Pregablin*	*–Tramadol*		*–Ketamine*
–Fluvoxamine	*–Lamotrigine*	*–Methadone*		*–Clonidine*
–Duloxetine	*–Carbamazepine*			*–Non-steroidal anti-inflammatory drugs*
–Venlafaxine				

NEUROMODULATION
–Deep brain stimulation
–Motor cortex stimulation
–Spinal cord stimulation
–Trancutaneous magnetic stimulation

INTRATHECAL MEDICATIONS
–Opioids
–Benzodiazepines
–Clonidine
–Ziconotide
–Baclofen

ABLATIVE/SURGICAL
–Cordotomy
–Myelotomy

SUMMARY

CPS is a painful and disturbing constellation of symptoms that result from an insult to the CNS. Recent research suggests that central pain states occur more frequently than previously estimated, and given the aging demographics in society, these conditions are apt to become even more commonplace. A diagnosis of central pain is made based primarily on a patient's medical history and physical exam, which may be supplemented by diagnostic studies. The treatment of CPS should ideally involve a multimodal approach combining psychological, physical, pharmacological, and, in refractory cases, surgical treatment methods.

REFERENCES

1. Merskey H, Bogduk N. Classification of chronic pain In: Merskey H, Bogduk N, eds. *IASP Task Force on Taxonomy*. 2nd ed. Seattle, WA: IASP; 1994.
2. Wasner G. Central pain syndromes. *Curr Opin Headache Rep*. 2010;14:489–496.
3. Finnerup NB. A review of central neuropathic pain states. *Curr Opin Anaesthesiol*. 2008;12:586–589.
4. Canavero S, Bonicalzi V. Central pain syndrome: elucidation of genesis and treatment. *Exp Rev Neurother*. 2007;7:1485–1497.
5. Wrigley PJ, Press SR, Gustin SM, et al. Neuropathic pain and primary somatosensory cortex reorganization following spinal cord injury. *Pain*. 2009;141:52–59.
6. Ofek H, Defrin R. The characteristics of chronic pain after traumatic brain injury. *Pain*. 2007;131:330–340.
7. Nampiaparampil DE. Prevalence of chronic pain after traumaticbrain injury. *JAMA*. 2008;300:711–719.
8. Alviar MJM, Hale T, Dungca M. Pharmacologic interventions for treating phantom limb pain (review). *Cochrane Database Syst Rev*. 2011;12:CD006380.
9. Defrin R, Ohry A, Blumen N, Urca G. Characterization of chronic pain and somatosensory function in spinal cord injury subjects. *Pain*. 2001;89:253–263.
10. Brummett CM, Raja SN. Central pain states. In: Benzon HT, Raja SN, Liu SS, et al., eds. *Essentials of Pain Medicine*. 3rd ed. Philadelphia, PA: Elsevier-Saunders; 2011: 370–377

11. Klit H, Finnerup NB, Jensen TS. Central post-stroke pain: clinical characteristics, pathophysiology, and management. *Lancet Neurol.* 2009;8:857–868.
12. Boivie J. Central pain. In: McMahon SB, Koltzenburg M, eds. *Wall and Melzack's Textbook of Pain: Central Pain.* 5th ed. Philadelphia, PA: Elsevier, Churchill-Livingstone; 2006: 1057–1074.
13. Hanagasi HA, Akat S, Gurvit H, Yazici J, Emre M. Pain is common in Parkinson's disease. *Clin Neurol Neurosurg.* 2011;113:11–13.
14. Ford B. Pain in Parkinson's disease. *Mov Disord.* 2010;25(Suppl 1):S103.
15. Nurmikko TJ, Gupta S, Maclver K. Multiple sclerosis-related central pain disorder. *Curr Pain Headache Rep.* 2010;14:189–195.
16. Nair DR, Najm I, Bulacio J, et al. Painful auras in focal epilepsy. *Neurology.* 2001;57:700–702.
17. Young GB, Blume WT. Painful epileptic seizures. *Brain.* 1983;106:537–554.
18. Todor DR, Mu HT, Milhorat TH. Pain and syringomyelia: a review. *Neurosurg Focus.* 2000;8:1–6.
19. Fattal C, Kong-A-Siou D, Gilbert C, et al. What is the efficacy of physical therapeutics for treating neuropathic pain in spinal cord injury patients? *Ann Phys Rehabil Med.* 2009;52:149–166.
20. Wassermann EM, Zimmermann T. Transcranial magnetic brain stimulation: therapeutic promises and scientific gaps. *Pharmacol Ther.* 2012;133:98–107.
21. Attal N, Cruccu G, Baron R, et al.; European Federation of Neurological Societies. EFNS guidelines on the pharmacological treatment of neuropathic pain: 2010 revision. *Eur J Neurol.* 2010;17:1113–e88.
22. Dyson-Hudson TA, Kadar P, LaFountaine M, et al. Acupuncture for chronic shoulder pain in persons with spinal cord injury: a small-scale clinical trial. *Arch Phys Med Rehabil.* 2007;88(10):1276–1283.
23. Norrbrink C, Lundeberg T. Acupuncture and massage therapy for neuropathic pain following spinal cord injury: an exploratory study. *Acupunct Med.* 2011;29(2):108–125.
24. Dworkin RH, O'Connor AB, Audette J, et al. Recommendations for the pharmacological management of neuropathic pain: an overview and literature update. *Mayo Clin Proc.* 2010;85:S3–S14.
25. Bastrup C, Finnerup NB. Pharmacological management of neuropathic pain following spinal cord injury. *CNS Drugs.* 2008;22:455–475.
26. Frese A, Husstedt IW, Ringlestein EB, Evers S. Pharmacologic treatment of central post-stroke pain. *Clin J Pain.* 2006;22:252–260.
27. Canavero, Bonicalzi V. Neuromodulation for central pain. *Expert Rev Neurother.* 2003;3(5):591–607.

20

Fibromyalgia and Other Central Pain States

DANIEL J. CLAUW

Case Presentation

The patient is a 45-year-old white male who initially presented to primary care with an episode of acute low back pain. Upon evaluation, he reveals that he has in fact had chronic pain in the back and neck, as well as issues with headaches, chronic prostatitis, and poor sleep. He has not received relief from non-steroidal anti-inflammatory drugs (NSAIDs) or the occasional use of opioids. Examination reveals diffuse tenderness. The patient was diagnosed with fibromyalgia (FM) and improved significantly on a regimen including cyclobenzaprine at bedtime, a serotonin-norepinephrine reuptake inhibitor (SNRI) during the day, and a daily exercise program.

After years of skepticism and questioning, FM is now a widely accepted medical disorder, with many years of research identifying the augmented pain and sensory processing and a distinct clinical phenotype. Like most chronic pain states, there is no definitive test, biomarker, or physical exam with which to make the diagnosis of FM. The diagnosis can be made by using one of several established diagnostic criteria and/or by using clinical judgment.

Although FM is now well accepted as a discrete diagnosis by many clinicians (i.e., this patient has FM), it is also useful to think of FM as a metaphor or construct that applies to many individuals with other chronic regional pain conditions for whom there is evidence of generalized pain amplification and thus "centralization" of their pain.[1] For example, for several decades FM has been known to frequently occur as a co-morbidity with a group of "central pain state" conditions such as irritable bowel syndrome, tension headache, temporomandibular joint disorder, chronic fatigue syndrome, and interstitial cystitis.[2] However, more recent work has shown that the same central nervous system (CNS) contributions to pain occur in subsets of individuals with nearly any type of chronic pain, including low back pain, osteoarthritis, and even inflammatory pain states such as rheumatoid arthritis.[3] Furthermore, this phenomenon is now understood to occur over a continuum rather than being "yes" or "no," and Wolfe and others have performed seminal work showing that the degree of "fibromyalgia-ness" predicts levels of pain and disability in any chronic musculoskeletal disorder, not just individuals with the "categorical" diagnosis of FM.[4]

There are a multitude of recent reviews that focus on the epidemiology, pathophysiology, diagnosis, and treatment of FM.[5] This chapter reviews the basics of FM, but special attention is paid to the implications for the non-pain physician.

DIAGNOSTIC CRITERIA FOR FM

The diagnosis of FM has been a source of confusion and frustration for clinicians for many years. It is widely accepted that chronic widespread pain (CWP) (pain above and below the waist, on both sides of the body, and involving the axial skeleton) is the hallmark feature of FM. The "widespreadedness" of any individual's pain, identified either via performing a history or using a body map as part of the initial evaluation, is a required element of FM. Traditional teaching required that in addition to having CWP, individuals also needed to have a tender point assessment, and the diagnosis of FM was made only when an individual also reported pain when 11 or more of these 18 discrete areas were palpated using 4 kg of pressure.[6] Whereas most female patients with CWP also satisfy the tender point criteria, it is unusual for males with CWP to have adequate numbers of tender points to meet these 1990 American College of Rheumatology (ACR) FM criteria (because women are inherently more sensitive to pain than men). Thus, using these older criteria, FM was an almost exclusively female disease.

In part because of this, in 2010 new diagnostic criteria for FM were developed and validated; these still require widespread pain but eliminate the tender point evaluation and instead query the patient about co-morbid symptoms that are commonly seen in FM and other centralized pain states (fatigue, trouble thinking, waking up tired, depression, abdominal pain/cramps, and headache).[7] Figure 20.1 shows the new ACR survey for FM with the 19 potential body areas and the symptom assessment. Scores can range from 0 to 31, and patients are asked whether the symptoms have been present at nearly the same level for the past 3 months or more. The presence of pain for 3 months or more with a score of ≥13 meets the survey criteria for FM.

EPIDEMIOLOGY

Epidemiologic approaches to the FM population have enhanced the understanding of the disorder and led to further hypothesis

Using the following scale, indicate for each item your severity **over the past week** by checking the appropriate box.

0: No problem
1: Slight or mild problems; generally mild or intermittent
2: Moderate; considerable problems; often present and/or at a moderate level
3: Severe: continuous, life-disturbing problems

Fatigue	☐ 0	☐ 1	☐ 2	☐ 3
Trouble thinking or remembering	☐ 0	☐ 1	☐ 2	☐ 3
Waking up tired (unrefreshed)	☐ 0	☐ 1	☐ 2	☐ 3

During the past 6 months have you had any of the following symptoms?

Pain or cramps in lower abdomen:	☐ Yes	☐ No
Depression:	☐ Yes	☐ No
Headache:	☐ Yes	☐ No

JOINT/BODY PAIN

Please indicate below if you have had pain or tenderness over the past 7 days in each of the areas listed below.
Please make an X in the box if you have had pain or tenderness. Be sure to mark both right side and left side separately

☐ Shoulder, Lt. ☐ Shoulder, Rt.	☐ Upper Leg, Lt. ☐ Upper Leg, Rt.	☐ Lower Back ☐ Upper Back ☐ Neck
☐ Hip, Lt. ☐ Hip, Rt.	☐ Lower Leg, Lt. ☐ Lower Leg, Rt.	
☐ Upper Arm, Lt. ☐ Upper Arm, Rt.	☐ Jaw, Lt. ☐ Jaw, Rt.	☐ No pain in any of these areas
☐ Lower Arm, Lt. ☐ Lower Arm, Rt.	☐ Chest ☐ Abdomen	

Draft

Figure 20.1. The 2011 American College of Rheumatology survey criteria for fibromyalgia (FM) is a validated self-report measure that assesses widespread body pain from a pre-specified check list or body map (0–19 points) and a comorbid symptom severity index (0–12) to give a total score from 0 to 31. Patients scoring ≥13 (or ≥12 depending on the distribution of widespred pain and symptoms) are categorized as FM positive. More importantly, the scale can be used as a continuous scale as a surrogate of the relative degree of centralization and sensitivity. Modified with permission from *The Journal of Rheumatology;* Wolfe F, Clauw DJ, Fitzcharles MA, et al. Fibromyalgia criteria and severity scales for clinical and epidemiological studies: a modification of the ACR Preliminary Diagnostic Criteria for Fibromyalgia. *J Rheumatol.* 2011;38(6):1113–1122.

generation and ongoing research. The historical component of FM (i.e., CWP) is remarkably constant in different countries and cultures, afflicting approximately 8 percent of men and 12 percent of women.[8] Thus, the older ACR criteria for FM had unintentionally transformed a condition that affected slightly more women than men into one that almost exclusively affected women by also requiring that individuals have 11 or more tender points. There is a strong family predisposition for developing FM, but again this now is more broadly understood to occur across virtually all chronic pain conditions.[9] The first-degree relatives of FM patients have eight times the risk of developing FM and much higher risks of developing any type of chronic pain, and they are much more tender than the first-degree relatives of controls.[10]

ALTERED SENSORY PERCEPTION AND CENTRAL NEUROTRANSMISSION

Pain is the most common complaint of FM patients. Patients with FM demonstrate altered noxious thresholds (the point at which a sensory experience such as pressure, heat, or sound becomes bothersome) for virtually every type of sensory testing.[11] This can be easily understood by patients and clinicians alike when the phenomenon is likened to "an increased volume control in the brain for any sensory stimuli." Because of this, individuals with FM or other central pain states will often note that they find noises, odors, and bright lights very bothersome, and this sensory sensitivity likely even explains many of the visceral symptoms these individuals experience (e.g., indigestion, heartburn, abdominal pain, urinary urgency and frequency). Sometimes merely highlighting this physiological understanding of FM can be extremely helpful to patients, because when they develop new symptoms that follow this same pattern they are less concerned that "there is something wrong," a fear that would often trigger a frustrating "search for the cause of the pain."

Although there are a number of ways to determine how pain sensitive an individual is, current evidence suggests that assessing one's pressure pain threshold (i.e., tenderness to palpation, in contrast to assessing one's heat or cold pain threshold) is the most reliable and reproducible method. Routine testing of the pressure pain threshold is not yet available as a routine test in clinical practice, so methods of assessing tenderness in practice include performing a tender point count and incorporating alternative methods of assessing pain threshold into routine practice. For example, one way to assess patients' overall pain threshold while also getting other valuable diagnostic information is to assess pain thresholds in the hands and arms of all chronic pain patients. A rapid examination in which one applies firm pressure over several inter-phalangeal (IP) joints of each hand, as well as over the adjacent phalanges, and then moves centrally to include firm palpation of the muscles of the forearm, including the lateral epicondyle region, is one way to assess overall pain threshold and get additional diagnostic information about the patient. If the individual is tender in many of these areas or in just the muscles of the forearm, he or she likely is diffusely tender (i.e., the patient has a low central pain threshold). However, if the individual is tender only over the IP joints and not in the other regions, and especially if there is any swelling over these joints, one should be more concerned about a systemic autoimmune disorder (e.g., rheumatoid arthritis, lupus). Alternatively, sometimes individuals are tender only over the phalanges, and in these instances one might suspect a metabolic bone disease or a condition causing periostitis (e.g., hypothyroidism, hyperparathyroidism).

This type of musculoskeletal examination, along with judicious laboratory testing (erythrocyte sedimentation rate [ESR] and C-reactive protein, thyroid stimulating hormone [TSH], chemistry profile; *not* antinuclear antibodies and rheumatoid factor, unless specifically indicated), can essentially rule out most alternative causes of CWP.

These findings of augmented sensory processing noted on exam have been confirmed through quantitative sensory studies and many types functional and structural neuroimaging studies that identify augmented pain processing (i.e., increased volume control), as well as by "objective" structural and chemical evidence of why this augmented pain processing might be occurring.[12,13] In addition, approximately 80 percent of FM patients, and comparable proportions of individuals with other chronic pain syndromes with prominent CNS contributions, demonstrate abnormal or absent descending analgesic activity.[14] Of note, although historically some have questioned whether FM is fundamentally a psychiatric disorder with pathophysiology similar to depression, neither diffuse pain sensitivity nor decreased descending analgesic activity is found in individuals with depression.[15]

A fuller understanding of the pathophysiology of FM, as well as the likely explanation for the frequent co-morbid symptoms such as fatigue, pain, insomnia, memory, and mood difficulties, is gained by assessing the associated neurochemical variations. FM patients have higher levels of CNS neurotransmitters associated with the facilitation of pain than do controls, including glutamate, substance P, and nerve growth factor.[16] Although most of these studies have examined cerebrospinal fluid (CSF) levels of neurotransmitters, Harris and colleagues have performed a series of studies using proton spectroscopy to demonstrate that glutamate levels are elevated in the insula of individuals with FM (a finding also noted in CSF), and that insular glutamate levels are closely related to pain sensitivity *in both FM patients and controls*.[17] These studies add additional biological support to the "fibromyalgia-ness" construct, because the relationship between insular glutamate was the same in both FM patients and controls, but the FM patients were more pain sensitive because their mean glutamate levels were higher.

Levels of neurotransmitters associated with down-regulation of pain transmission tend to be lower, including norepinephrine, serotonin (presumably acting at the $5HT_{1a,b}$ receptors), and γ-aminobutyric acid (GABA). The only neurotransmitter system that does not follow this pattern (i.e., increased levels of neurotransmitters that increase pain sensitivity, and decreased levels of neurotransmitters that reduce pain sensitivity) is the endogenous opioid system. Current evidence suggests that endogenous opioid levels in FM are elevated, and positron emission tomography studies show that μ-opioid receptors in pain processing areas in the brain have increased occupancy, giving a potential biological reason that opioids seem to be ineffective or less effective in centralized pain states than in nociceptive pain conditions.[18] Thus, despite the lack of a definitive clinical biomarker or test for FM, these findings have largely validated the complaints and symptoms of FM patients, altered the treatment recommendations (see the section "Treatment of FM" below), and led to an explosion in new pain research applying "lessons learned" regarding FM and centralized pain states to nearly every chronic pain disorder.

CO-MORBID PSYCHOPATHOLOGY

Psychological diagnoses, especially depression and anxiety, are common in the FM population, as they are with any chronic pain condition. Although some have suggested that psychopathology is the "cause" of FM, at any given time a minority of individuals with FM will display an active Axis I or II psychiatric disorder, and psychological variables do not fully explain the widespread body pain and symptoms seen in this population.[19] It is likely that some of the same neurotransmitter abnormalities that contribute to pain amplification (e.g., high substance P and glutamate; low serotonin, norepinephrine, and GABA) also contribute to the fatigue, sleep, memory, and mood symptoms experienced by individuals with FM or fibromyalgia-ness.

OTHER CO-MORBID CONDITIONS AND SYMPTOMS

Although FM remains an independent medical diagnosis, co-morbid clusters of other pain conditions are often seen. When individuals present with several of these conditions that have been previously diagnosed over the course of their lifetime (and/or if they have a family history of same), it makes it much more likely that the individual is suffering from FM or another centralized pain state. These symptoms include multifocal pain, fatigue, memory problems, and sleep and mood disturbances, and conditions include tension and migraine headaches, temporomandibular joint disorder, chronic neck and low back pain, functional gastroenterological disorders (irritable bowel syndrome, esophageal dysmotility, non-cardiac chest pain), interstitial cystitis, chronic prostatitis, vulvodynia, chronic fatigue syndrome, and "chemical sensitivity" (likely sensory sensitivity misnamed). Just as with any other disease, patients do not uniformly manifest all symptoms or disorders, and the pathophysiology behind the clustering is still an area of ongoing research.

GENETIC PREDISPOSITION

Supporting the notion that there is a strong familial contribution to FM, as well as more broadly chronic pain and tenderness, several genes have been identified that occur more commonly in FM patients than in controls. As is commonly seen in genetic studies, these genes are not found in all studies, but those involving the regulation of serotonin and norepinephrine are the ones most commonly identified, including the serotonin receptor polymorphisms and catechol-O-methly transferase.[20,21] As some of these same genes that lead to decreased availability of serotonin or norepinephrine have also been shown to put individuals at risk for developing major depressive disorder, a better understanding is developing regarding why psychiatric conditions such as depression, posttraumatic stress disorder, obsessive-compulsive disorder, and other disorders occur more commonly as co-morbidities in central pain states.

TREATMENT OF FM

There are multiple recent reviews and meta-analyses that provide a more complete picture of the chronic management of FM.[22] Although many clinicians assume that our treatments for FM are less effective than those we use for other chronic pain conditions, data suggest otherwise, and the overall efficacy of the current drugs for FM is comparable to that of pharmacological therapy for other chronic pain states.[23]

Opioid and NSAID Therapy

Although NSAIDs and opioids are very effective analgesics for acute pain and are amongst the first-line agents selected for many patients with long-standing nociceptive pain states (i.e., conditions in which the pain is caused primarily by damage or inflammation of peripheral tissue), there is no evidence that either of these treatments is effective in individuals with "just" FM. This is a point of emphasis because recent studies show that ongoing peripheral nociceptive input (as might occur due to osteoarthritis) might lead to further "centralization" of pain, and thus in this setting it might be useful to use an NSAID (or even an opioid) in an individual with FM if he or she has such a co-morbid pain state. Despite the general recommendation against the use of opioids in FM, as well as the (largely anecdotal) concern that these patients might preferentially be at risk for opioid-induced hyperalgesia that would actually lead to worsening of their pain with these agents, the use of opioids for the condition is still widespread.

Antidepressants

Many of the recommended and U.S. Food and Drug Administration (FDA)-approved drugs were originally developed as antidepressants, but it is important to recognize that not all antidepressants are effective in pain or FM. It is more appropriate to use the term SNRI to describe two such drugs, duloxetine and milnacipran. Duloxetine was tested in doses as high as 120 mg/d and is approved in doses of up to 60 mg (Cymbalta, Eli Lilly Co., Indianapolis, IN), and milnacipran was studied at doses of up to 200 mg/d and is approved for doses of up to 100 mg/d (Savella, Forest Pharmaceuticals). The tolerability of this class of drugs can be increased by warning individuals of the risk of nausea and assuring them that in most cases this is transient, and by starting at a low dose and increasing slowly.

Prior to these FDA-approved drugs, tricyclic compounds such as amitriptyline (10 to 70 mg a few hours before bedtime) and cyclobenzaprine (5 to 20 mg a few hours before bedtime) were the best studied and most commonly used class of drugs for FM.[24] Although this group does not carry official FDA approval, they also likely work by blocking the reuptake of serotonin and norepinephrine. The anticholinergic side effects of tricyclics often limit their tolerability, especially in older patients. Nortriptyline has less anticholinergic effects and is generally the tricyclic antidepressant (TCA) of choice. The benefits of TCAs are that they are inexpensive and can improve sleep. Although package inserts warn of the risk of serotonin syndrome when using SNRIs and TCAs together, this occurs very rarely, and this is a commonly used combination (e.g., TCA at night and SNRI in the morning) in clinical practice.

The SNRI venlafaxine has had mixed results in FM trials, with one trial using the drug at a high dose showing efficacy, but with two other studies at lower doses not. This is in line with studies of selective serotonin reuptake inhibitors (SSRIs) in FM. It appears as though both venlafaxine and the older, less serotonin-specific SSRIs (sertraline, fluoxetine, paroxetine) all can become analgesics when used at relatively higher doses, where they begin to have more effect on noradrenergic reuptake. For example, one study showed that a mean dose of 45 mg of fluoxetine was effective in FM (a dose much higher than most would use as an antidepressant). Two important clinical points bear emphasis. First, the efficacy of antidepressants in FM and other chronic pain conditions seems to be independent of their antidepressant effects.[25] Second, it appears as though norepinephrine is the more important of the two neurotransmitters for relief of chronic pain, in that a pure norepinephrine reuptake inhibitor (es-reboxetine) has been shown to be quite effective in FM (although it is not currently available in the United States), whereas highly-selective SSRIs (e.g., citalopram, es-citalopram) have not been shown to be effective in preclinical or clinical chronic pain conditions.[26]

Gabapentanoids

Another class of medications used in FM is the gabapentanoids, or α-2-δ calcium channel ligands. The only medication in this class that carries FDA approval is pregabalin (Lyrica, Pfizer), which was tested at doses as high as 600 mg/d and is approved for use in FM at doses up to 450 mg. However, a randomized controlled trial in FM showed similar efficacy using gabapentin at doses of 1800 to 2400 mg/d.[27] Although there might be some unique dosing and pharmacokinetic properties of pregabalin relative to gabapentin, their efficacy and side-effect profiles are not significantly different.

Emerging Therapies

Because of the approval of three drugs for FM and the fact that the majority of trials that have been performed in the past decade in this condition have been "positive," there has been significant work in developing even better therapies for FM. Sodium oxybate (also known as γ-hydroxybutyrate) is an example of a compound that has recently been shown to be very efficacious in FM.[28] However, in spite of the strong efficacy data, this drug was not approved by the FDA because of safety concerns. Nonetheless, the prominent simultaneous salutary effects on pain, sleep, and fatigue strongly suggest that low GABA is an important therapeutic target in FM and related conditions. Similarly, although there are no cannabinoids approved for use in chronic pain in the United States, this class of drugs has displayed efficacy in both FM and other chronic pain conditions.[29] Another neurotransmitter system that is clearly involved in FM and more broadly in pain is the glutamatergic system, as evidenced by the fact that an intravenous ketamine infusion seems to be predictive of subsequent responsiveness to dextromethorphan in FM but is not efficacious itself as long-term therapy.[30]

Another exciting development in the pain field that is being partially led by work in FM is the explosion of interest and knowledge in the use of central neurostimulatory therapies in FM and related conditions.[31] These therapies, which include transcranial direct current stimulation and magnetic stimulation, have been shown to have impressive effects on pain and a number of other domains in FM, and in some cases the effect of therapy has lasted well after the cessation of treatment.

Non-pharmacological Therapies

Non-pharmacological therapies should be a key component in the overall treatment of FM, as well as that of any other chronic pain condition, but they are often under-utilized in clinical practice. The treatments of this type with the most consistent effects include patient education, cognitive-behavioral therapy (CBT), and exercise. Although the treatment of depression and anxiety seems obvious to most clinicians, CBT and biofeedback are specific techniques that demonstrate effect sizes that are often greater than many of the pharmacologic treatments. These techniques are unique to standard methods of counseling and are not offered by all psychiatrists and psychologists. Despite the documented efficacy of CBT and exercise, many patients cannot find trained providers in their local communities, and more commonly insurance providers do not pay for the service. Because of this, many groups are moving toward showing that Internet-based programs that incorporate education, CBT, and exercise can be quite effective in FM and other chronic pain states.[32] The content of these programs is also being scrutinized and refined, as studies are demonstrating that even simply becoming more active (in contrast to formal exercise) can be beneficial in FM, and that CBT that encourages individuals to identify stressful early life events and "disclose" and work through these events might actually cure some individuals with chronic pain, instead of offering palliation as occurs with typical CBT.[33] Additional details regarding behavioral therapies can be found in Chapter 4.

SUMMARY

Figure 20.2 shows a suggested algorithm for diagnosing and treating FM. This diagnosis should be considered when an individual presents

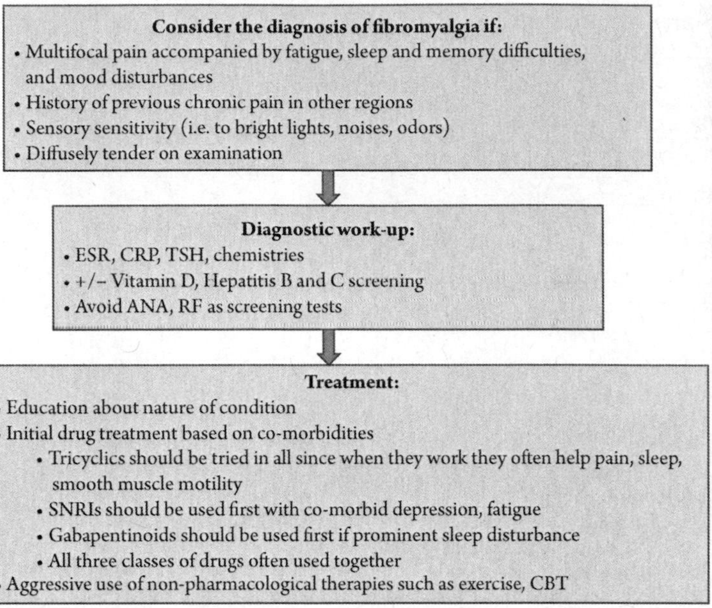

Consider the diagnosis of fibromyalgia if:
• Multifocal pain accompanied by fatigue, sleep and memory difficulties, and mood disturbances
• History of previous chronic pain in other regions
• Sensory sensitivity (i.e. to bright lights, noises, odors)
• Diffusely tender on examination
Diagnostic work-up:
• ESR, CRP, TSH, chemistries
• +/– Vitamin D, Hepatitis B and C screening
• Avoid ANA, RF as screening tests
Treatment:
• Education about nature of condition
• Initial drug treatment based on co-morbidities
• Tricyclics should be tried in all since when they work they often help pain, sleep, smooth muscle motility
• SNRIs should be used first with co-morbid depression, fatigue
• Gabapentinoids should be used first if prominent sleep disturbance
• All three classes of drugs often used together
• Aggressive use of non-pharmacological therapies such as exercise, CBT

Figure 20.2. Clinical diagnosis, diagnostic work up, and treatment of fibromyalgia.

with chronic multifocal pain, especially if other symptoms such as fatigue, memory problems, and sleep and mood disturbances are also noted. The diagnosis is more likely if the patients have had a family and/or lifetime history or multiple other episodes of chronic pain, and if they also have symptoms (sensitivity to touch or wearing tight clothing; sensitivity to light, noises, odors) and signs (tenderness to palpation in multiple body regions) of sensory sensitivity.

Once the diagnosis is considered, some minimal diagnostic testing can be helpful in ruling out other conditions that might be confused with FM. In most instances, this consists of an ESR and C-reactive protein test to rule out inflammatory or autoimmune disorders, a TSH panel to exclude hypothyroidism, and routine chemistries and a complete blood count to screen for other systemic disorders.

Some also now recommend vitamin D testing, because levels of this vitamin are very often low in chronic pain patients; it is not yet clear whether vitamin D therapy leads to any improvement in pain, but at a minimum it is likely to be useful for bone health.

Before embarking on a treatment program, it is very important to educate the patient about the condition, emphasizing that like most diseases FM can be managed but not cured, and that most patients can function quite well if they play an active role in their therapy, which will likely contain a combination of drug and non-drug therapies. Often initiating pharmacological therapy prior to non-pharmacological therapy is helpful because patients might be more compliant with exercise and cognitive-behavioral techniques if their symptoms are somewhat improved by medications.

The classes of drugs with the most evidence of efficacy include the TCAs, SNRIs, and gabapentinoids. Often patients will benefit from all three classes of drugs when they are used together, whereas in other cases individuals respond to (or need) only one of these. All individuals should probably be tried on one or two TCAs until arriving at the best therapeutic algorithm (e.g., cyclobenzaprine, amitriptyline, nortriptyline); these drugs are inexpensive, and when they do work, they often improve sleep, pain, and visceral motility issues. An SNRI is a good first choice when the patient suffers from co-morbid depression or fatigue, whereas a gabapentinoid might be a better first choice when the individual is experiencing significant co-morbid sleep issues (especially if these drugs are given just at bedtime or with a higher proportion of the dose at bedtime). Many other classes of drugs (described under "Emerging Therapies") have shown some evidence of efficacy and would be considered "second-line" agents.

Once the patient has noted some improvement in his or her symptoms with pharmacological therapies, the clinician should aggressively advocate for the use of non-pharmacological therapies, such as education, exercise, and cognitive-behavioral approaches.

Many types of therapy that combine exercise and relaxation, such as yoga and Tai Chi, have also been shown to be helpful.

Using this suggested approach, most individuals with FM note a significant improvement and can continue to function normally in spite of this condition. Some individuals, especially those with long-standing symptoms and functional consequences (e.g., disability, compensation), those on high-dose opioids, those with significant psychiatric co-morbidities, and those who have had multiple "failed" surgical procedures, will not respond to this simple "primary-care-centric" approach and will need interdisciplinary care.

REFERENCES

1. Ablin K, Clauw DJ. From fibrositis to functional somatic syndromes to a bell-shaped curve of pain and sensory sensitivity: evolution of a clinical construct. *Rheum Dis Clin North Am.* 2009;35(2):233–251.
2. Aaron LA, Buchwald D. A review of the evidence for overlap among unexplained clinical conditions. *Ann Intern Med.* 2001;134(9 Pt 2):868–881.
3. Lee YC, Nassikas NJ, Clauw DJ. The role of the central nervous system in the generation and maintenance of chronic pain in rheumatoid arthritis, osteoarthritis and fibromyalgia. *Arthritis Res Ther.* 2011;13(2):211.
4. Wolfe F. Fibromyalgianess. *Arthritis Rheum.* 2009;61(6):715–716.
5. Arnold LM, Clauw DJ. Fibromyalgia syndrome: practical strategies for improving diagnosis and patient outcomes. *Am J Med.* 2010;123(6):S2.
6. Wolfe F, Smythe HA, Yunus MB, et al. The American College of Rheumatology 1990 Criteria for the Classification of Fibromyalgia. Report of the Multicenter Criteria Committee. *Arthritis Rheum.* 1990;33(2):160–172.
7. Wolfe F, Clauw DJ, Fitzcharles MA, et al. The American College of Rheumatology preliminary diagnostic criteria for fibromyalgia and measurement of symptom severity. *Arthritis Care Res (Hoboken).* 2010;62(5):600–610.
8. McBeth J, Jones K. Epidemiology of chronic musculoskeletal pain. *Best Pract Res Clin Rheumatol.* 2007;21(3):403–425.
9. Diatchenko L, Nackley AG, Tchivileva IE, Shabalina SA, Maixner W. Genetic architecture of human pain perception. *Trends Genet.* 2007;23(12):605–613.
10. Arnold LM, Hudson JI, Hess EV, et al. Family study of fibromyalgia. *Arthritis Rheum.* 2004;50(3):944–952.

11. Geisser ME, Strader DC, Petzke F, Gracely RH, Clauw DJ, Williams DA. Comorbid somatic symptoms and functional status in patients with fibromyalgia and chronic fatigue syndrome: sensory amplification as a common mechanism. *Psychosomatics.* 2008;49(3):235–242.
12. Nebel MB, Gracely RH. Neuroimaging of fibromyalgia. *Rheum Dis Clin North Am.* 2009;35(2):313–327.
13. Foerster BR, Petrou M, Harris RE, et al. Cerebral blood flow alterations in pain-processing regions of patients with fibromyalgia using perfusion MR imaging. *AJNR Am J Neuroradiol.* 2011;32(10):1873–1878.
14. Yarnitsky D. Conditioned pain modulation (the diffuse noxious inhibitory control-like effect): its relevance for acute and chronic pain states. *Curr Opin Anaesthesiol.* 2010;23(5):611–615.
15. Paul-Savoie E, Potvin S, Daigle K, et al. A deficit in peripheral serotonin levels in major depressive disorder but not in chronic widespread pain. *Clin J Pain.* 2011;27(6):529–534.
16. Dadabhoy D, Crofford LJ, Spaeth M, Russell IJ, Clauw DJ. Biology and therapy of fibromyalgia. Evidence-based biomarkers for fibromyalgia syndrome. *Arthritis Res Ther.* 2008;10(4):211.
17. Harris RE, Sundgren PC, Craig AD, et al. Elevated insular glutamate in fibromyalgia is associated with experimental pain. *Arthritis Rheum.* 2009;60(10):3146–3152.
18. Harris RE, Clauw DJ, Scott DJ, McLean SA, Gracely RH, Zubieta JK. Decreased central mu-opioid receptor availability in fibromyalgia. *J Neurosci.* 2007;27(37):10000–10006.
19. Xiao Y, He W, Russell IJ. Genetic polymorphisms of the ²2-adrenergic receptor relate to guanosine protein-coupled stimulator receptor dysfunction in fibromyalgia syndrome. *J Rheumatol.* 2011;38(6):1095–1103.
20. Epstein SA, Kay GG, Clauw DJ, et al. Psychiatric disorders in patients with fibromyalgia. A multicenter investigation. *Psychosomatics.* 1999;40:57–63.
21. Lee YH, Choi SJ, Ji JD, Song GG. Candidate gene studies of fibromyalgia: a systematic review and meta-analysis. *Rheumatol Int.* 2012 Feb;32(2):417–426.
22. Schmidt-Wilcke T, Clauw DJ. Fibromyalgia: from pathophysiology to therapy. *Nat Rev Rheumatol.* 2011;7(9):518–527.
23. Clauw DJ. Pain management: fibromyalgia drugs are "as good as it gets" in chronic pain. *Nat Rev Rheumatol.* 2010;6(8):439–440.
24. Arnold LM, Keck PE Jr., Welge JA. Antidepressant treatment of fibromyalgia. A meta-analysis and review. *Psychosomatics.* 2000;41(2):104–113.
25. Hauser W, Bernardy K, Uceyler N, Sommer C. Treatment of fibromyalgia syndrome with antidepressants: a meta-analysis. *JAMA.* 2009;301(2):198–209.
26. Arnold LM, Chatamra K, Hirsch I, Stoker M. Safety and efficacy of esreboxetine in patients with fibromyalgia: an 8-week, multicenter, randomized, double-blind, placebo-controlled study. *Clin Ther.* 2010;32(9):1618–1632.

27. Arnold LM, Goldenberg DL, Stanford SB, et al. Gabapentin in the treatment of fibromyalgia: a randomized, double-blind, placebo-controlled, multicenter trial. *Arthritis Rheum.* 2007;56(4):1336–1344.
28. Russell IJ, Holman AJ, Swick TJ, Alvarez-Horine S, Wang YG, Guinta D. Sodium oxybate reduces pain, fatigue, and sleep disturbance and improves functionality in fibromyalgia: results from a 14-week, randomized, double-blind, placebo-controlled study. *Pain.* 2011;152(5):1007–1017.
29. Lynch ME, Campbell F. Cannabinoids for treatment of chronic non-cancer pain; a systematic review of randomized trials. *Br J Clin Pharmacol.* 2011;72(5):735–744.
30. Cohen SP, Verdolin MH, Chang AS, Kurihara C, Morlando BJ, Mao J. The intravenous ketamine test predicts subsequent response to an oral dextromethorphan treatment regimen in fibromyalgia patients. *J Pain.* 2006;7(6):391–398.
31. Mhalla A, Baudic S, de Andrade DC, et al. Long-term maintenance of the analgesic effects of transcranial magnetic stimulation in fibromyalgia. *Pain.* 2011;152:1478–1485.
32. Williams DA, Kuper D, Segar M, Mohan N, Sheth M, Clauw DJ. Internet-enhanced management of fibromyalgia: a randomized controlled trial. *Pain.* 2010;151(3):694–702.
33. Hsu MC, Schubiner H, Lumley MA, Stracks JS, Clauw DJ, Williams DA. Sustained pain reduction through affective self-awareness in fibromyalgia: a randomized controlled trial. *J Gen Intern Med.* 2010;25(10):1064–1070.

INDEX